SO-FBW-869

# SEX, SICKNESS, AND SLAVERY

# Sex, Sickness, and Slavery

## Illness in the Antebellum South

MARLI F. WEINER
with MAZIE HOUGH

UNIVERSITY OF ILLINOIS PRESS
URBANA, CHICAGO, AND SPRINGFIELD

RA
418.3
. U6
W44
2012

© 2012 by the Board of Trustees
of the University of Illinois
All rights reserved
Manufactured in the United States of America
C 5 4 3 2 1
∞ This book is printed on acid-free paper.

Library of Congress Cataloging-in-Publication Data
Weiner, Marli Frances, 1953–
Sex, sickness, and slavery: illness in the antebellum South /
Marli F. Weiner; with Mazie Hough.
p.   cm.
Includes bibliographical references and index.
ISBN 978-0-252-03699-6 (cloth : acid-free paper)
1. Diseases—Social aspects—Southern States—History—19th century.
2. Diseases—Social aspects—Southern States—History—19th century—Sources.
3. Medicine—Practice—Southern States—History—19th century.
4. Physicians—Southern States—History—19th century.
5. Human body—Social aspects—Southern States—History—19th century.
6. Sex differences—Social aspects—Southern States—History—19th century.
7. Slavery—Social aspects—Southern States—History—19th century.
8. Race—Social aspects—Southern States—History—19th century.
9. Southern States—Race relations—History—19th century.
10. Southern States—Social conditions—19th century.
I. Hough, Mazie. II. Title.
RA418.3.U6W44      2012
614.4'27509034—dc23      2011046500

*For my mother and Elizabeth,*

*who shared their dying*

*and*

*For my father and Judy,*

*who share my life*

University Libraries
Carnegie Mellon University
Pittsburgh, PA 15213-3890

The academic discipline . . . closest to being a clinician is not a science, however, it is history. Clinicians and historians are always going into the past in order to dig out recordable, archival facts. Yet both must attempt to get inside the people whose history they seek in order to understand the world in terms of that person.

—Eric J. Cassell, MD, *The Nature of Suffering
and the Goals of Medicine*

# CONTENTS

## ACKNOWLEDGMENTS

Like all historians, I have depended on an array of friends, family, colleagues, librarians, and students in the process of writing this book. While researching and writing are often solitary pursuits, they have been informed and enlivened by the crowd of people surrounding me in many parts of my life.

I want first to thank the many people who have listened to me talk about this book in endless detail and still were willing to read drafts of this book over the years. The members of the scribbling women writing group have helped enormously, reading draft after draft, particularly of the early chapters: Mazie Hough, Kristin Langellier, Pauleena MacDougall, Amy Fried, Sue Estler, and Elizabeth Allan. In addition, Judy Thornton read every word, some of them more than once, and offered suggestions on everything from interpretation to punctuation.

I also want to thank the many members of the Literature and Medicine seminars at Maine Coast Memorial Hospital in Ellsworth, at Mayo Regional Hospital in Dover-Foxcroft, and at Eastern Maine Medical Center in Bangor and the hospitals for sponsoring them. My understanding of all aspects of the medical profession is far deeper and more nuanced as a result of our discussions. Thanks are particularly due to Charlie Alexander, Sherrie Downing, Marie Langlois, Christine diPretoro, and Jean Johnson at Maine Coast and to Tom Lizotte at Mayo for organizing and sustaining interest in these seminars over the years.

Literature and Medicine would not exist without the hard work and visionary leadership of the staff and board members at the Maine Humanities Council, particularly Deedee Schwartz, Victoria Bonebakker, Lizz Sinclair, Erik Jorgensen, and Geoff Gratwick. I have worked closely with them and the rest of the staff and board members on this and other projects; they have directly and indirectly shaped my thinking about the issues discussed in this book. I am grateful to them for the opportunities they have given me, along with fine discussions, important work, good food, and the chance to explore all parts of Maine.

I am also grateful to several medical people who patiently answered the multitude of questions that arose for a historian with no formal training in medicine: Kathryn Rensenbrink, Sherrie Downing, and Jean Curran. They helped me to understand in twentieth-century terms what nineteenth-century doctors described. In addition, I am grateful to the twenty-first-century doctors and other medical personnel who provided good care during the last stages of work on this book: Geoff Gratwick, Kathryn Rensenbrink, Moritz Hansen, and Seth Blank, among others.

Librarians at several institutions have made this work possible, including Chris Hoolihan at the History of Medicine Library at Strong Memorial Hospital, University of Rochester; Jane Brown and Kay Carter at the Waring Historical Library at the South Carolina Medical University in Charleston; Elizabeth Dunn and Bill Irwin at Special Collections, Perkins Library, Duke University; Barbara Busse and Gayle Elmore of the History of Medicine collection at the Duke University Medical Center Library; Richard Shrader at the Southern Historical Collection, Wilson Library, University of North Carolina at Chapel Hill; and Mel Johnson and especially Libby Soifer and Barbara Jones at Inter-Library Loan at the University of Maine, who found materials for me that I never imagined possible.

Several students helped with various aspects of research, including Dena De-Marco, Kristen Gwinn, Marilyn Costanzo, and Michelle Isham. Other students listened patiently as I sometimes offered far more gory details of nineteenth-century medicine than they wanted to hear. Only one student has ever fainted on me, although others I am sure were tempted. At the University of Maine, Ann Schonberger and Mazie Hough of the Women in the Curriculum and Women's Studies Program have created a supportive community in which to work, learn, and teach. I have also benefited from audience comments on the papers I've given on aspects of this material at conferences in Mississippi, New York, and Maine and from the suggestions of anonymous readers for the University of Illinois Press.

Financial help to travel to libraries in the South was provided by Duke University and by the Women in the Curriculum and Women's Studies grant program at the University of Maine.

I also want to thank the friends and family who have kept me going, who somehow knew when to ask about my progress and when it was better to talk of something else, who listened to my struggles and helped to put them into perspective. Thanks are particularly due to Peggy Muir, Mazie Hough, Laurie Osher, and Andrea Hawkes. Noam and Zivi Osher giggled with me and laughed at my jokes. I treasure them all.

My mother and Elizabeth Kelly Ebitz died while I was working on this book. I wish more than I know how to say that they were alive to share it with me. My father has always been there for me, even though he might have wanted me to write a different book. Judy has transformed everything, bringing sunshine and a cabin by a pond and a new kind of joy into my life. This book is for them.

These acknowledgments would not be complete without my deep thanks to Marli Weiner, mentor, colleague, and friend, who entrusted me with seeing this manuscript through its publication. She called on all of us to maintain the highest standards as historians and at the same time offered us the support and guidance that enabled us to achieve them. She is sadly missed.

SEX, SICKNESS, AND SLAVERY

# The Political Body

In the July 1860 issue of the *Oglethorpe Medical and Surgical Journal,* William C. Bellamy published an article entitled "History of a Case of Insanity with Hemorrhage from Some Unknown Source Escaping from the Urethra." Bellamy, who had an AB degree and was a medical student from Alabama, published the description of a patient, Ben, whom he had never seen because he thought the man "no less singular than interesting." Diagnosing what was wrong with him was perplexing even to eminent local physicians, so Bellamy wrote his account in order to share a "new and interesting" case and to ask his colleagues for advice about how best to understand it. Clearly unable to decide which aspects of Ben's experience were most significant, Bellamy presented it in great detail.[1]

Bellamy described the patient as a thirty-seven-year-old man, a slave sawyer near Columbus, Georgia, who had been injured eight years earlier. While working in the mill, he had apparently fallen twelve feet through the floor onto "a solid granite rock below" and lost about half a gallon of blood. When discovered, Ben was "under the mill insensible, bloody, and dying," with blood "running in a continuous stream from the urethra." The doctor his owner called could not tell where the blood came from for certain, but he was sure it did not come from Ben's bladder. Blood "continued to escape at intervals, sometimes spontaneously, at others with the urine." Although he appeared "quite rational and apparently comfortable" at first, two or three days later when the master visited he found Ben "with a wild unnatural expression, and giving utterance to various incoherent expressions such as we are likely to hear from an insane man." Later that day, Ben left home but was found and confined. He was released when his owner realized "that he would kill himself rather than submit to confinement." For the eight years since the accident, Ben "would not stay at home," instead "wandering about" and "studiously avoiding his master and every member of his family, although quite free and friendly with others."[2]

According to Bellamy, Ben's "principal hallucination is in imagining himself a woman, and subject to the diseases peculiar to women." He was "very much afraid of dying" and of thunder and lightning, which Bellamy presumably associated with women. He also still experienced occasional hemorrhages, "though he seems in all respects sound and healthy except" for that and "the wandering of his mind." Ben "ignores his master's control and will not come near him or any of his family for food, raiment, or any thing else." Ben earned a living doing odd jobs in town, which his owner tolerated. Ben was unable to explain the cause of his injury, nor was Bellamy able to explain the cause of the hemorrhage, why it came on "at intervals," and why it did "not exhaust his strength." Bellamy was certain that Ben was "non compos mentis," but wondered how the injury "affect[ed] his mind" since "there is no apparent cephalic [head] injury." He asked readers to tell him about any similar case they might have seen, with "its history, diagnosis, treatment and result."[3]

Ben's story as related by soon-to-be doctor Bellamy offers a window into the experience of illness and injury and the practice of medicine in the antebellum South. In some senses, Ben's experiences of work and medical care were typical of those shared by slaves in long-settled areas of the South. Ben did laborious work under difficult conditions, which left him physically vulnerable to harm. His injury was serious enough that his master called a physician. Although the injury was physical, it affected Ben emotionally. Ben was unable to work at his assigned task while he was injured. Bellamy's behavior likewise reflected that of many antebellum physicians. He was eager to understand a case that he found perplexing and hoped to learn from it. He asked his peers for advice. He apparently believed what he had heard about Ben and showed no sign of questioning the truth of the story. He was curious about the links between Ben's physical injury and his mental disorder. He tried to define what was normal and was curious about its limits.

At the same time, neither man's experience was particularly like that of others, especially Ben's. Unlike many slaves, Ben was skilled at a demanding trade. He lived in a city, which allowed him to support himself doing odd jobs, which would not have been possible in the countryside where most slaves lived. His injury enabled him to avoid both his master and the work his master would otherwise have required him to do. Suffering slaves wanted respite from work but were not always granted it; very few were able to manage Ben's relative autonomy. Bellamy was also somewhat atypical, in that by 1860 few doctors were willing to report on a patient whom they had not seen personally. Doctors increasingly insisted on observing and touching their patients' bodies in order to know how to treat them, as part of their growing commitment to scientific medicine. Ben's owner, Colonel L., who was scarcely mentioned in Bellamy's account except as the person who sent a messenger for a doctor, apparently believed he had little choice but to allow his occasionally hemorrhaging and insane slave to earn his own living, which was certainly atypical behavior for a slaveholder.

Both Ben the slave and Bellamy the doctor shared a web of assumptions that would have shaped their interactions, were Ben ever actually to become Bellamy's patient. Their assumptions were rooted in their bodies. Both would have understood Ben's race as black or African, Bellamy's as white or European or Caucasian. Both would have understood themselves to be male, at least until Ben's fall and consequent bleeding caused him to question his sex. They both understood sex to be a fundamental determinant of identity, along with race. They also would have recognized that the biological characteristics of bodies had social consequences in the antebellum South. Neither would have questioned that white men could be doctors and black men could not,[4] and while Ben successfully challenged slavery as an institution shaping his daily life, both would have recognized that blacks were slaves and whites were not. Both might also have considered that Ben's injury was as much emotional as physical, that the injury to his body had caused harm to his mind, and that to cure one successfully would cure the other. Both possibly realized that Ben would have no interest in being cured as long as he was a slave, although Bellamy offered no such insight in his account. They both certainly would have recognized that their interactions were shaped by a set of oppositional relationships that was the consequence of the status of their bodies, as slave and free, victim and expert, subject and authority, although they would not have used this language.

Ben and Bellamy's experiences reflect contested aspects of antebellum southern society that will be explored throughout this book. As a trained doctor, Bellamy was part of an increasingly professionalized practice of medicine that often was rewarded cultural authority. This was a national phenomenon, reflecting a growing definition of medicine as a science and acceptance of science as an arbiter of truth. Southern doctors were active participants in this endeavor. However, in the South it took on a distinctly political cast, different from the rest of the nation. As slaveholders became ever more anxious about defending the peculiar institution on which they depended, southern doctors' claims of scientific authority sometimes took the form of providing anatomical and physiological arguments to support it. They increasingly argued that race carried with it bodily differences that justified the subordination of those of African descent, who were deemed biologically inferior to those who enslaved them. Doctors' growing contributions to the defense of slavery simultaneously enhanced their own prestige and that of the science in which they wrapped their claims.[5]

At the same time that southern physicians located themselves on the front lines of defending slavery, their peers throughout the nation sought to justify the social subordination of women on the basis of their biological differences from men.[6] At least in the North, the conventions that separated the spheres of men and women were increasingly challenged by women eager to legitimize their fuller participation in society. Medicine became a key arena for debate about male and female bodies and minds and consequently about their places in society. Many physicians defined women by their bodies. While their arguments varied to some extent, they believed that women's reproductive functions rendered them fundamentally different from men, physically vulnerable and in need of protection. While white

women in the South offered fewer challenges to the social order than their northern counterparts, the region's doctors shared the belief that women's bodies were
weaker than men's, justifying their subordination. Thus the occasional bleeding
from Ben's urethra caused by his injury led him to fear that he had become a
woman, which Bellamy believed was the chief cause and symptom of his insanity.

Debates about the implications of race and sex differences came together in
the South, where they were so closely intertwined as to make it impossible to
generalize about black and white bodies without considering male and female
and vice versa. In order to be consistent, those doctors who sought to define black
bodies as inferior to white bodies, and female bodies as inferior to male bodies, also had to consider that some black bodies were male and thus supposedly
superior and that some white bodies were female and thus supposedly inferior.
In other words, simply pronouncing male bodies superior did not allow for the
subordination of black men; simply pronouncing white bodies superior did not
allow for the subordination of white women. Outside the South, where debates
about slavery were political rather than medical, doctors had a lesser need to
reconcile race and sex differences. There, medical attention could focus on sex
alone, or sometimes on the connections between sex and class differences. But
since class was not defined as biologically fixed, the need to reconcile contradictory positions was far less urgent than it was in the South.[7]

Like Bellamy, one way doctors sought to understand race and sex was to define
what was normal, which they conceptualized in terms of the ideal. They believed
that medical truths were timeless and objective, needing only to be discovered
and implemented to improve human lives. Drawing on the growing cultural authority of science, doctors began to appropriate the prerogative once claimed by
ministers to define the ideal life, a role physicians have not relinquished to this
day. Doctors believed that they held a privileged position in relation to the truth
about bodies. They thought that their knowledge could ensure the well-being of
individuals and thus create a society that was not marred by strife. Only if people
stayed in the literal and figurative places for which their bodies were best suited
could they achieve happiness and society become more perfect. Only doctors
could define those places. They defined those who rejected their proper place
as suffering from physical and mental illnesses, assuming that body and mind
interacted to produce people who did not behave as they should.

Laypeople of both sexes and races did not necessarily agree with all of the truths
about bodies offered by physicians. The cultural authority claimed by physicians in
the name of science was new in antebellum America, and not everyone was convinced by it. Laypeople knew that bodies suffered and died and that physicians did
not always bring significant relief. Neither could they always save lives. Laypeople
were not about to cede explanatory power to doctors without measuring doctors'
views against their own bodily experiences or evaluating them according to their
own beliefs. Blacks in particular had their own explanatory models to account

for bodily differences and for illness, rooted in cultural traditions and religious beliefs brought from Africa. Doctors may have wished to claim cultural authority but were not automatically granted it by their patients or society in general.

In the antebellum period, lay skepticism about medicine's explanatory powers was legitimized by medicine's obvious disunity. The old truths inherited from the Greeks about health being a state of balance of the four bodily humors were no longer convincing, although language referring to them continued to pervade medical writing. The germ theory of disease that would revolutionize medicine was still decades away, leaving both ordinary practitioners and medical theorists without a widely accepted system for understanding disease and how to cure it. Instead, a variety of what have come to be known as medical sects shared the practice of medicine with regular (or allopathic) physicians, each group offering a different set of explanations and remedies and each loudly proclaiming that the others were ineffective at best, dangerous at worst. Allopathic physicians were most common, but they practiced alongside Thomsonian, homeopathic, botanic, and eclectic physicians, among others.[8]

Physicians concerned with defining the parameters of the normal and abnormal body and mind did so in an increasingly professionalized context. During the antebellum period, medical schools, many with their own journals, appeared throughout the nation, each teaching a particular sect's version of the truth. While most doctors were trained by the traditional method of apprenticeships, increasing numbers of aspiring physicians and their patients began to want the benefits of a more formal medical education.[9] Journals added to this education, offering their readers both the latest information and a forum for discussion of theory and practice. In addition, physicians of the various sects regularly encouraged one another to subscribe to codes of medical ethics that would establish definitions of appropriate practice; many of these included statements about appropriate behavior for patients as well.[10] The existence of codes defining proper practice did not prevent physicians from deriding the efforts of their rivals, sometimes even to their white patients. Those patients were then left to choose the practitioner whose views corresponded most closely to their own or who made the most convincing promises—or who was available. Slaves were routinely denied the opportunity to choose at all but secretly sought the advice of their own practitioners. In an era of intense competition between sects and practitioners, professionalization was an appealing goal, but it had its limits. Nevertheless, physicians of all sorts were committed to healing their patients. Their efforts to professionalize were among the most visible signs of their desire to ameliorate suffering and save lives, even as they quarreled with one another about how best to do so.

No matter what medical sect the doctors belonged to, their views about the body often reflected those of significant segments of the white public, and sometimes of blacks as well. Doctors were, after all, embedded in their culture and shared many of its fundamental assumptions. In many cases, it was not so much their practices that were controversial as the language and authority with which they proclaimed them. Their training and specialized knowledge did not prevent them from defining the body in ways that were familiar to most southern whites. Their medical claims were often compelling precisely because they were based on widely accepted truths. In particular, doctors in the South were influenced by the race and gender beliefs of their society. Often, preserving those beliefs meant that they had to struggle to maintain medical consistency. The social hierarchies of race and sex were too deeply entrenched for them to question.

Southern doctors shared more than just the beliefs about race and sex of their society. Virtually all of them also thought that disease was different in each ailing body. Cholera was always cholera and smallpox always smallpox, but that did not mean that everyone afflicted with either ailment had the same experience or reacted the same way to treatment. The race and sex as well as the temperament of the ailing body mattered. In addition, one disease could easily transform itself into another, further complicating diagnosis. For example, there was no way to know when a patient's diarrhea was cholera or whether it would become cholera, nor was it possible to distinguish between a simple cold, a long list of different fevers, pneumonia, and consumption, any of which could easily slide into another. Physicians struggling to diagnose their patients' ills had to take the inconclusiveness of diseases into account as well as the individual body. H. R. Easterling, an Alabama physician, noted, "We find but seldom the same treatment applicable to each similar case of disease, because we have to administer to patients of different temperaments, habits, and different strength of constitution."[11] Another physician warned his colleagues to be careful when treating women patients: "It is with herself, only, *when in health,* that we can rationally compare her if diseased."[12] Furthermore, southern physicians increasingly believed that diseases, like the bodies they affected, were regional as well, requiring them to consider not just race and sex, but also place. They thought fevers were particularly local in nature. While physicians may have wished to rely on the authority of science, the science of medicine remained remarkably imprecise.

Medicine's imprecision, at least by modern standards, was the result of the complex relationship between theory and practice. Elite physicians were becoming quite skeptical of empiricism, claiming that understanding disease demanded explanatory theories and Baconian analysis, not anecdotal accounts. Gunning Bedford, professor of obstetrics, the diseases of women and children, and clinical midwifery at the University of New York, warned physicians "to be cautious in your diagnosis; all successful treatment depends upon it. . . . It makes our science one of philosophic truth, and gives it the impress of certainty." He added, "[N]o such light guides the empiric; he is lost in darkness and doubt, and floats in a sea of conjecture, whilst the scientific physician proudly claims for his profession a basis firm and impregnable."[13]

Physicians in actual practice appreciated the importance of theory but were also concerned with the daily demands of curing their patients and sustaining their reputations. Those demands required observation, insight, and experience, which brought them dangerously close to empiricism in the eyes of the elite. These tensions were reflected in the attempt of many physicians, including Bellamy, to define the parameters of what was normal. Empiricism may have been derided by those physicians in a position to shape professional medicine, but understanding the truths of the body as well as the exceptions to those truths remained an important undertaking for all physicians.[14]

Doctors who sought to understand the bodies of their patients also sought to define what was abnormal—that is, sickness. For midcentury physicians, that sometimes included identifying new diseases and medicalizing conditions not previously considered part of their terrain, such as most reproductive functions. This reinforced their cultural authority, as it enabled them to claim all bodies, women's in particular, as in need of their specialized expertise and care. It also allowed them to enhance their definition of medicine as science, for even when sick individuals could not recognize themselves as sick, doctors could and thereby might restore them to health.

Physicians committed to understanding the ailing bodies of their patients recognized that they had no choice but to consider their patients' own views of what was wrong with them and how to cure it. The resulting tensions inspired doctors to consider the ways bodies and minds influenced each other. While religious thinkers and philosophers had long considered such questions as the physical location of the soul and the mechanisms of consciousness, questions that were given new immediacy by Enlightenment philosophers, doctors were relative latecomers to the discussion of mind and body.[15] Joining in, they quickly realized that they could turn the conversation to their advantage by attributing their patients' failure to get better to the diseased actions of their minds. While never expressed in such crass terms, physicians nevertheless self-consciously traced a circular route between mind and body, suggesting that a wise healer had to pay attention to both, as well as to the connections between them, in order to cure disease and restore health.

Physicians' debates about mind and body most often focused on women, who were presumed to be weaker than men in both dimensions. Women's inability to willfully control the workings of their reproductive bodies led physicians to assume that women experienced a similar lack of control over their wills, both of which they believed could cause disease. They did not think that sick women could will themselves to health. But in their efforts to explain women's illnesses and their failure to respond to treatment, doctors found the malignant workings of women's minds on their weak and diseased bodies a helpful ally. Nowhere was this link more clear than in physicians' diagnosing of hysteria, an old disease that seemingly reappeared with renewed vigor in the nineteenth century. They believed that insanity in all its forms could have organic causes, just as a deranged mind could lead to bodily decay. Women were perceived as far more vulnerable than men to both sources of affliction. For example, physicians worried that the influence of mind over body led women to a false sense of modesty that caused them to reject examination and treatment. At the same time, women's reproductive functions could cause them to engage in erratic and dangerous thinking and behavior. Doctors exhorted women to try to control their minds, but with little hope of success because they were convinced that women's weaknesses prevented them from doing so effectively.

These general trends in the history of medicine were complicated in the South, where some people could be recognized as sick while others had to be pronounced well according to the demands of race-based slavery. As we will see in the first two chapters, what was increasingly defined in the South as normal for white bodies might not be accepted as normal for black. Similarly, what was normal for male bodies could not be considered normal for female. Yet southern physicians bent on developing theories of medicine worked hard to develop plausible theories about race and sex that met the region's ideological needs while remaining consistent with the biological truths they observed. Defining bodies was tricky business that demanded social and cultural sensitivity as well as scientific rigor. However, few southern doctors worried very much about Native Americans, perhaps because by the antebellum period relatively few native people remained within the Old South and those who did seldom called upon their services.

Doctors who tried to define health and sickness for men and women, black and white, also had to contend with the realities of a slaveholding society. Slaveholders often defined slaves as healthy enough to work when the slaves considered themselves to be sick. At the same time, slaveholders wanted to protect their financial investment in the bodies of slaves and so had incentive to provide medical care for them. Slaves had their own beliefs about bodily differences and the causes of sickness as well as how to cure them, but their beliefs were seldom validated or their practices respected by slaveholders and doctors. Doctors had financial as well as class-based incentives to agree with slaveholders, yet they were sometimes willing to set themselves up as guardians of slaves' well-being by insisting that they be treated with sufficient care to preserve or restore health. That care, of course, included calling on the services of physicians when slaves were sick, along with appropriate food, clothing, and shelter. In the process, some physicians advocated for a more humane version of slavery, even as they remained important defenders of it.

Southern physicians did not limit themselves to defining the meanings of black and white bodies; they also considered the bodies of men and women, the focus of chapter 2. Believing reproductive processes were inherently dangerous to women's health, doctors throughout the nation sought to extend their authority by proclaiming that menarche, menstruation, pregnancy, childbirth, lactation, and menopause often required medical attention. In the South, these vulnerabilities had to be ascribed to white women's bodies at the same time that doctors rejected them for black women. But doctors eager to expand their practice and willing to acknowledge black women's suffering could not reject them too vehemently. While never completely successful at resolving these contradictions, southern doctors utilized the familiar trope of the dangers of modern civilized life to explain white women's vulnerable bodies and reproductive suffering in contrast to the relative absence of such weakness in black women. They argued that black women lived closer to a state of nature and thus were healthier than their mistresses, even though biologically inferior. But this left doctors scrambling to explain why civilization was harmful to white women's health, since it was also considered beneficial because it lifted them out of benighted subservience to men and offered them protection from the demands of earning a living. Their ingenious answer was to accuse white women in modern society of leading unhealthy lives. Doctors could thus claim jurisdiction over the bodies of women of both races, but for very different reasons. They felt less need to compare the bodies of black and white men. Both were assumed to be physically strong because they were male, while black men's assumed mental inferiority was ascribed to their race.

In the increasingly contested political arena of the antebellum years, southern physicians knew that their work would most likely be received favorably if it reinforced the region's distinctiveness, the subject of chapter 3. Developing the concept of place helped them to reconcile the complexities of race and sex when defining bodies and their health and sicknesses. The belief that medicine was regional enabled the white South to lessen its anxieties about itself as provincial and to proclaim its superior understanding of black bodies. Even beyond race, however, doctors were well aware that southerners fell victim to different diseases and had to be treated differently from people elsewhere in the nation. Therapeutics appropriate in the North could have devastating consequences if prescribed for southern bodies even when the disease appeared to be the same. Regional diseases and treatments in turn demanded the development of separate southern medical schools and journals. Thus, doctors argued that a specifically southern medical theory and practice was necessary.

Physicians who developed ideas about placed bodies neatly allied themselves with the prevailing beliefs of their society. Southerners of all sorts believed that their bodies were directly influenced by all of the attributes of location: climate, atmosphere, smells. Whites believed that changes in weather influenced a body's susceptibility to disease and that travel could cure it. Those who could do so fled low-lying plantations in the spring and did not return until the first frost. Laypeople recognized that malaria and other fevers were far more common in the South than elsewhere and worried about epidemics of yellow fever, a specifically southern disease. In this sense, laypeople shared doctors' convictions that medicine was specific to place and that bodies were shaped by their environment.

Southern physicians who recognized race, sex, and place as essential aspects of bodies had little choice but to acknowledge that these categories were not always precisely defined. People could move from the North or from Europe to the South or from one place to another within it. Although custom and law defined all slaves as black, medicine recognized that interracial sex led to many bodies that combined the blood and thus the characteristics of the two races. Far less common, but certainly compelling to doctors, were bodies that exhibited aspects of both male and female. Undeniably female bodies presented their own ambiguities. Physicians determined to conceptualize a typology of bodies recognized that using oppositional categories did not satisfy the demands of their everyday experience. Determined to define what was normal, they recognized that studying bodies that fell between categories could help them understand health and sickness. Their efforts to understand various types of anomalous bodies are the subject of chapter 4.

Southern physicians believed that the bodies they examined and sought to cure were not simply subject to the physiological rules defined by race, sex, and place. They knew that bodies were also influenced by the beliefs, attitudes, and behavior of individuals, which they sometimes termed *mind*. Minds, too, were subject to the influence of race, sex, and place, but they also evinced a troubling inclination to defy what physicians considered appropriate behavior. In the South, where appropriate behavior was even more rigidly prescribed by race and sex than in the rest of the nation and where white men considered deviations from those norms dangerous to the social order, physicians struggled to disentangle the influences of minds and bodies for each group in the population. They asked themselves how best to treat women of both races suffering from gynecologic disorders as well as pregnant and birthing women whose ideas about their bodies did not match those of their physicians. They asked whether black men as well as women of both races could be diagnosed with hysteria. They wondered how to reconcile their patients' own views of what was wrong and how to treat it with their own, which could lead to conflicts about modesty, use of the speculum, and the very nature of health and disease, among others. Doctors' views of the interactions of mind and body in their patients are the subject of chapter 5.

Ordinary southerners who tried to make sense of their illnesses turned to physicians for their expertise, but they also relied on their own understandings of their bodies, minds, and illnesses, which are the focus of chapter 6. Physicians' claims to scientific authority were only as good as laypeople's willingness to grant it to them. In the antebellum South, that willingness was partial at best. Laypeople of both races preferred to define health and sickness for themselves, although slaves also had to contend with their owners' interference. Slaveholders were concerned about shamming, the deliberate invocation of illness on the part of healthy slaves to gain respite from hard labor. Slaves had very different explanations for the origins and meaning of disease than whites did, which further complicated their efforts to define their own bodies' experiences. Women, especially white women, struggled to maintain the attitudes they believed would protect them and their babies from harm during pregnancy and childbirth. Illness itself could be a form of resistance, by slaves against their owners and, less obviously, by white women against pregnancy and patriarchal authority. Physicians who sought to define bodies and minds did so in an arena crowded with opinions.

Lay views were, of course, also important in their own right. Members of both races and sexes sought ways to be healthy and to find meaning in the suffering of their bodies. For white people, the meaning of their bodies was expressed as commonsense truisms that linked body and mind in a web of responsibility for health and sickness. Blacks had an alternate paradigm from that of whites, one that held them less personally responsible for the state of their health and instead recognized the importance of the physical conditions imposed upon them by their owners. Both races were influenced by the teachings of Christianity, although the messages they took from it differed; some blacks retained significant aspects of African beliefs about the body as well.

Lay views about bodies were important to doctors because they defined the parameters of what was possible within the daily practice of medicine, the subject of chapter 7. Doctors knew that laypeople were not reluctant to voice their opinions or critique their doctors' diagnoses and treatments. The sick individual and his or her family, friends, and, in the case of slaves, owners contested doctors' advice when it was not consistent with their own beliefs. They were likely to try to cure themselves before calling for help, which physicians complained caused greater sickness. Sick people also switched physicians or the kind of physician when it suited them and it was possible to do so. Doctors were constantly evaluated by their patients, even as they constantly evaluated them.

Southern physicians' efforts to define ideal lives, health and sickness, and the differences between categories of bodies were important not only for their practices and the cultural politics of the region, but also because illness itself seemed so dangerous. There could be no doubt in the minds of doctors and laypeople alike that disease was ubiquitous. People were often sick, and sick people often died. Life was uncertain; danger lurked everywhere. Dogs could be mad, a change in the weather could bring disease, teething was dangerous to babies, the progress of epidemics could be watched but not halted. There was no way to know whether even the most innocuous-appearing illness would end in death. Every pregnancy brought the possibility of injury or death to mother and child. Slaves could be sold, with loved ones separated forever even more cruelly than when deaths were caused by illness and injury. As a result, understanding the nature of bodies was important for everyone.

Ways of understanding the body and mind were different for black and white, men and women, physician and layperson. Along each overlapping line of difference, the body became a deeply politicized arena of contest, in which the nature of suffering and the definition of health and sickness became part of the larger tensions that stretched the fabric of southern society. As southerners struggled with one another over the consequences of slavery and subordination, they relied most directly on definitions of the body as raced, sexed, and placed to give meaning and substance to their politics. Those definitions played themselves out in very specific and often highly charged ways, as Ben, the slave man who used his periodic bleeding to gain a degree of autonomy from his master, and Bellamy, his erstwhile physician, surely recognized.

This book examines medical and lay perspectives on the political body in the antebellum old South, focusing primarily on those states from Virginia to Alabama. More recently settled and frontier areas would have had fewer physicians, and they would have had less investment in elite theorizing and medical education than those on the seaboard. Memphis and New Orleans were exceptions to that pattern, and the writings of physicians from those cities were widely reprinted in the medical journals published farther east. The book relies on a range of sources to understand physicians' thinking and practice, including medical journals and texts, the theses and other writing of medical students, and physicians' diaries, daybooks, and letters. It also explores laypeople's views, using a range of private documents from whites, primarily letters and diaries, and the slave narratives and folklore for slaves. Each of these sources has limits that have been carefully explored by historians, but together they remain the best windows into the thoughts, feelings, and experiences of people in the past. The views represented are skewed toward the elite among both doctors and the lay white public. Wealthy whites were most likely to own slaves and were overwhelmingly literate, enabling them to leave records of their experiences. Elite doctors were most likely to publish in medical journals, which were typically affiliated with medical schools and edited by their faculty. However, journal editors eager—sometimes desperate—to fill their pages often printed material from more ordinary practitioners, including accounts of interesting cases such as Bellamy's. As a result, both regular and sectarian medical journals reflected a conversation among physicians searching for the best ways to understand ailing bodies. That conversation is reflected in these pages as well, as elite doctors developed theories of race, sex, and place that their less abstractly inclined peers sought to integrate into their daily practice. In fact, even those physicians most interested in defining bodies spent time at the bedsides of patients; doing so was necessary both for their livelihoods and for their identities as physicians.

Although Eric Cassell would see doctors as historians, even with the best of sources historians cannot turn themselves into modern-day clinicians. Not only do diseases change over time, so too does the language with which people describe their subjective experiences and the labels doctors attach to them. Similarly, the social meanings of disease change in different contexts.[16] The historian's responsibility is to understand bodies, sickness, and health in peoples' own time, not to translate their experiences or diagnoses into modern terms.

# CHAPTER 1

# Constructing Race

For mid-nineteenth-century white southerners, race was a biological category so deeply rooted that determining whether the group of people variously called black, African, or Negro were even of the same order of being as those who were white, European, or Caucasian was a fundamental question. Scientists, physicians, clergymen, and more ordinary observers questioned whether God had created all human beings according to one design or whether humans were of different species, the results of separate creations, a belief known as polygenesis. Making a determination between the theories supporting the unity of human beings from the time of creation and those that emphasized racial differences as a result of separate creations was no easy undertaking, in part because the consequences were profound. Those arguing for the unity of the human race from the time of creation generally founded their thinking in Christian teachings and claimed that no matter what the color of their skin or other physical characteristics, all human beings could be saved. Medical and scientific observers, by contrast, tended to argue for racial diversity. They claimed that like horses and donkeys that were distinct types of animals but yet could mate and produce offspring, albeit sterile ones, Negroes and Caucasians were distinct orders of being. They viewed Africans as closer to apes than to Europeans, justifying their position by a variety of scientific observations of skulls, genitalia, and other body parts. Adherents of both positions were convinced of the inherent inferiority of Africans and the superiority of Caucasians. Even those who believed that all peoples were created at the same time agreed that the influence of the environment on subsequent generations had resulted in profound differences.[1]

The origins of race were of more than theoretical or political interest for those who were concerned with caring for the sick. If those of African descent were of a different species from Europeans or Americans,[2] then their bodies experienced disease differently and responded differently to treatment. Not acknowledging the implications of those differences could have serious, even fatal, consequences. As a result, white southern physicians and slaveholders believed it was important to study the disease consequences of differences and to apply that knowledge in ways that would ameliorate suffering and save lives.

Slaves had their own understandings of the origins of race and their implications for bodily suffering. Far less elaborately developed at least in surviving sources than the ideas of whites, slaves' theories nevertheless sought to explain not just the origins of the visible differences between the races, but also the bodily consequences of those differences. Some of their explanations were built upon Christian imagery, such as those that viewed Africans as the descendants of Ham, cursed but still human. Others referred to God as a baker who burned one attempt at creating humans and undercooked another, resulting in dark and light skins; the implication was that those of mixed race were God's ideal.[3] Whatever their explanation for racial diversity, slaves could not help but be immediately aware of the consequences, legal as well as medical. Slaves recognized not only the close ties between their skin color and subordination, they also knew that their race was vulnerable to physical as well as emotional suffering as a result of that subordination.

Members of both races who sought explanations for and control over suffering and disease had to grapple with the nature of illness itself and its racial context. For whites in particular, this was a problematic undertaking, for explanations of disease causation were very much in flux in the mid-nineteenth century. Medical authorities still spoke of imbalances in the four humors familiar from ancient medical writings, but their explanatory usefulness was compromised by newer ideas that attributed disease not just to the peculiarities of the individual body but also to its race, sex, wealth, housing, diet, work, and location. Diseases did not present the same symptoms or follow the same trajectory from person to person or even in individuals of the same race, sex, or body type.[4] The individual course of the disease in the body demanded individualized treatment; what was therapeutic for one person was not necessarily so for another. In addition, one disease could easily shade into another, making distinctions even more difficult to determine for physicians hoping to cure their patients' ills. Physicians sometimes did not even bother to try to name a specific disease in a suffering individual, since diseases and bodies were so specific. If nothing else, allopathic physicians intent on validating their professional credentials could point to this extreme specificity as a means of justifying their own knowledge and importance. Since few generalizations were possible, only experts could determine what was best for the individually suffering body.[5]

At the same time that physicians were bent on coming to grips with the racialized characteristics of bodies, they also needed to find generalizations so that they could build their profession upon an agreed-upon body of knowledge that could be transmitted to students in medical schools. To describe their undertaking as exclusively political or mercenary is unnecessarily harsh, although such factors certainly entered into their deliberations. Mid-nineteenth-century physicians of all sorts were engaged in a wide-ranging struggle for professional definition, and such considerations were unlikely to be excluded from their thinking. Southern physicians, however, were additionally concerned with constructing theories of the body that had explanatory power in the sickrooms of both slaves and whites. In their efforts to do so, they developed theories of race and disease that directly influenced their analysis of individual suffering bodies as well as lay understanding of the meaning of health and illness. The solutions they devised affected individuals' experiences of illness, the treatment of the sick, and the South's racial politics.

Physicians' interest in exploring the differences between black and white bodies was more than simply medical. In addition, physicians sought to claim a place for themselves in the increasingly shrill national debate about slavery. By offering their expertise as impartial observers of immutable biological truths, doctors hoped to demonstrate the inevitability and benefits of slavery and, at the same time, enhance their own reputations. Some might wish to contest the implications of race and the legitimacy of slavery, but southern doctors were united in their belief that the truth could be known by studying the laws of science and nature. While thus positioning themselves above the political fray, doctors insisted on the primacy of race in defining bodies, which allowed them to speak with a new kind of authority in defense of slavery. The success of their efforts to do so, closely tied to strategies for developing their own professional status, inspired yet even more searching for scientific truth in a circular process. While some physicians were able to critique the practices of individual slaveholders and call for a more humane slavery, none was able to recognize the politics that was at the heart of science as they perceived it. Instead, those who sought national recognition for their conclusions about raced bodies and slavery ended up simultaneously defending a particular southern science of medicine, one far less objective than they were willing to admit.

## Defining the Differences between Races

Physicians concerned with the bodily consequences of race differences typically grounded their thinking in observation. Empiricism was a common strategy of midcentury medical practice that effectively served the needs of those whose culture and society led them to view race as paramount in explaining human variation.[6] Confronted with multiple challenges to and defenses of slavery, southern doctors could rarely see beyond race as a way of defining bodies. Instead, they turned their attention to studies of comparative anatomy as a means of determining for themselves the meanings and consequences of race for the body.

Midcentury southern physicians were unlikely to ask themselves whether the differences between whites and blacks were no more than skin deep. To do so would have required them to acknowledge the possibility that slavery was immoral, because the human beings inside those skins were essentially the same.

As a group, physicians were quite unprepared to do this, although many called for improvements in the treatment of slaves. Instead, assumptions about race differences were so ingrained as to be beyond question; the only significant issue had to do with the meanings of those differences, not their existence. Their studies of comparative anatomy, then, were built on the presumption that there were significant race differences, differences that led them to consider the medical meanings of race.

Inspired in part by a new scientific interest in accurate measurement, physicians and natural scientists made a variety of efforts to quantify physical difference. Their interest in comparative anatomy was influenced by the work of such men as Samuel Morton and Louis Agassiz, non-southerners whose work was much admired in the South. After studying medicine in Edinburgh, Morton studied fossils and tuberculosis, practiced medicine, taught anatomy at the Pennsylvania Medical College, collected skulls, and became well known among American scientists through his position as corresponding secretary of the Academy of Natural Sciences. At his death in 1851, he had amassed over a thousand skulls. Even more prestigious was Louis Agassiz, the Swiss-born Harvard professor widely acknowledged to be America's premier scientist. He founded and directed Harvard's Museum of Comparative Zoology; later he would become the "only major scientific opponent of evolution." Agassiz' personal repugnance toward blacks influenced his belief in polygenesis and his theories of racial differences.[7] He lectured repeatedly in Charleston between 1847 and 1853 and held a chair in comparative anatomy at the Medical College of South Carolina in 1852–53. He thus influenced many southern naturalists, scientists, and physicians to share both his scientific approach to race and his interest in comparative anatomy.[8]

Medical interest in comparative anatomy and racial difference was aided in the 1830s and 1840s by scientific and popular interest in phrenology, which sought to understand personality by reading the shape of individual skulls. While phrenology's claims to scientific validity were diminished by its reputation as a parlor curiosity, efforts to measure the comparative size, weight, and volume of skulls retained an aura of legitimate science long after the public's enthusiasm for phrenology had dimmed. Led by Morton, natural scientists collected as many skulls as they could from different races and sought to measure their volume by filling them with sand, millet, pepper seed, or buckshot. As expected, they found that Caucasian skulls were the largest while "Ethiopian" the smallest.[9] They found it easy to move from measuring skulls to assertions about brain size; smaller skulls could only mean smaller brains and therefore lesser intelligence.

Southern physicians shared this interest in brain size. In 1838, the *Southern Botanic Journal,* one of the most successful of the Thomsonian[10] journals, reprinted an article by Andrew Combe, a leading theorist of phrenology, in which he argued "that de facto the negro brain is inferior in intellectual power to that of the European." While Combe grudgingly conceded in response to critics that in some measures the two categories of skulls might appear to be equal, still he concluded that when the parts of the brain that mattered most for intelligence were measured, Europeans enjoyed "a decided superiority . . . over the negro."[11]

In addition to measuring skulls, those determined to prove white superiority paid close attention to the angle of the face. They argued that the more nearly vertical the plane of the face (orthognathic) from forehead to jaw, the greater the intellect and the more highly developed the category of people. Those whose jaws jutted out and foreheads receded had a more horizontal (prognathic) facial angle and were considered less attractive, less intelligent, and less developed. Proponents of this theory relied on both observations of individual subjects and images of characteristic types, including Greek statuary. Not surprisingly, they found what they expected, although they were never successful in offering a coherent explanation. At best, they argued from history: Because the Greeks were highly developed and had vertical faces while Africans were primitive and had jutting jaws, they assumed a correlation. They appeared not to notice the tautology in their thinking. The most extreme proponents of this view extended the analogy even to animals, sometimes including drawings of chimpanzees, apes, or baboons to demonstrate the similarity between their faces and those of Africans.

As subjects of study, physiognomy, comparative anatomy, and ethnology all sought to explain race differences. As a result, they drew the attention of clergymen and physicians as well as those who would today be considered anthropologists, natural scientists, and sociologists.[12] One of the key voices in the debate belonged to Josiah Nott, who was particularly well known throughout the nation and abroad for his writings on race theory. Nott, a physician, was educated at South Carolina College, the University of Pennsylvania, and in Europe. He practiced first in Columbia, South Carolina, and then in Mobile, Alabama. Deeply interested in science and natural history, Nott argued in a series of articles and books published from the mid-1840s to the late 1850s and beyond that blacks and whites were the result of separate creations. His racial theories were influenced by his medical training, but Nott was not primarily concerned with the medical consequences of racial differences. His concerns were more related to classifying humanity and refuting the clerical position regarding the unity of human creation than about the specifics of medical care. Nott argued that blacks and whites were created separately and amounted to separate species; mulattos[13] were, in his view, a hybrid species sharing characteristics of both parent races.[14] His writing, and those of others who shared his concerns, would set the stage for an extensive debate regarding comparative anatomy and race differences. While Nott sometimes appeared to present his views in the most obstreperous manner possible in order to goad his clerical opponents, his views were taken seriously by many physicians and laypeople who saw in them convincing explanations for race differences.

Nott published widely in the medical journals of the day while sustaining a busy and lucrative medical practice. His chief work, published jointly with the peripatetic lecturer George Gliddon, was *Types of Mankind; or, Ethnological Researches,* published in 1854. An immediate sensation, the book secured Nott's reputation as a racial theorist. Here and elsewhere, Nott argued that the Bible's account of the creation of Adam and Eve applied only to Caucasians. Humanity was divided into many different types or races, each biologically distinct and each best suited to the specific geographic area in which it had first existed.[15] Further, Nott argued, the races of the world were ordered hierarchically, progressing roughly from the darkest-skinned and most geographically southern races to the lightest and most northerly ones. He also considered the implications of orthognathic and prognathic facial angles to be telling evidence of African inferiority to other races. *Types of Mankind* contains dramatic images of these differences and features a foldout engraving that places African skulls on a continuum alongside those of animals. Perhaps most important, Nott claimed to base his conclusions on the inescapable foundation of scientific fact, independent of theology or the chronology of human history offered in the Bible.[16]

For Nott, the key questions for scientific inquiry concerned the "primitive organic structure of each race," its "moral and psychical character," how it was "modified by the combined action of time and moral and physical causes," and its "position in the social scale" as assigned by Providence. He argued that race differences were both original, dating from the Creation, and permanent. The history of the world showed "that human progress has arisen mainly from the war of races." He had no doubt that some races were superior, others far inferior.[17]

In his effort to be precise and scientific, Nott refused to posit a direct relationship between climate and the world's diversity of races, but he did argue that "a black skin would seem to be the best suited to hot climates" while "the strictly white races lie mostly in the Temperate Zone, where they flourish best." According to Nott, the Caucasian races have "the largest brains and the most powerful intellect . . . [and] are by nature ambitious, daring, domineering, and reckless of danger"; only they "have extended over and colonized all parts of the globe" in order to "carry out their great mission of civilizing the earth." Nott described the many varieties of Caucasians to be found in Europe, the eastern Mediterranean, and Egypt, tracing their histories as far back in time as he could.[18]

Nott similarly described the "African types," which were "as varied as those of Europe or Asia." He portrayed them in "a regular gradation" from the lowest Hottentot and Bushmen in the southern part of Africa to the highest Egyptian and Berber in the northeastern parts of the continent.[19] The former were "the lowest and most beastly specimens of mankind, . . . but little removed, both in moral and physical characters, from the orang-outan." In general, Nott remarked, Africa "shows a succession of human beings with intellects as dark as their skins" and with heads that offered little hope of future improvement. Those brought to or born in America were "more intelligent and better developed in their physique generally than their native compatriots of Africa; . . . but such intelligence is easily explained by their ceaseless contact with the whites, from whom they derive much instruction . . . [and] increased comforts." In the United States, where "they are regularly and adequately fed, they become healthier, better developed, and more humanized," compared to those who remained in Africa. Like the wild animals they resembled, Africans were "greatly improved . . . by domestication." That improvement, however, reached its limit after one or two generations. Central to Nott's argument was the concept of permanence within the races,[20] which made them specific and separate: "[N]o causes . . . can transmute one type of man into another . . . any more than they could change a horse into an ass." In order to prove his argument, Nott pointed to evidence derived from skulls, which he used to demonstrate the prominent characteristics of each race.[21]

Some of Nott's writings on the medical consequences of separate creations of the various types of mankind were inspired by his work for the insurance industry. In attempting to help insurance companies quantify risk, he carefully investigated mortality rates for white individuals and slave property. Much of this work was based on his own extensive practice, including at the hospital he founded for slaves in Mobile. In this, Nott was in the forefront of the use of statistics for the insurance industry and in public health. He compared the mortality rates among blacks in Charleston, Baltimore, and several northern cities and concluded that the rate of death compared with that in Charleston was double in Philadelphia and triple in Boston.

Nott attributed these differences largely to "the influence of climate and social condition," adding that there can be no question "that many [free blacks] die in the Northern cities, because they have neglected to provide those comforts which are necessary to protect them[selves] against the cold." He added that "when left alone" they were "indolent and improvident, and consequently subject to greater mortality, than they should be."[22] Nott warned that freedom and climate were the cause of high rates of death among Boston blacks. In contrast, blacks in Charleston and the rest of the South enjoyed a lower rate of mortality than any population in continental Europe. To explain these statistics, Nott argued that, unlike whites, people of African descent did not require acclimation to the South because they were "originally natives of hot climates."[23] Overall, Nott claimed that living in slavery was beneficial to blacks, who otherwise suffered undue rates of illness and death. Many physicians shared his conclusions, although few were willing to undertake his rigorous data collection and statistical analysis to support them.

Another outspoken participant in this debate was Samuel Cartwright. Cartwright was a controversial physician whose writings were widely published and reprinted in southern medical journals and *DeBow's Review*. Well trained, he had studied with America's premier physician, Benjamin Rush, at the University of Pennsylvania and practiced medicine in Natchez, Mississippi, and New Orleans, where he developed expertise in battling cholera as well as diseases peculiar to the South. His reputation inspired the Louisiana State Medical Convention to appoint him to chair a committee reporting on diseases of blacks, which led to his best-known and most widely reprinted articles.[24] An avid defender of slavery and polygenesis, Cartwright used the opportunity to define the differences between the races to justify blacks' continued subordination. While his views were considered outlandish by many of his colleagues and recognized as extreme even among southern physicians, Cartwright nevertheless vigorously defended himself in print and influenced the terms of debate among southern physicians.

Cartwright argued that there were "two distinct races of people" in the South, "differing widely in their anatomy and physiology, and consequently requiring a corresponding difference in their medical treatment." According to Cartwright, it had been known for centuries that Africans' blood was blacker than that of whites: "[T]he negro is not only a negro on the skin, but under the skin." He called upon a range of authorities to demonstrate that not only was the blood of Africans darker, but so were their brains, membranes, and muscles. In addition, their bones were harder, their brains smaller, and their nerves larger than those of whites. These differences were the cause of blacks' "debasement of mind," which was "imprinted by the hand of nature" and not, as some northerners suggested, the result of slavery. As a result of these differences, "the same medical treatment which would benefit or cure a white man, would often injure or kill a negro, because of the differences in the organic or physical characters."[25] Cartwright urged physicians to pay careful attention to race differences in order to provide effective care to their patients.

Cartwright particularly urged southern physicians to pay attention to the "external" and "physical difference[s] between the races" at "the dissecting table" and by "daily observation." He challenged the assumption that "the color of the skin constitutes the main and essential difference between the white and black races"; other differences were "more deep, durable, and indelible." These differences extended to "the membranes, the muscles, the tendons, and . . . all the fluids and secretions" as well as the "brain and nerves, the chyle and all the humors," all of which were "tinctured with a shade of the pervading darkness." Cartwright cataloged a long list of anatomical differences, extending to every part of the body.[26]

According to Cartwright, blacks' anatomical differences from whites had a variety of consequences, some medical, others social. For example, differences in blacks' brains and nerves caused them to be more sensual than intellectual; thus "music is a mere sensual pleasure with the negro," without "addressing the understanding." Similarly, their extensively developed nervous systems "would make the Ethiopian race entirely unmanageable," except that they were "associated with a deficiency of red blood" caused by "defective atmospherization . . . of the blood in the lungs." This ineffective breathing, "an excess of nervous matter," and "a deficiency of cerebral matter in the cranium" together "rendered the people of Africa unable to take care of themselves." In other words, anatomy and physiology were the cause "of their indolence and apathy, and [explained] why they have chosen, through countless ages, idleness, misery, and barbarism, instead of industry and frugality."[27] For Cartwright, the characteristics of the raced body explained historical and social differences.

Cartwright was particularly concerned about the consequences of defective atmospherization and hematosis, which "impart to the negro, a nature not unlike that of a new born infant of the white race." In other words, improper breathing (atmospherization) caused blacks' blood to be improperly oxygenated (hematosis), which left them like children. In infants of both races, "full and free respiration of pure, fresh air in repose, so far from being required, is hurtful and prejudicial."[28] However, what was beneficial for babies was "the identical kind of respiration most congenial to the negro constitution, of all ages and sexes," demonstrated by "the universal practice among them of covering their faces and heads, during sleep, with a blanket, or any kind of covering they can get hold of." The inevitable result of this "instinctive and universal method of breathing during sleep" was "defective hematosis and hebitude [*sic*] of intellect."[29]

The sluggishness caused by sleeping with blankets over their heads was not the only similarity between blacks of all ages and white children, according to Cartwright. In addition, they resembled one another "in the activity of the liver" and in their thick but sensitive skin, which caused them to "fear the rod." Blacks of all ages and white children were most alike because "they are very easily governed by love combined with fear, and are ungovernable, vicious and rude" without such attention. Both were "constrained by unalterable physiological laws, to love those in authority over them, who minister to their wants and immediate necessities, and are not cruel or unmerciful." For both, "defective hematosis . . . produces . . . an instinctive feeling of dependence on others, to direct them and to take care of them." Cartwright attributed both children's love of their parents and the "love [slaves] bear to their masters" to these "physiological laws." "Anatomy and physiology have been interrogated," he concluded, and had demonstrated that "the Ethiopian . . . is unfitted from his organization, for the responsibilities of a freeman, but, like the child, is only fitted for a state of dependence and subordination."[30] Cartwright had no sense of irony regarding the convenience of his conclusions for slaveholders, although he would become an important defender of slavery.

Professional identification did not prevent physicians from disagreeing with one another, and southern physicians found plenty to challenge in Cartwright's arguments, even when they accepted his commitment to slavery. Not everyone was convinced by Cartwright's description of the nature and consequences of race differences for the body. One unidentified southern physician writing in the *Charleston Medical Journal and Review* challenged him "to distinguish between two specimens of blood taken respectively from the white and black man" or between specimens of other body parts. This unidentified physician claimed his own experiences of dissection did not reveal "variations of color in other tissues than the skin." He considered those who vouched for such differences "aspirant[s] in the race for fame" and possessed of "imaginative brain[s]." He also did not accept

Cartwright's view that "the negro hears more acutely than the white man" or that his sight is stronger, nor was he convinced by Cartwright's arguments regarding blacks' musical sensibilities. As proof, he offered the complaints of slaveholders whose slaves claimed not to have heard what they were told. He said the only reason that few field hands wore spectacles was that they rarely performed close work; slave cooks and seamstresses were usually "incapacitated by impaired vision." He compared blacks' musical tastes with those of "the rude Irish laborer" and "our own plain, honest backwoods farmers," suggesting that none of them would appreciate "an orchestra in full blast," just as Americans did not appreciate "the monotonous screeches of a bagpipe" or native Chinese music.[31]

Cartwright's critic expanded his objections in the next issue of the journal. The unnamed physician challenged Cartwright to demonstrate with his scalpel his assertions regarding anatomical differences between the races. Even if Cartwright were able to do so, however, he thought little would be proved: "[W]e see no ground here on which to base the idea that [the Negro] is governed by separate and distinct physiological laws." He wondered whether "every little variation which comparative anatomy shall declare to exist between animals belonging to the same species is to give rise to a special system of physiology" and suggested that if this were so, "we are but entering a labyrinth, the intricate windings of which it is but folly to attempt to penetrate." He asked whether "the physiology of a black sheep differ[s] from that of a white one," a question he clearly regarded as absurd.

This same critic viewed Cartwright as "biased by political prejudices" and again warned that mingling "medicine and politics is an unholy contamination of the former" and a danger to science, truth, and virtuous ambition. He was most critical of Cartwright for using the notion of defective hematosis to argue that blacks preferred slavery and were similar to white infants. He suggested that the same could not be said of blacks in Africa and accused him of being "guilty of the most palpable contradictions imaginable."[32] Another critic countered Cartwright by suggesting that "the reason why negroes cover their heads is . . . not to obtain an impure atmosphere, . . . but in cold weather for the purpose of warming themselves . . . and in warm weather to ward off the attack of insects."[33]

The disagreements between Cartwright and his critics were important because they forced southern physicians to clarify their positions regarding the medical construction of race. Southern physicians were demanding for themselves a legitimate voice in the national debate regarding race, arguing that as scientists they were committed to a level of objectivity based on empirical observation that allowed them—and only them—to define truth and reality. Earlier, the right to define race and its consequences had been claimed by political philosophers, legislators, and jurists, who sought to define and encode legal categories of race first in colonial and then in state statutes. Now physicians were increasingly laying claim to this territory, in the name of scientific objectivity.[34] By defining race in medical terms, physicians could argue that slavery was rooted in biology and thus not open to question or interpretation. Yet Cartwright was not merely an apologist for slavery. In his efforts to define the consequences of differences in the anatomy and physiology of the races, he was also trying to advance the boundaries of medicine and the legitimacy of science. That he did not do so to the satisfaction even of those who could easily have been his allies does not negate the significance of his effort to define race in medical terms and at the same time enhance the role of physicians as social arbiters.

Many physicians shared Nott and Cartwright's interest in the medical, moral, and political consequences of race differences. While members of the clergy attacked Nott for rejecting the authority of the Bible, physicians used his findings and those of others interested in race differences to pursue ever more elaborate ideas about the medical consequences of race. In particular, they were interested in understanding the consequences of race differences on a body's susceptibility to disease. There was little doubt in most physicians' minds that the race of a sick body mattered; the question was how. However, most doctors were unable to separate the biological differences they observed and that were so carefully elaborated by men like Nott and Cartwright from the consequences of social conditions, namely slavery and freedom. The result was a confused blend of scientific precision and racial assumption that usually sought to justify slavery in terms of blacks' biological inferiority. The race of bodies mattered in medical terms because it forced doctors to consider its implications for the bodies they treated, even as it allowed them to justify the subordination of slavery.

## Disease Consequences of Raced Bodies

Physicians interested in the biology of race differences were inspired by these theories to explore their medical consequences. If differences rooted in the body caused such dramatic differences in the histories and social experiences of the races, then surely they led to different experiences of disease as well. Physicians who demonstrated anatomical and physiological differences between the races turned their attention also to the disease consequences of those differences. As a result, they asked whether black and white bodies suffered from different diseases or experienced the same diseases differently.[35] The result of their investigating and theorizing added another layer of meaning to their understanding of raced bodies.

As physicians debated the fundamental differences between black and white bodies, they turned to the relative susceptibility of blacks and whites to disease. Physicians wondered whether disease followed a different course and reacted differently to treatment in black and white bodies and whether blacks and whites were subject to entirely different diseases. Answers to such questions would help them resolve the debate about separate creations and blacks' bodily suitability for slavery as well as improve their practice of medicine.

The debate about the disease consequences of raced bodies turned on two major questions. One was simply whether blacks and whites experienced the same diseases in the same way and at the same rates, which had significant implications for medical practice. The second, of particular interest to polygenesists, was whether blacks were subject to specific diseases that could help explain their inferior natures. Even physicians for whom the task of defining race differences in the abstract seemed irrelevant to the daily practice of medicine sought to understand the ways different bodies experienced disease.

Much of the debate centered on blacks' relative susceptibility to diseases commonly found in the South. Not surprisingly, Josiah Nott believed that "negroes are comparatively exempt from all the endemic diseases of the South." Other physicians disagreed. According to one of Nott's critics, "every planter knows that his negroes suffer equally with the whites, annual attacks of intermittent and remittent fevers,[36] dysentery, malarial pneumonia, &c."[37] According to another, Erasmus Darwin Fenner, the issue turned on the question of acclimation, "the habituation of a person to a special climate."[38] If the races were fixed and best suited to the climate in which they first appeared, then acclimation was neither possible nor necessary for blacks in the American South. But if races could adapt to different climates and diseases, then perhaps the categories of race were not quite as fixed as Nott believed.

Fenner entered into the debate in spite of or because of his affiliation with his "talented and esteemed friend" Josiah Nott; both taught at the New Orleans School of Medicine. Fenner had been educated at Transylvania University, where he studied with a pupil of Benjamin Rush, and as the editor of the *New Orleans Medical and Surgical Journal,* he first published Samuel Cartwright's work, although not without qualms.[39] Fenner argued that when truth "cannot be satisfactorily demonstrated, we have to receive as truth the concurrent observations and conclusions of the largest number of equally competent observers and thinkers." He drew on the authority of "thousands, not only of physicians, but planters, too, who differ" with Nott's conclusions. This anonymous majority, according to Fenner, believed that blacks not only needed to become acclimated to various diseases in the South, but that, like the horse, ox, milch cow, and even dogs, turkeys, and chickens, blacks could do so. Fenner took Nott to task for his hedging and ambiguity and called on a range of experts to support his own belief in black acclimation. However, like Nott, Fenner hedged his own conclusions, arguing "malaria is certainly a poison to the negro as well as the white, but it is less deleterious to the former, and he more readily becomes seasoned to it."[40] While much of the debate's confusion stemmed from the vague characteristics and indistinguishable diagnoses of different fevers, it is important because it directly addressed the proslavery argument that only blacks could labor successfully in the South's hot and pestilent climate.

Doctors and planters had long recognized that Africans were less likely to fall victim to malaria and other fevers, although they could not have understood modern explanations.[41] But this conclusion became increasingly contentious in the antebellum period, and many physicians remained perplexed about fever's prevalence among the populations they served. In 1849, Thompson McGown asserted that there was "no difference" in black and white liability to malaria's severity or danger, "when both are placed under the same circumstances." Other diseases did distinguish between the races. He thought that typhoid pneumonia was "more common and fatal" for blacks, particularly black men, while yellow fever was more common among whites.[42] Tomlinson Fort agreed that "neither age, sex, color nor condition, will protect from attacks" of intermittent fever. He thought that "for obvious reasons the colored population in countries holding them as slaves . . . are most subject to typhus" because "their habitations are too densely peopled."[43] Like many physicians, John Stainback Wilson believed that the "physiological peculiarities of the negro . . . tend to unfit him for the endurance of cold."[44] He thought "in health or disease, there is ever present that want of vital resistance, characteristic of the race" that left them vulnerable to "acute or chronic disease, or from the premature decline of the physical powers."[45]

Relative susceptibility was not the only way blacks and whites experienced disease differently from one another. Their response to its dangers was also a factor. One Thomsonian physician from Charleston, Dr. D. F. Nardin, claimed to have proved that "indolence and carelessness are characteristic of the African, and this constitutes the great mark of the diminutive intellect of that race." Whites confronted by a cholera epidemic would try "to secure themselves" and take "measures to avert the calamity"; the implication was that blacks would not. He disagreed with those who claimed that differences in the rate of death from cholera could be attributed to "a peculiarity in the miasma[46] which had some affinity for the African race, more than for the European descendant." Instead, he believed it could be demonstrated that "the fatal effects of Cholera among the blacks, is owing to their indolence and manner of living," which were themselves rooted in biology.[47] Nardin did not, of course, consider that slaves' response to cholera and other dangers was circumscribed by the control their owners held over them.

Physicians did not limit their inquiry to questions of affinity or susceptibility to disease. In addition, they explored whether blacks were liable to specific diseases that did not afflict other races. This, too, would simultaneously shed light on the significance of race differences while improving medical care. Doctors who wanted to provide the best care for their slave patients had to be able to recognize their diseases in order to cure them. The most ambitious sought also to prevent illness in the first place.

Physicians were especially intrigued by several diseases that they identified as unique to Africans. First recognized in the West Indies, where "it has excited considerable interest," cachexia Africana,[48] or dirt eating, was brought to the attention of southern physicians by W. M. Carpenter, physician and professor at the Louisiana Medical College.[49] According to Carpenter, the "essential feature" of the disease, whose very name delimited its victims, was "a depraved appetite causing an invincible craving for earthy substances." Sufferers from the disease ate "clay, mud, dried mortar, plaster, lime, dust, ashes, chalk, tobacco pipes, slate, bricks, sand, rotten wood, rags, hair and some other unnatural substances." In the United States today, eating such things is labeled pica and considered the sign of a nutritional deficiency; then it could also have been the result of hookworm.[50] Carpenter noted that blacks made "crafty and cunning plans" to procure these forbidden items. Their desire was so strong "that it generally triumphs over every effort to prevent the practice; and such is the indomitable force of the habit, that neither bolts, nor bars, nor punishment, nor the certainty that it will inevitably end in death, can in any measure prevent [Africans] indulging in it."[51]

In the early stages, according to Carpenter, a patient suffering from the disease of dirt eating avoided "effort of any kind [and] skulks from work." Later, sufferers became "excessively dull; sometimes stupid almost to idiocy" as "function after function becomes deranged [and] physiological balance is completely destroyed." Diagnosis was often difficult, especially since patients and their masters "deny the existence of any such habit, and [patients] often evince a degree of cunning in their attempts to evade detection, in remarkable contrast with the stupidity which usually characterizes the subjects of this unnatural appetite."[52] Carpenter seemingly did not notice the contradiction between sufferers' determined efforts to acquire the objects they craved and the lack of effort that he said was a symptom of the disease.

Carpenter acknowledged that cures for this "generally fatal" disease were rare, "owing to the inveterate obstinacy with which the habit is persevered in." Cures were only possible when doctors broke the disease early, before too much bodily damage had occurred. He endorsed the West Indian practice of having the patient "wear a close wire mask, secured by a lock" as more humane than the alternative of confining them in a room. He also recommended establishing "an appropriate system of diet." Physicians did not agree about what caused the disease; possible explanations included "unwholesome food, prolonged abstinence, and irregularity in eating"; mental derangement; and "a depraved state of the digestive organs, brought on by long exposure to a malarious atmosphere." Carpenter believed "an unwholesome atmosphere [was] a predisposing cause" of the disease, but he did not consider it necessary to point out that whites living in the South did not suffer from it.[53] Dirt eating in his view was a disease exclusive to Africans. The journal's editor lauded Carpenter for bringing to public attention a disease resulting "from the peculiar physical constitution of the negro race."[54]

S. L. Grier, a Mississippi physician who acknowledged Carpenter's influence, also included cachexia Africana in an account of "The Negro and His Diseases." Grier thought slaves brought "this groveling propensity" from Africa and warned that "sometimes a dirt-eating mania will seem suddenly to take possession of the inhabitants of a place, and rage with almost epidemic violence." Likening it to "the passion for alcoholic drinks," he believed that some slaves were moderate dirt eaters, while others "seem to have no control over their appetite, and indulge in the pernicious practice with all the eagerness and relish of the incorrigible topers." Those who could not exert "control over the groveling taste" were "the sots in this species of intemperance" who "with an awful rapidity anticipate their doom." Grier believed that the disease's effects and symptoms were well known: "[A]ll have noticed and can recognize at a glance, the peculiar physiognomy, the livid and ghastly expression of countenance" typical of its sufferers. He warned that the disease was "mainly a moral rather than a physical disorder" and that "drugs will not be found of any service," although physicians were "expected to furnish a remedy." The only solution, Grier argued, was to break the habit, which could best be accomplished by "a proper attention to the discipline of negroes, and the employment of all those means calculated to improve their morale."[55]

Physicians evidently heeded Carpenter and Grier's warnings about the disease, although not without some confusion. In an accounting of "the diseases of the colored population of the South and West," Daniel Drake included both "consumption, or cachexia Africana," which was "prevalent and always fatal," and "the strange habit . . . of eating dirt or clay, the common soil of the fields, . . . producing serious and fatal diseases." In addition, "a disease of the heart, conjectured to arise from dirt-eating, destroys quite a number." He reported that on one plantation in Alabama fourteen slaves died from dirt eating, while on a Red River plantation more than thirty died from the heart disease caused by it.[56] A Mississippi physician reported on a case in which a slave woman who had fainted and was nauseous and feeble for several days was charged with dirt eating, which she denied. The true nature of her illness was only revealed when she vomited a worm; when treated she expelled 156 of them.[57]

The southern medical profession not only recognized the disease, it also evidently accepted its racial identification. Only a few physicians described it without reference to race. Tomlinson Fort suggested that it was "commonly witnessed in the childhood and youth of persons who have resided in unhealthy localities, and been exposed to hardship and privation."[58] John Stainback Wilson said the desire for "the most unwholesome and disgusting things, as dirt, ashes, and even insects" was one symptom of chlorosis, or greensickness, which he considered "connected with the various disorders of menstruation." He also attributed longings for "spiders and other disgusting insects . . . chalk, ginger, spices, spirits, vinegar" and even human flesh to "a disordered condition of the stomach" during pregnancy.[59] Laypeople also recognized the existence of the disease and were no more successful at treating it than were the physicians. John Evans wrote about his "misfortune" in losing a slave woman, who "got to eating dirt again & bloted [sic] up & I could not save her she died with a fit on her she complained of a shortness of breath all the time."[60]

Like Carpenter, Samuel Cartwright, who had argued so vehemently for the bodily differences between blacks and whites, identified several diseases that were unique to blacks, specifically drapetomania, "the disease causing negroes to run away" and "Dysoesthesia Ethiopis, or hebitude of mind, and obtuse sensibility of body, a disease peculiar to negroes, and called by overseers 'Rascality.'" In labeling both diseases, Cartwright defined unacceptable behavior in medical terms, as diseases "of the mind" from which only slaves could suffer. He acknowledged that drapetomania was "unknown to our medical authorities, although its diagnostic symptom, absconding from service, is well known to our planters and overseers." A form of "mental alienation," it represented a "troublesome practice" that "can be almost entirely prevented" even "within a stone's throw of the abolitionists."[61] Cartwright's definitions reflected contemporary ideas of the mind and body. Neurology and other systematic efforts to separate the brain and nervous system from other bodily functions did not yet exist as medical specialties.

Cartwright so intertwined racial anatomy and disease with their social and political context that he located the cure of drapetomania in the biblical label for the African as "submissive knee bender." The biblical term echoed the "physical structure of his knees, they being more flexed or bent, than in any other kind of man." Whites ignored this evidence of the knees to their peril; "trying to raise [the Negro] to a level with himself" or "abus[ing] the power which God has given him over his fellow man" had created the disease. Whites who kept blacks with bent knees, in "the position of submission," would discover that "the negro is spell-bound and can not run away." Cartwright warned those who would keep their slaves from falling victim to the disease and running away to watch them carefully. If there were some who were "inclined to raise their heads to a level with their master or overseer, humanity and their own good require that they should be punished till they fall into that submissive state which it was intended for them," that of "submissive knee bender."[62]

Cartwright's effort to medicalize what others would consider an individual or political or even moral problem suggests both the power of anatomical difference as an explanatory trope and the extent to which at least some physicians believed that race differences manifested on the body determined social as well as bodily experience. But not everyone agreed. One of his critics, James T. Smith, warned "if a strong desire to do what is wrong be a disease, the violation of any one of the ten commandments will furnish us with a new one . . . all of which shall no longer be treated by the Penitentiary, but by calomel, capsicum, etc." He saw this as "the greatest step in the progress of philanthropy in modern times."[63]

Like drapetomania, the disease of dysoesthesia Ethiopis, or "rascality," also affected mind and body. Like cachexia Africana, or dirt eating, it was named for the category of body that could be affected by it. Unlike "every other species of mental disease," Cartwright said, dysoesthesia Ethiopis "is accompanied with physical signs of lesions of the body, discoverable to the medical observer." More prevalent among free blacks than slaves, the disease was responsible for the "history of the ruins and dilapidation" found in Haiti and Africa. The disease caused slaves "to do much mischief, which appears as if intentional, but is mostly owing to the stupidity of mind and insensibility of the nerves" it induced. That mischief included breaking, wasting, and abusing objects and animals; wandering at night; slighting work; and raising disturbances, none of which was "premeditated." Instead, individuals who behaved in this way showed "an almost total loss of feeling." Cartwright attributed it to what he called the defective atmospherization, or improper breathing characteristic, of blacks: "hebitude [*sic*] . . . of intellect, . . . slothfulness, torpor, and disinclination to exercise" were the result of their blood being insufficiently "vitalized" in circulation because they slept with blankets over their heads.[64]

Fortunately, dysoesthesia Ethiopis was "easily curable, if treated on sound physiological principles," including stimulating the liver, skin, and kidneys "to assist in carbonizing the blood." This could be accomplished by anointing the patient's skin with oil and slapping it "with a broad leather strap," then setting him to hard work in the open air, thus compelling him to expand his lungs. Patients should be given opportunities to rest, wholesome food and drink, and clean beds. The patient would be cured as soon as the blood felt "the vivifying influence [of] full and perfect atmospherization." As a result, "the negro seems to be awakened to a new existence, and to look grateful and thankful to the white man whose compulsory power . . . has restored his sensation and dispelled the mist that clouded his intellect."[65]

Cartwright attributed both drapetomania and dysoesthesia Ethiopis exclusively to blacks, which inspired him to wonder why the "African race . . . has not been made the subject of much scientific investigation." He was particularly surprised that their diseases "should have escaped the attention of the medical profession." Northern physicians had "noticed the symptoms, but not the disease from which they spring," attributing them instead to "the debasing influence of slavery on the mind." Rather than being the result of slavery, Cartwright considered them "the natural offspring of negro liberty—the liberty to be idle, to wallow in filth, and to indulge in improper food and drinks." Southern physicians' knowledge of them, limited as it was, was derived "from facts learned from their own observation in the field of experience." He urged doctors and abolitionists to pay attention to the "radical, internal difference between the two races, so great in kind as to make what is wholesome and beneficial for the white man, viz: liberty, republicanism, free institutions, etc., not only unsuitable to the negro race, but actually poisonous to its happiness."[66] Once again, Cartwright mingled the medical construction of race differences with the political defense of slavery in a manner designed in part to enhance the legitimacy of medicine as a social arbiter. By creating disease out of what he considered unacceptable behavior, he pathologized race and assigned to physicians the key role in curing it, thus claiming for them a central role in the defense of slavery and southern society.

Cartwright was not content merely to identify racially specific diseases. He also was concerned with the ways in which the races differed in their experience of the same illnesses. Even when blacks and whites developed what seemed to be the same disease, anatomical and physiological differences caused them to experience it differently. He wrote in particular of blacks' vulnerability to "pulmonary congestions" and pneumonia, to various fevers, to scrofula, yaws, and "negro consumption." In each instance, the disease as suffered by blacks differed from similar diseases in whites. "Negro consumption," for example, "has no form or semblance of the phthisis of the white race, except in emaciation." Even though "negro consumption" resembled dyspepsia,[67] "dyspepsia is not a disease of the negro." Instead, dyspepsia "selects its victims from the most intellectual of mankind, passing by the ignorant and unreflecting"—that is, blacks. Like drapetomania and rascality, "the seat of negro consumption is . . . in the mind; and its cause is generally mismanagement or bad government on the part of the master, and superstition on the part of the negro."[68] Even diseases with the most seemingly organic causes that afflicted members of both races, he argued, were experienced differently by different bodies.

According to Cartwright, illness could never be separated from race, and both were tied to social context. Blacks developed illnesses when they were insufficiently subordinated by whites; only good treatment within the bounds of slavery could keep them healthy. Given the racial assumptions of the time as well as widespread uncertainty as to the cause of disease, his views were convincing to many of his readers, even if they might disagree with the details. Only the most independent-minded physicians were likely to demand experimentally based confirmation of what the vast majority would consider the self-evident truth of race differences in the experience of disease. Instead, many southern physicians were likely to applaud Cartwright for the scientific rigor with which he systematized what they understood to be true, even though the extremity of his views left some of them uneasy.

Other physicians built on Cartwright's foundation, without necessarily sharing all of his conclusions. Among them was A. P. Merrill, who in 1856 published a three-part essay in the *Southern Medical and Surgical Journal.* Merrill was concerned with the "distinctive peculiarities [of the Negro constitution], requiring the adoption of habits of life in health, and the application of remedial measures in sickness, differing . . . from those which are applicable to the white race." Like many others, including Cartwright, Merrill cataloged the anatomical and physiological characteristics of blacks and attributed their differences from whites to the hot African climate, observations regarding their brains, and "forty or more centuries of constant decline." Like Cartwright, too, Merrill viewed American slavery as best suited to "the improvement and elevation in the scale of being, of this degraded race."[69] Merrill, however, focused his attention on the effects of moving Africans to a more temperate climate, partly because they had "less resiliency of constitution, and self adaptation to change" than whites. He urged planters to provide slaves with sufficient food and blankets and to avoid exposing them to cold, especially during the winter, lest they become ill due to "the inability of the negro constitution to generate heat."[70] He warned that most of their illnesses "are caused by a want of proper attention" to their need for heat and fresh air. Merrill used blacks' constitutional vulnerabilities to argue for the importance of minimal standards of living to ensure their well-being.[71]

Merrill was not the only physician to use blacks' medical differences from whites to justify trying to improve their material conditions. John Stainback Wilson, whose plans to publish a book on black health were interrupted by the Civil War, also urged planters to consider slaves' physiology when providing for them. He warned that blacks' "feeble heat generating powers should be strictly regarded" when giving them food and clothing. He warned that they should be given breakfast before going to the fields to work to fortify their systems against "marsh exhalations" and given overcoats to protect against "general chilling of the surface of the body." Such protection was necessary because "there is ever present that want of vital resistance, characteristic of the race . . . which incapacitates them for excessive toil, and causes them to sink under it." Wilson warned that "the natural stamina, the vital resistance, the enduring and recovering powers of the negro are inferior to those of the white man." He added: "Negroes are troublesome customers any way you can fix them."[72]

Merrill was also concerned with the diseases that afflicted blacks because of their bodies' vulnerabilities. He believed that "physicians are apt to take it for granted, that the negro race undoubtedly has its peculiar and distinctive diseases, which require equally peculiar and distinctive plans of treatment." But Merrill was unwilling to accept such an "extreme view," suggesting that while "peculiarities undoubtedly do exist . . . the differences between the white and colored races . . . consists, not so much in the existence of any distinct class of negro diseases, as in the modifications of the same diseases as they affect the different races." While there were some race-based differences in disease experiences, "the disease itself is ordinarily characterized by the same, or very similar pathological conditions, indicating the application of similar therapeutical measures." Merrill noted that diseases "very rarely" prevailed among one of the races but not the other.[73]

Since the diseases themselves were not racially distinct, Merrill explained, physiological differences between the races accounted for their different experiences of disease. Blacks' vitality was "of a less vigorous and normal character, than in white persons," which caused "less activity and acuteness in their nervous susceptibilities." This, in turn, required differences in treatment of their diseases. At the same time, because slavery kept them from vices such as alcohol and tobacco, blacks were protected from "the attacks of many diseases to which [they] would otherwise be subject, and moderate the violence and frequency of others to which [they are] constantly liable." As a result, "the slaves of the south are probably subject to a less number and variety of diseases, and enjoy a longer average duration of life, than the white population of any large section of our country."[74]

Merrill's efforts to provide a more moderate view of racial medicine led him to conclude that blacks' "habits and character" and "bodily and mental constitution" rendered "inapplicable . . . the teachings of medical authors, whose study and practice have been confined to the white race," even though he rejected the notion of an exclusively race-based disease pathology.[75]

Merrill adopted a similarly moderate tone in his description of the specific illnesses suffered by blacks. He believed that fevers accounted for the majority of their ailments, remarking, "[T]he two races differ in their susceptibilities to the influence of the cause of fever, only in degree." Furthermore, those differences could largely be explained by the locations in which the two races lived. When their homes were "in close proximity with each other," "the difference in the susceptibility of the two races to attacks of febrile disease, has been less distinctly marked." In Africa and to a lesser degree in the South, blacks were "much less liable to the more violent and fatal forms of fever" than whites, because blacks were "prepared by nature and habit for the enjoyment of health and comfort in hot climates." However, according to Merrill, the real differences between the races were "in the extent to which [fever] endangers the life of the patient, rather than in any peculiar pathological characteristics of the disease."[76] Merrill claimed to base his conclusions on a third of a century of experience as a physician, which may well account for his willingness to acknowledge fundamental similarities in the bodies of blacks and whites as well as their differences. As a practicing physician, he clearly struggled to reconcile southern racial beliefs with his observations of suffering individuals, whose bodily ailments seemed to follow similar patterns regardless of race.

Doctors who sought to understand the medical implication of race were convinced that black bodies suffered from the same diseases as whites, even if not always at the same rate or with the same severity; some thought they had their own peculiar illnesses as well. No matter where they stood on these matters, however, doctors agreed that race differences rendered blacks vulnerable to illnesses that could best be kept in check by keeping them enslaved and thus subject to the protection and oversight of owners.

## Doctors and the Debate about Race and Slavery

For southern physicians, the question of how to understand the bodies that appeared before them could not be separated from the growing need to defend slavery that preoccupied the nation in the decades before the Civil War. Physicians concerned about enhancing the profession's credentials and their own importance as shapers of opinion in the South claimed the right to define racial characteristics and their consequences. Their eagerness to extend their cultural authority led many doctors to adopt views of black and white bodies that differed sharply from clerical views and white popular understanding, which acknowledged black and white unity before God even as it assumed black inferiority. Only physicians, they argued, could know the ways in which blacks and whites differed under as well as on the surface of the skin; only they could define the truth of racialized bodies because only they could lay claim to the science that allowed such truths to be known. That their writings emphasized difference rather than sameness should come as no surprise, given the cultural context in which they lived. What is perhaps surprising is the extent to which they blurred biological and cultural factors in their efforts to provide explanations for difference. Medicalizing ethnology and behavior, they constructed an argument about racialized bodies that depended on an astonishingly crude biological determinism. In the process, they added a new dimension to the defense of slavery.

One medical professor and journal editor, H. L. Byrd, used theories about blacks' bodily differences from whites' to urge the reopening of the international slave trade, which he considered a "necessity from a scientific stand-point." He believed that the black race was doomed to die out, "that its fate is fixed, without fresh African blood," because "each generation of the negro race in this country, has been shorter lived than its predecessor." Even though the black population was growing numerically, it was depreciating "longevically." In the "so called Free States," blacks were "rapidly dying out, notwithstanding hundreds . . . annually stolen from the South."[77] Byrd urged the reopening of the slave trade as beneficial for the Africans brought to this country. "Nature's God has proclaimed his inferior condition in the form of his face and head, as well as in the 'unchangeable color of his skin,' but has endowed him with sufficient powers of imitation to render him happy in contributing to the pleasures of a superior race."[78] Byrd's comments were published in the late 1850s; by then, the political uses of medicine wore only the thinnest of guises.

A. P. Merrill shared this view of the medical benefits of slavery for the African race, although he argued from a different demographic understanding. Were slaves suddenly emancipated, he argued, "instead of a progressive increase in numbers, as at the present time, there would undoubtedly be a rapid diminution of them, until extinction, as with some of the Indian tribes." He argued that "the indolent and sluggish nature of the negro, renders him more liable to such consequences than the Indian."[79] The dangers stemmed from "the inaptitude of the negro mind to improvement," Merrill noted, claiming that "in his native country he exhibits no signs of progression." Instead, "they are content with doing precisely as has been done by their progenitors for ages." The race had been "stationary . . . from the earliest times, tending more, perhaps, to deterioration than to improvement" unless it was "brought under a system of tutelage, in contact with a race vastly superior." Merrill hoped that, with time, blacks might be enabled "to recover [their] lost position in the scale of being." Slavery was the only way to accomplish "the enlightenment and regeneration of benighted Africa," although he remained doubtful whether "the negro will . . . ever be elevated in the scale of being" even in the "long and tedious future."[80]

Merrill believed "the negro race is physiologically constituted for the enjoyment of a hot climate"; the United States South was "much too far north for him." This was potentially dangerous: "[T]he evil influences upon his animal functions . . . must be counteracted by corresponding changes in his mode of living, or disease and an abridgement of the duration of life, must be the result." Blacks were possessed of "less resiliency of constitution, and self adaptation to change" than whites and thus needed to be provided with adequate care by whites in order to avoid disease. If well cared for and healthy, Merrill noted, "the negro is very enduring of labor . . . but he cannot be driven . . . beyond his natural or habitual movements; and any attempt to do it must always result in ultimate loss to the master." Should he be overworked, he "becomes exhausted and disordered . . . [and] he recovers from the effects much more slowly than the white man." These racial characteristics made slavery the ideal situation for "the negro, . . . [who] is ever ready to place himself under the guidance and instruction of the white man, the superiority of whose judgment and intellect he is always willing to acknowledge." Africans were "a submissive and yielding race, wholly incapable of bearing malice on account of their degraded condition as slaves; and equally incapable of forming and maintaining, an effective and permanent organization among themselves, to assert their freedom, or to avenge their wrongs."[81]

Samuel Cartwright was among the most vehement of those physicians who defended slavery by focusing attention on the biological differences between the races. Claiming to be rooted in careful observation of physiological differences, his arguments drew on the growing legitimacy of medicine and the objectivity of science to make their case. Unlike those who defended slavery for its economic contributions or its benefits to slaves, Cartwright relied on the seemingly infallible truths of bodily difference to demonstrate blacks' biological suitability to be slaves. Unfit for anything other than slavery, blacks' inferiorly raced bodies doomed them to subordination. "According to unalterable physiological laws, negroes . . . can only have their intellectual faculties awakened in a sufficient degree . . . when under the compulsory authority of the white man." If blacks are left on their own, "the black blood distributed to the brain chains the mind to ignorance, superstition, and barbarism, and bolts the door against civilization, moral culture, and religious truth." Only "the compulsory power of the white man" could force "the slothful negro" to behaviors necessary to avoid defective atmospherization and the diseases it caused. This, in turn, was beneficial to whites, blacks, and "the world at large," because "the very exercise beneficial to the negro, is expended in cultivating those burning fields in cotton, sugar, rice, and tobacco, which, but for his labor, would, from the heat of the climate, go uncultivated, and their products be lost to the world." Cartwright concluded that the African's "physical organization, and the laws of his nature, are in perfect unison with slavery, and in entire discordance with liberty—a discordance so great as to produce the loathsome disease that locks up the understanding, blunts the sensations, and chains the mind to superstition, ignorance and barbarism."[82]

According to Cartwright, slavery not only benefited society and its members, it was "a blessing instead of a curse" to the "slave race" because of the "different conformation of body, cast of mind, and turn of thought" that gave it "a fitness for that institution, and an unfitness for any other." In a direct appeal for the legitimacy of science to determine answers to political questions, he urged those debating slavery in the nation to study comparative anatomy, which could "put the question beyond controversy." Likewise, "physiology could say whether the laws governing the white and black man's organism be the same or different," while chemistry could answer similar questions about "the composition of the bones, the blood, the flesh, skin and the secretions," all of which would "leave the North and the South nothing to dispute about."[83]

The unidentified physician critic who rejected many of Cartwright's views regarding the differences between black and white bodies agreed with him about black inferiority and its implications for slavery, albeit for different reasons. His conclusions regarding the physiological foundation of African slavery rested on other assumptions, specifically their capacity for labor. He urged Cartwright to "be candid enough to admit" that slaves were brought here "because we knew that they could contribute to the promotion of our pecuniary interests . . . and no contortion of facts can ever make it appear otherwise." He took Cartwright to task for involving science in his polemics: "Science blushes—aye, she is indignant at the effort to make her a post against which to lean so frail an argument." He rejected Cartwright's theories of defective hematosis and suggested "the blacks imported to our shores would have been quite as well, or better off, if they had been left alone in their pristine state."[84]

This unidentified physician reserved his most scornful criticism for Cartwright's decision to wrap his views in the guise of medicine and publish them in a medical journal, based as they were on "an elaborate array of biblical evidence." He argued that Cartwright had "a political desire to depreciate the race," which he found objectionable since "medicine and politics are as incompatible as acids and alkalies." Any doctor who combined them "will be totally unfit to treat the sick negro: he will imagine his patient but little superior to the horse he rides, and he will 'drench' him accordingly."[85] The editors of the medical journal in which this critique appeared felt compelled to append a comment distancing themselves from the author's views. While they "consider it, as far as it goes, a complete refutation of Dr. Cartwright's most extraordinary and hypothetical assertions," the editors specified several key aspects in which they disagreed with the unidentified author.[86] The politics of defining black bodies were contentious indeed, even when all of the players supported slavery.

In thus defending slavery and subordination by emphasizing the ethnological origins and medical consequences of African inferiority, Merrill, Cartwright, and other physicians committed themselves to demonstrating that inferiority by scientific means. Unwilling simply to assert that blacks were lesser beings, perhaps because they recognized that such assertions were open to challenge in the increasingly contentious arena of racial politics in the antebellum years, they drew on the authority of science to buttress their support for slavery by emphasizing its racial and medical benefits. By appealing to scientific authority, they hoped to reposition the debate beyond politics. Politics, after all, could be debated, but in their view science was sacrosanct.

In part, these elite physicians' commitment to science as a means of ordering their views of society stemmed from their training, which for most took place in the North and sometimes continued in Europe. They were undoubtedly aware of growing perceptions of the South as an intellectual and scientific backwater, an awareness made more acute by their frequent complaints about their limited access to journals, books, and libraries.[87] Anxious to be taken seriously and to have the validity of their work respected, they were eager to be perceived as modern and attuned to the most current ways of thinking, which meant drawing on the legitimacy of science. Determined to defend the South's racial institutions and at the same time enhance their own professional standing, they never questioned the assumptions that informed their scientific work.

More ordinary physicians were not likely to share these physicians' commitment to science or their determination to explicate race differences and their implications for disease and slavery. Instead, physicians in everyday practice were likely to take for granted the subordination of blacks and the legitimacy of slavery, since everything in their culture did so. Their apparent reluctance to enter the fray was less a sign of disagreement than of a lack of concern for advancing the intellectual status of their profession. Most doctors, after all, probably did not read medical journals, much less write for them. There is, however, no reason to think that they did anything but support slavery. Nott, Cartwright, and the rest were bent upon carving out a sphere of authority for physicians, a position few in the practice were likely to defy.

## Slaves Explain Race and Slavery

African Americans have left far less elaborate explanations for the meanings of raced bodies. While to some extent this is a problem of sources, it also reflects lesser need. Some of the impetus for white theorizing about race was inspired by the growing urgency of defending slavery from the challenges of abolitionists; doctors were also inspired by the desire to professionalize medicine and science. Slaves had no such needs, nor did they have access to print to make their views known beyond their immediate community. Nevertheless, blacks have left some sense of their beliefs about the meanings of race and race differences in their folklore. While folklore has sometimes been a difficult source for historians to accept, it offers one of the few possibilities for exploring blacks' views of difference, if only indirectly. Historians' reluctance to consider folklore stems, in part, from concerns about its reliability. Much of the folklore material is obviously influenced by the assumptions held by the whites who collected it. In this, it closely resembles the Works Progress Administration (WPA) narratives of the Great Depression, also a problematic source. Sometimes folklorists' work veered perilously close to fiction, as in the collections of Brer Rabbit and other stories by Joel Chandler Harris and others. However, many of the folklore collectors were concerned with authenticity and made real efforts to ensure the legitimacy of their work. Often, even the most fictional stories penned by whites were drawn from tales told by blacks. Like any source, folklore demands careful evaluation from historians, but it is an effort worth making for the insights it provides.

Blacks revealed their thoughts about the meanings of race in the various stories they told about God's creation of animals and people.[88] In several of these stories, God created animals that were somehow incomplete. In one version, they lacked mouths, in another tails, in still another brains. According to the mouth version of the story, animals were better off without mouths, because they did not have to eat or work, fight, or steal to get food; they were "more peacable" because "dey aint hab to agonize so 'bout how dey goin' to git long," saving them "a heap o' trouble . . . [and] argifying,' an' 'sputin,' an' cussin,' an' fussin.'" But when the animals begged for mouths, God had Br' Dog make them, with predictable consequences. At first the creatures "aint know 'nough den to complain" and enjoyed hearing one another's different voices. But Dog "might ha' 'spicioned dat dey can't nebber git satisfy! . . . Dey ain' rightly understan' till dey been older dat de bigger dey mout,' de mo' harder dey is goin' to hab to work for fill 'em." In the tail version of the story, the animals appointed Sis' Nanny-Goat to ask God to give them tails. She reported that "he look at me again for a minute an' he kind o' grin an' say, 'Bery well, den, Sis' Nanny-Goat. But if I gi' dem tails you got to put 'em on dem all, an' I don't want to hear nothin' mo' about it.'"[89] Needless to say, adding tails caused the animals just as much pleasure and conflict as cutting mouths had, and left them no more satisfied.

African American explanations for the creation of difference and its troubling consequences also encompassed human beings. While many blacks presumably accepted biblical versions of the creation of Adam and Eve, others added details reflecting a sharper and more ironic sense of human history. In one version, Eve complained so often to Adam about her loneliness while he was away hunting and fishing that he reported his troubles to God. God offered to "make a few more people" to keep Eve company, shaping them of mud and "lean[ing] them against a rail fence to dry." God told Adam he would return later to "put some brains in them," but forgot "He had some other engagements that afternoon [and] did not return to finish His work until the next morning." God's absent-mindedness had serious consequences: [B]efore he returned, "the people with no brains had walked off! And they have been increasing and multiplying ever since!"[90] Each of these stories offers a view of an all too fallible God, albeit one with a wry sense of humor, whose inability to control the results of his creations accounted for their differences.

In a story recounted by former North Carolina and Alabama slave Gus Rogers, God was not as fallible as one of Noah's sons. According to Rogers, "when Noah got drunk on wine, one of his sons laughed at him," while the other two covered him with a sheet without looking. In response, "Noah told the one who laughed, 'You children will be hewers of wood and drawers of water for the other's two children, and they will be known by their hair and their skin being dark.'" Rogers concluded "that is the way God meant us to be. We have always had to follow the white folks and do what we saw them do, and that's all there is to it. You just can't get away from what the Lord said." But Rogers built a note of ambiguity into his comments when he claimed that God only gave religion to Noah after first giving and then taking it away from Adam, implying that God could change his mind.[91] Black people who sought to understand race and the subordination it brought did not view them as fixed, as did whites, even when they based their explanations on the authority of the Bible.

A more fanciful yet still biblically based explanation for race differences appeared in an extrapolation of the story of Cain. Sent into exile after killing Abel, Cain found himself watched by a hairy, black young girl. Deciding "to 'tice dat gal to stay roun' dere, an' at least mek some company for him," Cain was even more eager when he saw "she had de makin's o' a real good hoe-hand." He enticed her with food and little by little was able to draw her closer, supplementing his food offerings with "sweetmout' talk." Just as his efforts were approaching success and he began to consider marriage, the girl's mother appeared and tried "to run she off de place." Kicking and cussing, the two women fought until Cain ran the mother off and he "mek an grab an' ketch she. . . . He git dat gal for a wife den an' dere" and they became "a settle married couple." Years later, the serpent brought news of the marriage to Adam. When he told Eve, she wondered, "Who de debbil in dis worl' kin de boy be married to?" Adam, dissembling, told her "'Tis some kind o' 'oman from de Land o' Nod." They immediately went to visit, and Eve grilled Cain about "what kind o' 'oman kin de gal been," assuming she "aint wut a drat." When Eve first saw Cain's wife, the hair on her head "riz right up," but she was won over because "de yard is nice, an' swep,' an' eberyt'ing look deestent" and by the presence of a grandchild. When the rest of the children were called, "De fus' one is white, an' de nex' after dat been black, twelve head already. Half o' dem chillen been buckra like dey Pa, an' de res,' while dey ain' been hairy like dey Ma, been black as soot, an' burrhead! An' dat howcome dey been two kind o' people ebber since den."[92] The story is remarkable for the objections of both mothers, one white and one black, to the marriage of their children and for the suggestion implicit in it that Cain's hairy, black wife needed to be tamed like an animal. It is also significant that Cain wanted a wife to ease his loneliness and to work with him in the fields and in his home. In an interesting twist on the tale, the folklore collected by Frank C. Brown in North Carolina, predominantly among whites, showed him that "Many preachers believe the Negro is the descendant of Cain and a gorilla out of the Land of Nod."[93]

African Americans could never forget the consequences of race differences in their daily lives. They knew that according to slaveholders, their bodies existed as a source of labor to generate profits, and they recognized that they were sometimes considered little different from animals in that regard. As a consequence, they occasionally echoed some of the perceptions of their masters regarding race and difference. Pioneering folklorist Elsie Clews Parsons recorded a story in South Carolina in which the girls at a dance chose Ber Crane as their dancing partner because he was white. Their preference angered Ber Rabbit, who was still not chosen when Crane loaned him shoes, socks, coat, shirt, collar, and tie. Rabbit's anger led him to trick Crane into shedding all of his clothing, leaving Crane naked; "Ber Crane didn' choose [wasn't chosen] again dat night at all."[94] Another folklore collector, Newbell Niles Puckett, reported that for "antebellum Negroes . . . dreams of white [were] of good omen, while dreams of black pointed to evil. A white man in your dreams represents the Lord, and a black man the devil."[95] Blackness could be dangerous in real life as well as in dreams. Several people informed WPA interviewers that people with blue gums were dangerous. According to Annie Boyd, "blue gum[m]ed niggers is shon bad luck wen I sees one gits as far away as I kin foh if one bites you you is a ded nigger foh dey is pizen as er diamond back."[96] Even so, Carrie Pollard of Alabama reported that "you can't take a blue veined chile an' make a slave outa her."[97] Blue gums were not the only bodily difference associated with danger; so, too, were crossed eyes or having only one leg.[98] Less explanations for difference than warnings about behavior, such beliefs point to the ambiguity with which African Americans understood their circumstances. Living in a society that enslaved and tried to dehumanize those whose skin was dark, African Americans could not help but acknowledge the negative consequences of bodily difference even as they sought to avoid them in their lives in the quarters. While slaves did not medicalize bodily difference, speaking instead in the coded language of story and warning, neither could they ever forget its implications.

One of the most dramatic accounts of the dangers of blackness was attributed to Cato, a former slave who claimed to have come directly from Africa, the son of a prince. Cato explained that the "first man" was "a monstrous black man, with yellow hair" who descended from the clouds to the earth. His arrival caused the trees, flowers, and grasses to feel fear and destroyed peace, because his motion created the breeze and when he ran the wind "stirred up the waters" even though he was not evil. After a time, the "yellow-haired black man" became lonely, so he retreated to a cave for a week, then reappeared leading "by the hands a man and woman, black like himself, but ever so much smaller, who laughed and talked with him." They lived in happiness until the yellow-haired black man created a baboon, but as he "had forgotten to say one particular word . . . that creature was both mischievous and wicked." The baboon "practiced all manner of evil, taught [the small man and woman] lying and deceit, made them play tricks upon the black man, until . . . the patience and kindness of the black man gave way." He told the small man and woman "they must take care of themselves on the earth" and sent the baboon to live in the cave, suspected of being the devil. Then "the black man sorrowfully ascended the mountain and stepped up into the clouds and left the world to the inheritance of sinful man."[99] The white theorists of multiple creations were unlikely to have imagined such a story, never mind a yellow-haired black God who created human beings out of his own loneliness.

Yet another story of the time just after Creation, recounted by Harriette Kershaw Leiding of Charleston, has God placing one large and one small bundle before a black man and a white man. Given first choice, the black man "wid he greedy big eye: he tink de big bundle de best, so he tek dat. Den de white man he tek what was left,—de leetle bundle." When the two men unwrapped the bundles, the white man found "a pen an' a bottle of ink; an' dat's how come he do de writin' ob de worl'. An' de nigger he fin' de hoe an' de plough an' de aze in e bundle; an' dat's how come he hafter do de wuk in de worl.'"[100] Attributing slavery and subordination to the greed of blacks is certainly ironic but no less fanciful than the putative scientific theories of the medical doctors.

Another story drawing upon stereotypes of blacks, this time of their laziness, was offered by Joel Chandler Harris. When the little white boy who inspired many of Uncle Remus's stories asked his friend why his palms were white although his skin was dark, Remus offered "a piece of unwritten history that must prove interesting to ethnologists." Remus explained that "way back yander . . . we 'us all niggers tergedder." After a while, "de news come dat dere wuz a pon' er water some'rs in de naberhood" that washed anyone who entered it "nice en w'ite." The first to "splunge inter de pon' . . . come out w'ite ez a town gal." When people saw this, "dey make a break fer de pon.'" The first group to enter came out white, while the next "come out merlatters." But the crowd "mighty nigh use de water up," leaving only enough for the last group to "paddle about wid der foots en dabble in it wid der han's." Remus added that "de Injun en de Chinee got ter be 'counted 'long er de merlatter," adding that since the Chinese got to the pond in enough time to "git der head in de water, de water hit onkink der ha'r."[101] This is one of the few stories to offer an account of the creation of more than two races, perhaps a reflection of its distance from its slave origins. Levi Pollard, who had been a slave in Virginia, recounted a similar story that also explained that latecomers found the pond had become cloudy, so that "dey was comin' out kinda yellow an' dey named 'em mulatters. Some of de kinks was washed out of dey hair." Those who arrived still later found the water almost gone and so were only able to change the color of their palms and the bottom of their feet. Pollard noted "dat's de way hit is today, 'ceptin' when de whites has chillun by de blacks an' den dey might be any color from noon to midnight."[102]

In spite of their obvious differences, these stories of creation and human and animal foibles share a desire to explain the presence of variation and evil in the world. While all of them do not attempt to account for slavery, some offer explanations for black subordination; others simply take it for granted. Yet the stories also offer the possibility of alternate readings, as when Rabbit tricks the white Crane into disrobing at the dance, revealing him and thus rendering him less desirable. Similarly, the story of the monstrous yellow-haired black man attributes evil to the collusion of a black man and woman and a devilish baboon, but it also offers an image of an all-powerful black man as God. The ambiguities inherent in such stories point to the complexities of African American understandings of race. On the one hand, race differences were seen as clearly delineated and inviolate, while at the same time the presence of difference did not privilege one group over the other. Even the presence of evil in the world, whether represented by mouths and tails or attributed to greed or carelessness, did not necessarily condemn any category of being to subordination. Instead, difference was viewed with irony, sometimes also with humor, sometimes detachment. For such perspectives to arise out of slavery suggests a transcendent ability to make sense of the incomprehensible without bitterness or even the desire for imaginative retribution.

The absence of rancor is perhaps the most significant of the differences separating African American explanations for race and slavery from those of whites. While whites' justifications often assumed a defensive tone and served to advance the political, economic, and social interests of their proponents, African Americans were motivated by their desire to explain their circumstances to themselves. The results were far more revealing of the position of each group in society than they were of the relative status of science, medicine, and theology.

# CHAPTER 2

# Constructing Sex

There could be little doubt in anyone's mind in the mid-nineteenth century that men and women were different in every respect. Americans of all sorts believed that the obvious biological differences between men and women were significant far beyond the specific organs involved in reproduction. Those organs influenced every aspect of the individual body along with the mind. In the most simplistic formulations, women's reproductive organs shaped their nurturing, maternal personalities and determined their domestic roles in society, while men's bodies were biologically intended for the vigorous lives they led. Women's bodies rendered them weak and in need of protection, unable to compete in intellectual, political, or economic arenas; they were, instead, ideally suited for reproduction in both its biological and social meanings. Their biological limits were balanced by the far less biologically encumbered bodies of men, which were marked by strength and virility. Men's and women's reproductive organs influenced every other aspect of their bodies' functioning as well as determined their proper place in the social order. In the eyes of Americans, individual experience could not escape the limits of the sexed body.

In these beliefs, midcentury white southerners were little different from the rest of the nation. Yet white southerners could only perceive these fundamental sex differences as simple by ignoring race. Did male bodies share the characteristics of maleness in spite of skin color, with all of its implications? Was the biology of femaleness the same for black and white women? Which exerted a more powerful influence on the individual body, race or sex? Was it necessary to imagine a fourfold typology in order to encompass human variation: white men, white women, black men, black women? Southern physicians and laypeople alike struggled to find answers to these questions. In the process, they discovered that what had appeared to be simple was not. Understanding sex and gender in a racially polarized slave society required a difficult set of explanations and rationalizations. The bodily characteristics of black and white men and women had to be defined in a manner consistent with beliefs about both sex and race.

Given southern whites' assumptions about the inherent difference of black bodies that rendered them inferior to their own, they could easily have sidestepped the question of sex differences. Since race was seemingly the most important marker of difference, questions about black and white women's relative experiences of common biological processes like menstruation, pregnancy, and childbirth might never have occurred to them. However, for nineteenth-century southerners, sex was at least as important a marker of difference as race; no matter which an observer considered paramount at any given moment, both had to be considered, neither could be ignored. Black women's race might distinguish them from white women, but their sex also distinguished them from black men. White women could not be understood as having the same bodies and bodily experiences as white men, in spite of their racial identity. Indeed, nineteenth-century observers were the inheritors of long intellectual traditions that understood difference in terms simultaneously racial and sexual.[1] Simply raising the question of how best to understand bodily experience forced them to examine both the race and the sex of those bodies, however intellectually inconvenient it might be to do so at times. For southern physicians in particular, that inconvenience was partially offset by the potential advantage of viewing all categories of bodies as in need of their care, but the importance of recognizing bodies as both raced and sexed was widely understood.

White southerners struggled most directly with the consequences of what they understood to be the inherent unhealthiness of women's bodies, which they viewed as fragile and in need of care and protection. This forced them to consider how to think about black women's bodies, a subject for which they found consensus rather elusive. Sometimes, the dilemmas of thinking about sex and gender in a racial context inspired only silence. More often, they wrote about the category of "woman" as if it applied only to white women. The most thoughtful sought ways to resolve the apparent contradictions between sex and race.

For white southerners, the difficulty of reconciling ideas about race and sex was at heart an argument about superiority and inferiority. Whites were clearly superior to blacks, and men to women. The difficulty stemmed from the need to reconcile white women's perceived physical vulnerabilities with their racial superiority relative to black women. How, physicians asked themselves, could white women be less healthy than black women, suffer more from the consequences of their biology, and simultaneously be physically superior and more advanced? How could black women's bodies be both healthy and inferior? Either poor health had to be read as advantageous, a position no physician was willing to adopt, or race and sex differences had to be understood in some other manner that suited the ideological needs of a slave society. Southern physicians found that their uncertainty led them to engage in a host of complex, qualified generalizations and outright contradictions.

Physicians simultaneously found it necessary to consider the impact of women's minds on their bodies, a discussion just as liable to drag them into contradiction.

No one doubted that women's minds could make them sick, just as bodily ailments could have an impact on their minds. While this subject will be explored more fully in subsequent chapters, it is important to note that physicians found it most convincing to view all women's minds as subject to the influence of their bodies and thus liable to illness. The question they posed was whether black and white women were similarly vulnerable and, if so, what that might mean for understanding both race and sex. They were understandably reluctant to view white women as weaker than black in either mind or body, yet they somehow had to account for white women's greater vulnerability to mental as well as physical illness. At the same time, they recognized that black women's inferior minds also influenced their bodies in ways that could lead to physical illness; the question was whether the mechanisms and consequences were the same for both groups of women. Their answers were rarely consistent. They found explaining why white men were physically and mentally superior to black men far simpler.

Physicians in all parts of the country increasingly claimed sex and gender as their legitimate concern in the middle third of the century. Seizing cultural authority to define appropriate behavior from the hands of ministers reliant on the authority of the Bible, physicians claimed for themselves the right to preach the virtues of healthy living for men and women and to warn those who did not follow their advice about the dangers they faced. Wrapping themselves in the mantle of science, they wrote about women much more frequently than they did about men, in the process claiming women's bodies as their special purview. Women, the physicians declared, were biologically more vulnerable than men, and it was their responsibility as physicians to advise women how to live so as to maintain their fragile health. While southern physicians mainly turned their attention to white women, their explanations for women's special vulnerability allowed them to claim authority over black women as well, at least in some circumstances. The result was physicians' enhanced authority over all women as it perpetuated an identification of women with disease that would have important consequences for women of both races.

## Physicians Define (White) Women's Bodies

For nineteenth-century observers, women's bodies defined the scope of their destinies in a way that men's bodies did not. Women's bodily differences from men and their role in reproduction had earlier led them to be perceived as incomplete men, an idea that had virtually disappeared by midcentury, although echoes of it remained.[2] Instead, women were perceived to be ruled by their reproductive organs, which dominated their bodily processes and minds so thoroughly that no escape was possible. Gunning Bedford, a physician who was the author of a widely used textbook on gynecology, warned his students that what were once "regarded as idiopathic affections of the head, chest, abdomen, etc., are now recognized to be symptomatic disturbances, or merely effects of disease in the uterine organs." He marshaled the "facts" that declared "the complete subjection in which the uterine organs hold the general system."[3] Doctors believed that the uterus was the dominant organ in women's bodies, defining their personalities and their possibilities.

Southern physicians did not differ with this growing consensus. According to a Montgomery, Alabama, physician, "no subject . . . deserves more attention . . . than the pathological condition of the uterus . . . when we look upon the fair form wasting with disease." He argued that "some abnormal condition of the uterine functions" was the "most frequent" reason for "breaking down, and thoroughly perverting" woman's constitution and causing ill health.[4] Another asked how an organ "in perfect health" could produce problems like "vomiting, heart burn, salivation, sleeplessness, palpitation of the Heart, laughing, crying, and a variety of others?" According to his catalog of dangers, the uterus—and presumably the woman surrounding it—was not in perfect health during menstruation or gestation and was frequently diseased at other times as well.[5] The author of a volume on the diseases of women and children referred to menstruating women as "out of order," which "ought surely to put them upon their guard and to make them very circumspect in their conduct."[6] For these southern physicians, like their counterparts elsewhere, women's central role in reproduction influenced all aspects of their lives. By contrast, men's freedom from the organs necessary to gestating and nourishing children allowed them the greater health that made full participation in the public world their right and responsibility.

Physicians nationwide seemed intent on defining women's bodies as not only ruled by reproduction but also as diseased, so that even biologically natural processes were understood to be pathological. The author of a text on diseases of women and children noted: "Woman . . . is liable to disease and suffering; and it would, perhaps, appear to the careless observer, that God, for some wise yet mysterious purpose, had imposed on her penalties and afflictions far heavier than those which our sex is called upon to bear."[7]

Again, these views were shared by southern physicians. According to Larkin Jones in the medical thesis he wrote for the Medical College of South Carolina in 1829, woman's "contributions" to reproduction and her "peculiar structure and more complicated functions" made her "necessarily, the subject of many diseases, peculiar to Conception, Gestation, Parturition, and Lactation." Jones also noted the "less capacious" cavity for the brain in women and their "delicate and sensitive" nervous systems. Jones did grant woman slight advantage: Although she was "the subject of more diseases than men, in consequence of the delicacy of her organization and more complicated functions," she also possessed "more active recuperative powers" and had the "ability to bear more" than men.[8] Joseph Wright, author of a text published in Georgia on diseases of infants, children, and women, noted that "the structure and design of females . . . subject them to peculiar diseases, the chief of which are their monthly evacuations, pregnancy and childbearing . . . [which are] the source of numerous calamities."[9] These views increasingly dominated professional perceptions of women's bodies.

Physicians recognized that women's biological differences from men caused them to have different experiences of illness even beyond their reproductive functions. Samuel Jennings thought "the persons of women are more susceptible of injury, their nerves more readily take on irritation, than those of the males." Even "their ordinary diseases" were influenced by "their peculiarities," by which he meant the action of the uterus.[10] Tomlinson Fort thought that women were more likely to suffer from cancer than men, as they also were from "goitre—bronchocele" and what he called "eating cancer" or lupus. As Samuel Cartwright did for slaves, Fort identified a disease specific to women that was new to the medical profession: "excessive sensibility" or "hyperaesthesis." Sufferers "were females in the prime of life" who could not bear to be touched, recoiling from the possibility from a distance of two feet or more, and who were extraordinarily sensitive to sound.[11]

With the very functions of women's bodies defined as inherently unhealthy, physicians in all regions of the nation assumed women were intended by nature to need protection from the public world. A reviewer in the *Southern Medical and Surgical Journal* noted with approval Charles Meigs's comments on women's place: "She reigns in the heart; her seat and throne are by the hearthstone—The household alter is her place of worship and service."[12] A fledgling southern physician shared these beliefs, suggesting that in addition to the "delicacy" of woman's "structures subject[ing] her to diseases peculiar to herself," she "being of delicate & attenuate frame cannot master the rough & heavy labours that devolves upon man."[13] Samuel Cartwright noted that women in the South are "in a relation or state, in conformity to their nature, as the negroes are."[14]

Southern physicians who viewed women as unhealthy were as eager as their northern and European counterparts to gain legitimacy for themselves by claiming that their interventions offered relief from pain, debility, and death. Criticizing the ignorance of midwives and lay practitioners, physicians argued that only if women availed themselves of medical advice could they (and their families) hope to survive with a measure of health and happiness. In this way, they enhanced their own claims for professional standing and income.

Once again, southern physicians shared the views of those in the rest of the nation. In the thesis Lovick Hill wrote toward earning his medical degree from the South Carolina Medical College, he commented that women's structures and diseases were so peculiar and complicated as to "render them a special investigation of paramount importance to the practitioner."[15] According to the anonymous reviewer of a book on female hygiene, "as woman has peculiarities of organization and function . . . the part which she plays in the procreative process, renders her more peculiarly an object of attention, to the philanthropist and physician."[16]

However, such views did not fully take into account the peculiar circumstances of southern physicians, who could not easily expound upon the nature of women's bodies without addressing the consequences of race—and who were as eager to gain access to slave patients as to white.

In writing about women's bodies as inherently and increasingly unhealthy and as needing protection and care, southern physicians differed little from those in other parts of the nation, yet their intellectual task was different because of the racial context in which they lived. Gender was one of the key grounds upon which the cultural battles of the mid-nineteenth century were fought, and physicians everywhere claimed authority to define what they considered the scientific truths of women's bodies and minds. For them, the physical body carried its own truths that could not help but be mapped onto social relationships, including women's place in society. However, to do so in the South posed a specific set of problems and required a different set of arguments in order to meet the requirements of its peculiar social context.

Faced with such a complex undertaking, many southern physicians first focused their attention on demonstrating women's bodily vulnerability, implicitly defining those bodies as white. These ideas were new and controversial enough to have to be defended, and many southern physicians were dedicated to doing so without complicating matters by addressing race. They knew that white southerners' racial beliefs precluded defining black women as frail and in need of care; the demands of slavery were such that their bodies were needed in the fields and kitchens, not in sickbeds.

Yet southern doctors also knew that in order for their arguments about women as a category to seem convincing, they had to explain why white women's bodies were in so much danger, while not making the same claims for black women. Believing as they did that both blackness and femaleness pervaded the individual's entire being, physicians had to find a way to reconcile their views of race and gender with their assumptions of superiority and inferiority. If women's bodies were biologically vulnerable because they were ruled by their reproductive organs, doctors had to be able to explain why black women's bodies were not subject to the same laws of nature and so in need of the same care and protection—and medical attention. To claim that black women were not as vulnerable as white women to the depredations of biology was to run the risk of viewing them as inherently stronger and thus superior to white women, an untenable position in a slave society. Yet physicians and lay white southerners alike had no doubts that white women were more often sick, suffered more in childbirth, and in general were less healthy than the slave women among whom they lived, in spite of the advantages white skin conveyed. Reconciling these apparent contradictions became a necessity for southerners determined to enforce race and gender hierarchies in a manner that suited their ideological purposes and their way of life.

## Reconciling Sex and Race

Southern physicians and lay writers adopted a variety of strategies for addressing the contradictions in their explanations of race and sex differences. To some
extent, their strategies followed the lead of writers outside of the South, who
faced similar dilemmas explaining the health consequences of class differences.
Particularly in the urban centers of the Northeast, home of the most celebrated
medical schools in the United States, physicians had to explain why immigrants
and the poor were simultaneously sicker than their more well-to-do counterparts
and yet less vulnerable to bodily infirmity. Immigrant and poor women had to
be seen as less subject to derangements of the reproductive organs, so that they
could work in factories and sweatshops without attracting undue sympathy from
reformers, and yet also be considered under the bodily influence of those same
organs, so that they could be paid less than men because they were unable to
work as long or as hard. In the North, however, reconciling the conflicts between
these positions was less urgent in the thinking of physicians than addressing the
corresponding differences seemed in the South.[17] More secure in their professional status and less troubled by the contradictions of a class system still fluid
in its arrangements, northern physicians grappled only intermittently with the
medical consequences of reconciling class and sex.

One of the strategies southern physicians adopted to make sense of race and
sex was to think about the consequences of "civilization," by which they usually
meant modern society. Defined so as to encompass all aspects of fashionable
urban life, civilization was a flexible concept that referred to the pleasures of
opulence and refinement enjoyed by the wealthy. While committed to the benefits
of progress, physicians were not convinced that civilization was an unalloyed
blessing for the individuals who lived under its influence. Instead, they blamed
civilization for distancing women from what had originally been more natural
experiences. Civilization, they argued, changed women's bodies from effective,
naturally functioning organisms into weak and vulnerable objects unable to perform their expected biological tasks. The chief advantage of civilization as an
explanation for women's debility was that it was race specific: black women were
not civilized in the same way as white women.

Midcentury physicians frequently argued that women in the present were less
healthy than their grandmothers had been, a biological trade-off for the benefits
they enjoyed. While this argument would serve the needs of southern physicians
particularly well, even in the rest of the nation physicians believed that the general state of women's health had deteriorated over time. According to Gunning
Bedford, professor of obstetrics at the University of New York, "It was the pride of
the ancients to impart to their children robust constitutions and enduring health;
and could a mother of those sensible times again visit earth, look upon the present
condition of society, and witness its effects on the women of the present generation,

she would, indeed, think that human nature had nearly run its course."[18] This belief was shared by many women as well. Catharine Beecher, for example, surveyed women throughout the nation and found that very few considered themselves to be healthy, while believing that women in the past had been so.[19]

The dangers of civilization for women's bodies were perceived by southern physicians of all sorts. According to a writer in a Thomsonian journal published in Charleston, South Carolina, "a large portion of the bad health" of women "arises from the pernicious habits and fashions of the day."[20] Another Thomsonian agreed, noting that "the customs and the morality which are now popular, produce both vice and disease."[21] A regular physician shared their perspective but explained in more detail: "In the highest state of civilization and enlightenment, woman is more subject to disease, from the greater development of her nervous system, and the many unnatural exactions which society imposes." Joseph Wright wrote of the dangers of women's confinement indoors, which "besides hurting their figure and complexion, relaxes their solids, weakens their minds and disorders all the functions of the body."[22] A Columbia, South Carolina, physician noted simply, "our degenerate age is marked, to a very great extent, by a decline in the constitutional stamina of females."[23] Civilization, which physicians equated with modern life, clearly posed dangers to women.

Physicians believed that civilization posed particular dangers to women's reproductive organs—and thus to their entire bodies and minds. They found it convenient to distinguish between civilized women and those they categorized as savage or barbarous, terms they rarely defined with precision but that clearly referred to Africans and other dark-skinned peoples. Physicians were convinced that civilized women experienced worse suffering during menstruation, pregnancy, and childbirth than women of the other groups. One anonymous author noted that "the liability to disorders incidental on the changes brought about in women by puberty, increase daily as civilization increases." He explained the increase by arguing that those in "our high state of civilization . . . are amenable to greater variations, and must therefore accept the additional infirmities saddled upon us by civilization," especially when compared with "those who live in barbarous hardihood."[24]

Menstruation was not the only bodily function made more problematic by civilization. Childbirth, too, was widely perceived to be more painful among more civilized women. According to Joseph Eve, a distinguished professor of materia medica and obstetrics at the Medical College of Georgia, at least some of the pains of parturition had to be "the result of the unnatural and injurious habits and customs of civilized life; for we know that in the savage state and among those whose manner of living is more natural and conducive to the healthy performance of all the physical functions, there is comparatively little pain or danger."[25] Thomsonians were not immune from this argument. One claimed that "whatever may have been the happy condition of the human female during the early ages of the world, or whatever natural advantages may at present be possessed by the tawny mothers of the forest, it will be universally acknowledged that the original curse,—'in sorrow shalt thou bring forth children,'—still rests with unrelenting rigor upon the fair daughters of our own enlightened country." He was convinced that "woman, in a state of civilization, is exposed to the influence of a variety of casualties which tend to protract the process of parturition to more than ordinary length."[26]

Physicians who held such views recognized the centrality of women's reproductive organs to their overall well-being, yet they saw the impact of those organs as uneven. While civilization brought progress, it also brought debility. No observer urged returning to a state of savagery, but the dangerous consequences of civilization were clear to all. According to Gunning Bedford, "the scholar is gladdened by the triumphs of civilization, [while] the philanthropist . . . can not but lament the evils which necessarily follow in its train."[27] Samuel Jennings acknowledged that many women suffered during childbirth, but he did not "consider parturition, in its perfectly natural state, to be a disease." Women "in the Brazils, Calabria, and some parts of Africa" found it only "very moderately inconvenient" and so "scarcely regarded" it.[28] John Stainback Wilson thought civilized women, the "pampered daughters of idleness and luxury," were not "in a state of actual open disease," but he believed their habits "deranged the whole body, and especially the nervous system, thus rendering women preternaturally susceptible to pain," especially in childbirth. He noted that "the negro women of the Southern States, who are compelled to lead an active life, and to live on plain food, while their minds are undisturbed by corroding cares, have much easier labors, and are much less exposed to the accidents of child-bed, than their mistresses."[29]

For the majority of southern observers, civilization had caused women's health to decline, in spite of its apparent advantages. However, the dangers it brought did not fall evenly upon all women. Those who were most civilized were most likely to feel its harmful effects; by definition, such women were white and wealthy. Black women, poor white women, and those who lived in the countryside were deemed less civilized and thus less vulnerable to civilization's baneful health consequences. For physicians, such views offered both a way of reconciling their assumptions about race and sex—and class—and a convenient justification for their practices. Civilized women might be subject to more ill health than others, but they were also in a better position to pay for the services of a physician to attend them and more likely to live where one was close by. Physicians eager to cast themselves in the role of saviors of women and thus enhance their professional standing were quick to take advantage of the implications of this argument.

## Civilization and Women's Health

Physicians criticized all aspects of civilized women's lives as the sources of their poor health. One of their most frequent concerns was the danger posed by fashionable clothing, worn, of course, exclusively by white women. Thomsonians and other botanic physicians led the way, frequently railing against the dangers of tight corsets and fashionable styles that constricted internal organs and offered inadequate protection for the body. The editor of the *Southern Botanico-Medical Journal,* published in Georgia, was outraged by reports that a woman "laced herself to death" and warned of the "danger, deformity and consequent ill-health that must inevitably follow the practice of tight lacing."[30] Another writer warned that the "reprehensible practice" of dressing fashionably, "no matter how ridiculous or dangerous it may prove," was the cause of "indigestion, fainting, coughs, consumption and other complaints." He lamented that "by the present mode or fashion in dress, thousands of females are injured, if not killed."[31]

Regular physicians shared this sense of the harm women caused themselves by wearing corsets and other fashionable clothing. One physician identified clothing that compressed the belly as a cause of abortion, prolapsed uterus, and suppressed menses, another as the cause of "falling of the womb and . . . sick stomach, deranged bowels, nervousness, low spirits," along with derangements of the brain and spine.[32] Milton Antony was incensed by "the foolish—not to say criminal—sway of fashion over the intellects of some women" that caused their "reason [to be] reduced below intellect." He warned physicians to be alert to the dangers such clothing caused.[33]

Sometimes doctors, perhaps reluctant to alienate their fashionable patients, defended women's clothing. A faculty member at the Oglethorpe Medical College in Savannah, Georgia, praised the hoop skirt as a "light, graceful, and health preserving article of female apparel" that is "one of the most important *Hygienic* measures" of fashion. He praised it in comparison to the practice of wearing "from *half* a dozen, to *three* dozen petticoats, suspended from the hips," which was the cause of a "vast amount of injury . . . [to] the generative organs of the female." Nearly all physicians shared his view that clothing should allow "the free use of all the limbs."[34] John Stainback Wilson also endorsed hoop skirts, "which obviate the necessity for so many under-garments, and remove, to a considerable extent, the downward dragging weight" that caused "falling of the womb."[35]

Physicians who warned of the dangers of fashionable clothing knew that for the most part slave women did not wear the same garments. Only rarely did they report on cases like that of Eliza, a "mulatto" patient of D. T. Tayloe in Washington, North Carolina. Eliza "when quite a young girl, suffered from chronic ulceration of the umbilicus produced by the pressure of an oak split worn in her corsets."[36] More commonly, physicians warned of the dangers not of fashion but of inadequate clothing for slaves, particularly female slaves. Their reasons for doing so are complex, as they simultaneously sought to define black women as healthy enough to work and to extend the range of their own medical practices. One physician warned that slaves needed to be "specially protected from the depressing influences of cold, and from the influence of vicissitudes of the weather, in our capricious climate." He suggested that "the danger of loss of health and life, the loss of time, and the expense of medical aid, and of medicines, arising from a want of proper protection by warm clothing, is much more detrimental to the interests of planters, than the most expensive arrangements."[37]

H. W. Moore, in his thesis at the Medical College of South Carolina, argued that slave women were particularly susceptible to cold: "Exposure to cold and dampness gives rise to many of those diseases which belong alone to the female sex. Less protected by their mode of dress than the men, women should be furnished with woolen drawers and underclothes."[38] A Georgia physician, Robert Battey, was well aware of the discomfort inadequate clothing could cause. In his report of his treatment of a slave woman suffering from a gynecologic disorder, Battey remarked that after the operation he performed she was restless and "annoyed by flies." He added, "Had she been furnished with a pair of drawers, they would have materially added to her comfort, and relieved her surgeon and attendants."[39] It apparently did not occur to him to supply her with the undergarments himself. In spite of her misery, the woman eventually recovered.

Physicians like Moore and Battey who warned of the dangers of inadequately clothed slaves, particularly female slaves, did so in a different context from those who warned of the dangers of white women's fashionable attire. While white women harmed themselves by their behavior, slave women had little control over the garments they were given by their owners. In both cases, physicians believed that attention to proper clothing would improve health. However, they were more critical of white women, who caused their own illnesses and those of their daughters, than they were of slave women, who depended on others to provide adequate coverings. Civilized life was harder to cure than the neglect of slaveholders, for whom appeals to self-interest were assumed to be sufficient inducements to change. By contrast, white women could reject fashion, but only to a point, as prudent physicians acknowledged. As a result, white women faced illness to a far greater extent than did black, an unfortunate consequence of their advanced, civilized status.

Fashion was not the only cause of civilized white women's increased risk of illness. Southern physicians also railed about the dangers of lack of exercise associated with fashionable life. One warned that "the faulty physical education of girls may so pervert the play of the functions, that the mind and heart may become diseased as well as the body, thus totally incapacitating the sufferer from performing her part in society."[40] Another urged physicians to induce women "to take more exercise in the open air," suggesting specifically "the pleasant exercise afforded by dancing." Exercise "adds grace, and ease, to the carriage and manners of the young, and especially to females," and allows them to enjoy greater health.[41] John Stainback Wilson encouraged women to ignore the "moustached, Frenchified dandies" who called them "vulgar" for exercising, urging "the daughters of the heroes of '76" to "sternly resist any tampering with their birthright" and exercise to increase their breathing muscles. He wanted girls to become "a little more tomboyish," although he thought the best exercise for them was "combined with some useful occupation," such as housework.[42] Urging women to exercise was advice physicians knew needed only be directed at white women. Slaves, whose occupations normally required them to be out of doors and physically active much of the time, did not need to be told to exercise, nor did they suffer the bodily effects of not doing so. By defining civilized white women as sedentary and in need of exercise, physicians could justify portraying them as unhealthy as compared with black women and thus in need of medical care.

Physicians likewise worried about the consequences of civilized women's poor diets. One physician noted that "a country woman is robust and healthy, she eats a basin of sour milk and bread for breakfast." He asked, "Does this [not] prove it a good one for the luxurious and inactive town lady?"[43] The author of *The American Lady's Medical Pocket-Book* was more dogmatic in insisting upon the "temperate use of wholesome food" as the means of avoiding "the depraved and capricious appetite, the hysterical and nervous sensations, the feeling of langour and depression, the intense headach[e] and disturbed sleep, from which so many of those in the middle and more opulent ranks of society are almost continually sufferers."[44]

No less dangerous was the use of tobacco and alcohol. One physician was "incredulous" that "ladies of the greatest respectability, the most genteel and accomplished in one of our largest cities, carry their little jars, or boxes of snuff into the social circle, and with a delicate ivory spoon feed their *sweet* mouths with this most delicious and agreeable poison."[45] Another warned women that marriage to an intemperate man would draw "down upon her head the heaviest of curses"; it would be "better to embrace the sepulchre." Such a marriage would be "the wedlock of beauty and pollution; of purity and pestilence; the binding of the breathing form of life to the loathsomeness of death."[46] The "depraved tastes of 'modern civilization'" were just as dangerous when women imbibed the lighter alcoholic drinks intended for them, "containing various deleterious and even poisonous ingredients, which must be more or less detrimental to health, apart from the exciting effects of the alcoholic element."[47] Clearly, physicians saw civilization as mined with insidious dangers for the unwary woman.

Physicians who viewed civilization as dangerous for women's health were able to easily distinguish between the white women who enjoyed its benefits and the black women who did not. Unlike white women, black women were not likely to suffer the effects of tight lacing, lack of exercise, refined food, or other indulgences. Instead, because they lived in what physicians assumed was a more natural state, they were assumed to be more healthy. This was an effective, albeit rather circular, solution for the problem of understanding the consequences of sex and gender in a racialized context, while simultaneously offering physicians a legitimate mechanism for enhancing their cultural authority. Because their

arguments offered a convenient means of solving a perplexing dilemma, physicians' pronouncements about civilization were increasingly widely accepted
during the antebellum years.

Not content simply to point out the dangers posed by civilization to women's
bodies, physicians refined their analysis of the health consequences of sex by
distinguishing not just between black and white women's bodies, but also between different categories of whites. Never formally couched in the language of
class, physicians' writings about the health differences of what they typed as city
and country women deepened their understanding of civilization's dangers. City
women who succumbed to the demands of fashion and who spent most of their
time indoors avoiding exercise were widely recognized as being less healthy than
those who led more natural country lives. While such comments were found in
the writings of northern and European physicians, they were ubiquitous in the
South, where city women were assumed to be elite and country women, whether
white or black, were obviously socially inferior. These attitudes offered physicians
a way of medicalizing the bodily experiences of those women with the most access to and resources to pay for their services while still maintaining a posture
of scientific and social responsibility.

City women's greater bodily suffering and debility than their country counterparts' began with menstruation. A Virginia physician warned that women
"raised delicately in cities, have more difficulty and disorder of the menses than
those who enjoy the country air, and lead an active life."[48] A Savannah physician
agreed, noting that women "of the lower rank, inured to exercise and labor, and
strangers to those refinements which debilitate the system . . . are seldom observed
to suffer at these times"; in addition, "the full blooming country girl does not
discharge half the quantity that the pale-face lady of quality does."[49] The dangers
only increased at childbirth. One obstetrician recognized that it was impossible to
determine how much of the pain of childbirth was physiological and how much
was "the result of the unnatural and injurious habits and customs of civilized life."
He acknowledged that "in the savage state and among those whose manner of
living is more natural and conducive to healthy performance of all the physical
functions, there is comparatively very little pain or danger."[50]

Not only did overly civilized women suffer inordinately during childbirth,
they were unable to nurse their babies, according to the author of a volume
of medical advice aimed at southerners. Since it was "rare to find a woman of
fashion free from" health complaints who did not "deviate" from the "dictates"
of nature, few were able to nurse effectively. A "delicate female" might be able to
give birth to a child, "but it will be hardly fit to live."[51] By contrast, Joseph Wright
observed, women "chiefly employed without doors in the different branches of
husbandry, gardening and the like, were almost as hardy as their husbands, and
that their children were likewise strong and healthy."[52] Even beyond reproduction, city women suffered from disease to a greater extent than those elsewhere.

Prolapsed uterus, for example, "proves more or less inconvenient, according to the sensibilities of the patient," wrote the editor of the *Southern Medical and Surgical Journal*. "Hence, a degree of prolapsus which might pass unnoticed by those who are less irritable, may become a source of annoyance to the sedentary and nervous ladies of the city."[53] Clearly, civilization posed grave dangers to those women caught in the clutches of the indolent and irresponsible life of fashion demanded in southern cities.

Refined city life was not the only source of danger for civilized white women's health. Their lack of education, too, posed grave dangers. Unlike postwar northern physicians who would warn that educating women would draw vital energy away from their reproductive organs and thus cause severe illness, antebellum southern doctors advocated women's education as a means of improving their health and that of their families as well as humanity in general.[54] The ignorance associated with a lack of adequate information and wholesome pursuits was, according to southern physicians, a source of their poor habits and thus poor health.

Wright, who claimed that women who worked outdoors were as healthy as men, worried that "over anxious" mothers who wanted their daughters to have "a great number of accomplishments" deprived them of bodily exercise. He sought educated women who were "trained up to the spirit of the age" in "the higher, sterner qualities of the head and heart."[55] A Charleston physician concerned about hereditary disposition urged "females . . . be well educated, that their good qualities may be transmitted to their offspring."[56] Another physician told women not to feel any "violation of propriety in seeking modestly and conscientiously, information which shall fit them for the discharge of the sacred duties God sent them on earth to perform—that delicacy is not affected by a lady remembering that she is *a woman*."[57]

A professor of physiology at Oglethorpe Medical College in Savannah argued that his subject "ought to be taught in every school in the world, and to both girls and boys" in order to develop "the highest good of the race, physically, mentally, and morally."[58] An Alabama physician went even further, claiming that women should be educated "in certain branches of Medicine" so that "the blessings of scientific medicine may reach the fairest and best portion of the community," many of whom were currently "deprived of these, [and] subjected to numerous positive evils of the most grievous characters."[59] These physicians recognized that civilized city women rarely received the kind of education they believed would lead to healthy lives. They deplored the education women did receive, which taught them only to value "themselves upon the delicacy and tenderness of their constitutions" and made "a glory of imperfections."[60]

Some white women, however, were educated about their bodies. In 1855, sixty-year-old Mary Hort attended a "Lecture on Physiology" that she was informed enough to pronounce "very incomplete." The lecturer exhibited a skeleton and a mannequin, the latter "a complete representation of a sexless human body skinned every muscle of a side at least moveable & perfect in shape & colour the blood vessels & nerves—the skull & brain and cerebellum." Hort noted that the lecture also covered "the internal organs," many of which she named, including the "spleen of which the use lately discovered is to lodge the blood of the liver when that organ is diseased." She learned about the nervous and respiratory systems, pronouncing the whole "very instructive, very interesting" in spite of its incompleteness.[61] Dolly Lunt Burge attended "a course of PhrenolD gial Lectures," in which she pronounced herself "much interested." At one she learned about "the different organs how situated & their influence one with the other." She added "do not feel very well," but did not say whether this was the result of the lecture.[62] Both Hort and Burge were teachers, which may account for their curiosity about the human body.

Other women had contradictory feelings about one of the possible consequences of such knowledge. Although Martha Crawford deplored the "fanaticism" of northern women who were "holding conventions and 'resolving' such and such things," she wanted women to have "equal means of education." When she learned that "a female medical college is just chartered in Phila . . . it made my heart swell with joy and gratitude!" She added, "I have been praying for such times."[63] Eliza Clitherall was far less enthusiastic, commenting in her reminiscences: "How revolting to a refined mind of either sex, to hear of modern *female Physicians,* of *Ladies,* who profess to be acquainted with the diseases incident to both sexes, and competent to cure them!" She asked, "Is not the health too often sacrific'd to Popular Education?" and worried about the consequences for women of long hours of confinement a day, plus time needed to study.[64]

Physicians would have endorsed Clitherall's repugnance at the thought of women doctors, if only because of their reluctance to compete with them. Even when they wanted women's education to improve, doctors certainly did not want women to have that much knowledge. Instead, they focused their attention on women who lacked the education necessary to resist the temptations of fashionable life. Such women were all too well schooled in a set of attitudes about their bodies that was as dangerous as ignorance. Physicians lamented the false modesty taught by civilization that made women loath to engage their services. For example, a Thomsonian journal fretted about the "false delicacy" that led women to neglect the signs of consumption that "fearfully increases in our country."[65] John Stainback Wilson warned women that "modesty, though it is the brightest gem in the beauteous diadem of female loveliness, should not be prized above that knowledge which is necessary, in many instances, to health, and even life itself."[66] Samuel Cartwright thought physicians should study "the science of Prosoposcopia, or the physiognomy of disease," the ability to identify disease merely by looking at the patient, which he thought would be helpful for treating "females who often will not tell, what is the matter with them."[67]

Physicians of all sorts were particularly concerned about female modesty when it prevented them from conducting what they considered to be necessary gynecologic examinations. A physician writing for advice about a patient suffering from prolapsed uterus for more than four years, for example, noted she "could not be prevailed upon to employ a physician."[68] At other times, physicians complained that the dictates of fashion influenced women's reluctance to submit to their prescriptions. For instance, women sometimes avoided treatments that were prolonged or unpleasant or that interfered with their regular activities, which physicians assumed to be focused on pleasure.

Attributing such reluctance to the dictates of refinement, physicians once again deplored the ways in which civilization failed to deliver on its promise of better health. Here, too, southern physicians' arguments about the causes of elite white women's poor health enhanced their own roles as saviors of such women, as well as enabled them to interpret the race and gender context of illness. One Thomsonian physician made these connections explicit, recognizing that "the physician knows that the customs and the morality which are now popular, produce both vice and disease." He believed that "the honest and enlightened physician will tell you so." However, if you were to "ask him how it happens," his reply would address "the prudish severity with which society dooms one sex to unnatural restraints," as well as "the temporizing injustice with which she winks at the scarcely-veiled libertinism of the other." He continued: "Ask him what *he* thinks of popular morality, in itself; and he will tell you, that, *as a physiologist,* he disapproves and condemns it. But as a physician, he profits by it; unwillingly, indeed, if he be an honest and a worthy man, but yet positively and certainly." He concluded that "if society's customs, and society's morality, encouraged moderation in all things . . . men would be happier and better; but physicians would lose their practice."[69] While few allopathic physicians shared his perspective on their calling, most would have agreed with his views of the dangers of civilized morality and behavior, for elite white women in particular.

Only a few southern physicians thought that health problems were worse among slaves and poor whites than among more civilized women. In an essay on prolapsed uterus, a professor of obstetrics at a Savannah medical school noted that "aggravated cases are found" in women "whose condition in life demand the daily employment of labor for a livelihood, and negresses, whose employment often call for the lifting of burdens, more or less weighty."[70] The editor of the *Southern Medical and Surgical Journal* shared his view about the causes of this gynecologic problem and noted that "women should therefore abstain from great muscular efforts, and, in the case of our field hands, should not be allowed to use the axe nor to carry heavy baskets of cotton."[71] Joseph Eve noted that ulcers of the cervix were less commonly found in "ladies in respectable life and comfortable circumstances, who generally apply for assistance sooner, and in whom inflammation of the cervix is very much moderated in its intensity, and kept from producing ulceration by frequent ablutions, which are very much neglected among the lower classes."[72]

Slave women were also prone to miscarry as a result of their occupations, according to E. M. Pendleton, a Georgia physician interested in comparing the fecundity of the races. "Over-exertion at the wash-tub, scouring mop and plough, will be made to produce the great majority of cases, and not a few are induced by constant elevation of the arms, as in pulling fodder, warping cloth, etc." When he compared the condition of both races of women, "the one being doomed, in many instances, to perform the severe labor of the sterner sex, and that, too, during gestation, while the other enjoys the ease and quietude of indoor employment," he was not surprised by the results. However, he noted that "if the conditions of the two races were reversed, there would be triple the number of cases among the Caucasians that there is now among the Africans."[73]

Other physicians also attributed the health difficulties of working white women to hard work and neglect, not inherent weaknesses. A Georgia physician deplored the fact that a "labouring woman" who "had to perform all the domestic drudgery of a large poor family, the mother of seven children" suffered protracted and painful complications from the mumps. He lamented that "during the major part of the time *she had no treatment, or perhaps, more properly speaking, she was allowed to have no treatment, not even that of decent* HUMANITY."[74] Another physician wrote of a woman who had been in labor for five days with a child weighing seventeen pounds. The labor "had worn off, leaving the woman languid and exhausted, and insusceptible of a renewal of labor." He commented, "[T]his case was twelve miles from town, and amongst unenlightened people in the country—hence its neglect for so long a time."[75] Concerned and sympathetic physicians were convinced that such neglect could be far more easily resolved than the dangers posed by civilization.

With only limited exceptions, physicians attempting to explain why elite women suffered worse health than their slave and white country counterparts found blaming the evils of civilization a useful ideological strategy. It allowed them to argue that the women most able to pay for their services were also those most in need of care. More important, it allowed them to explain why women who were unquestionably superior by virtue of their race and class would suffer worse and more frequent illnesses than those inferior to them in every other respect. Perhaps most important of all, identifying civilization as the source of elite women's poor health contained within itself the essence of a powerful counterargument: If the refined lifestyle associated with civilization caused women to suffer, its benefits could also be turned to their advantage. Physicians attempting to understand why those women whose race (and class) placed them at the top of southern society suffered more than their inferiors could explain their afflictions as a temporary imbalance, easily rectified by educating women to healthier habits—and by proper medical care.

Physicians were convinced that their expertise could help women make better choices and thus lead healthier lives. Their prescriptions went far beyond abandoning corsets, late nights, rich diets, and indolent habits, although these were ubiquitous in the manuals for domestic medicine they wrote for a popular audience. Convinced that the first duty of the physician was disease prevention, they claimed for themselves that crucial task. According to one, physicians ought to instruct their patients in "the science of *Hygiene,*" as it was "the noblest . . . [and] the first duty of the physician to point out the means by which disease may be prevented."[76] For many, the key element in helping civilized women live healthier lives was to teach them when to enlist the aid of a physician. By enhancing women's education in this manner, physicians hoped women would recognize their limits in providing care for themselves and their families.

Fledgling physician Larkin Jones hoped his work would be responsible for "prolonging the life, or relieving the pain, of some amiable sufferer."[77] A more experienced physician saw it as the duty of the profession to "impress on the minds of mothers the importance of seeking medical counsel when the first indication of deranged function is presented, and to insist . . . that each day and each occasion of deviation from nature on the part of any organ, render less certain the chances of a speedy and effectual cure."[78] Another physician was even more blunt, claiming that "in the vast majority of diseases, both the welfare of the patient and pecuniary consideration, demand that the physician should be sent for at the onset of the disease."[79] By teaching women to avoid the pitfalls of refinement and encouraging them to take advantage of the promise of modern medicine, physicians hoped women's lives would be saved and improved.

The benefits of civilization for white women were not limited to their medical care. White women were widely perceived to be the bearers of civilization, both literally and figuratively, and as such were the recipients of its blessings. Commentators of all sorts expounded on the elevated status of women in a state of civilization as opposed to savagery or barbarism. In civilization, women were protected by men, who revered their nurturing abilities enough to shelter them and their children from the harsher aspects of life. By contrast, savage or barbarous women were forced by necessity to engage in the struggle for subsistence, with no allowances made for their assumed vulnerabilities during pregnancy or while nursing. Only civilization offered women protection from the harsh demands of earning a living. If society simultaneously sought to impose upon them the demands of fashion that led to ill health, the trade-off was worth the price—and could be remedied. White women were exhorted to resist the imprecations of a fashionable life even as they were repeatedly reminded of the benefits civilized society had bestowed upon them.

Perhaps not surprisingly, one of the benefits of civilization was the right to impart those benefits to the next generation. Women were freed from the burdens of public life and work in order to nurture their children in a manner that would advance the progress of civilization. As civilizers, white women were to tame more than just the unformed natures of their children; in addition, they were to extend their influence over their husbands and, through them, influence society as a whole. According to one newly minted physician, woman, "by her varied excellencies becomes the great civilizer of the entire family of man."[80] Civilization thus was both a blessing and a responsibility for white women: a blessing to the extent that it offered them protection from the rigors of earning a living so that they might focus on their reproductive functions, even as it imposed a responsibility to share those blessings with their families. If poor health sometimes accompanied civilization, it was only because women had strayed from its true path by exaggerating its meanings, becoming overcivilized or overrefined—and thus unhealthy—in the process.

Neither the blessings nor the responsibilities of civilization were shared by black women. Black women were too close to a state of savagery to be considered civilized, although they could be seen to be moving in that direction under the beneficent influence of slavery. As a result, there was no need to protect them during pregnancy, no justification for entertaining their sentimental attachments to their children. Just as their more robust and vigorous lives meant that they often enjoyed greater health and easier deliveries than the white women among whom they lived, at least according to the pronouncements of southern physicians, so, too, did black women escape the pitfall of ill health civilization could bring. Since black women were neither bearers nor beneficiaries of civilization in white eyes, not surprisingly their suffering was all too often simply not recognized outside of their own families and communities.

## Bodily Sympathy

Civilization was not the only trope southern physicians developed to explain the bodily consequences of race and gender differences, although it was the dominant one. A second strategy drew upon the medical concept of sympathy. Mid-nineteenth-century physicians did not recognize the existence of distinct disease entities that operated more or less identically in the various bodies that might suffer from them. Instead, they believed that each body reacted differently, according to its peculiar constitution. The concept of sympathy refined this argument, allowing physicians to claim that an illness in one part of the body could influence and extend to other parts. John Stainback Wilson called this vicarious action "the power of one organ to act for another . . . when the functions of an associated organ are suspended." For example, he noted that pregnant women sometimes suffered from toothaches that resulted from "a general nervous excitement of the jaw through sympathy with the womb."[81] Most of the time, physicians discussed sympathy in terms of women's reproductive organs; their often unspoken assumption was that the women under consideration were white and the reproductive organs those required for generation. Diseases of women's reproductive organs could be manifested elsewhere in the body; the digestive and nervous systems were considered especially vulnerable. The concept of sympathy enabled physicians to argue that nearly any ailment in nearly any part of a woman's body, including mental illness, originated in disturbances of the uterus or ovaries, even if the organs did not appear to be diseased. Sympathy complicated diagnosis, since even pain was not a reliable indicator of the source of the problem, encouraging the sick and their families to rely on the expertise of physicians. It also powerfully underscored women's bodily vulnerability.

Physicians found the concept of sympathy useful far beyond enhancing the scope of their practices. In addition, it helped them explain the differences between black and white women's bodies in another manner that suited the ideological needs of a slave society. Sympathy allowed physicians to claim that while all women's bodies were ruled by their reproductive organs, white women were more influenced by their generative organs (cervix, uterus, ovaries) while black women were subject to their genitalia (vagina, vulva, buttocks). As a result, the two races of women had different bodily experiences of sympathy and suffered differently as well.

Europeans had long viewed black women as thoroughly sexualized beings, their bodies representing all the aspects of sexuality that white men denied their wives and daughters and ostensibly themselves. Africans were viewed as the embodiment of dangerous sexuality: tantalizing and exotic, yet frightening.[82] Such views intensified in the New World as white men enacted into the laws of slavery their perceptions of the dangers Africans posed to public and private morality.[83] Although by the nineteenth century, white women were increasingly being viewed as passionless, black women were not; white men saw them as lascivious and enticing and in need of controL. A. P. Merrill, the physician who wrote so extensively about anatomical and physiological differences between the races, noted that in blacks, "the genital organs of both sexes are more largely developed, and the breasts of the females are more conical, with a less extent of base."[84]

For midcentury physicians, these views of black women's sexuality had become so commonplace as to be part of their mental landscape. However, they became newly significant when combined with the concept of sympathy in explaining the bodily implications of race and sex differences. Physicians defined black women by their vaginas, white women by their wombs. Both vagina and womb caused the women surrounding them to be diseased, but the diseases were different: Black women's vaginas carried diseases associated with filth and contagion, such as syphilis, that afflicted everyone they came into contact with, while white women's wombs caused only individual suffering and debility. For example, when North Carolina physician J. B. Hughes sought to explain the causes and cure of syphilis in newborns, every example he offered was of a black or mixed-race child, most of whom had contracted the disease from their mothers.[85] Defining black women by their genital and white women by their generative organs offered a way of viewing both groups as women, yet with bodies organized so differently that their roles in society and their medical needs could scarcely be compared. Physicians sometimes explained this difference in terms of white women's more civilized bodies; civilization had erased the taint of sexuality from them, freeing them to devote their energies to reproduction. Black women's sexualized bodies, caught in a state of savagery or barbarism, simply did not need the same kind of care as white women's reproductive bodies did, even during menstruation, pregnancy, and childbirth. In this view, civilization only explained what were fundamental biological differences between the two groups of women; the workings of their bodies and the concept of sympathy rendered them biologically distinct.

Physicians who explored the consequences of bodies that were sexed as well as raced believed that women's reproductive organs, both genital and generative, influenced their entire beings according to the concept of sympathy. Quite literally, black and white women's bodies and minds reacted differently to basic biological experiences due to the particular organs most influential upon them. Not insignificantly, the organs most dominant in white women were also categorized as the most dangerous. The English author of a popular textbook on midwifery remarked: "We are well aware of the sympathy which subsists between the uterus and the constitution generally; but the connection is less intimate between the vagina and the constitution."[86] The dangers the uterus could cause for (white) women's bodies were extensive. A southern physician noted that "displacement of the uterus is usually accompanied by a considerable number of sympathetic affections which are often looked upon and treated as independent disorders"; he specified "spinal diseases, liver complaint, [and] neuralgia" among them.[87] Another commented that "in the female we have an almost countless catalogue of disordered sensations, arising from the peculiarity and extended sympathies of their procreative system." His list included irritable breasts, "the excruciating pain felt by (mostly) barren women in the act of coition, perhaps the tortures of dysmennorhoea, [and] the torments of labour."[88] Clearly, white women whose bodies centered on their reproductive organs were biologically vulnerable in a way that black women, who were more sexually defined, were not. Only one physician, E. M. Pendleton of Georgia, attributed slave women's worse physical circumstances to their owners' reluctance to employ medical assistance and their inadequate living conditions, and not to any inherent differences in their bodies compared with white women.[89] Pendleton was a pioneer in the effort to apply statistics to mortality and morbidity, which perhaps helps explain his startling conclusions.

Physicians who viewed women's bodies as centered on their reproductive organs, like those who explored the consequences of civilization on them, concluded that race created differences between women. Even though women of both races shared the biological functions associated with reproduction, those functions did not have the same meanings or consequences. For antebellum physicians, shared biology did not mean shared experiences; the same anatomy did not mean the same physiology. Women of both races were subject to debilitating suffering that frequently warranted medical intervention. However, in order to accommodate the complex requirements of their society, physicians maintained that the bodily context of women's suffering was different according to race. In spite of appearances, black women were neither inherently healthier nor stronger than white women. Instead, they suffered less in pregnancy and childbirth and succumbed to fewer illnesses because they worked hard and lived healthy lives. These views, of course, were quite satisfactory to slaveholders, for whom preserving the health of slaves was of pecuniary as well as moral concern. And if following the dictates of fashionable refinement made white women appear to be less healthy than black women and thus biologically weaker, that could easily be remedied by following the advice of physicians; appearances were not realities. All women's roles in reproduction rendered them biologically inferior to men, but white women were still blessed with bodies that represented the peak of function and beauty, or at least possessed the potential to be so. For antebellum physicians, sex, as much as race, shaped human bodies, with hierarchies of the superior and inferior carefully preserved.

Tracing the ways in which women understood their gendered and raced bodies is much more difficult than analyzing the views of physicians. Southern white women were profoundly reticent about such intimate matters even in their most personal writings, while black women left few direct sources at all in which to discover their feelings.[90] As a result, there is simply no way to know how ordinary women of either race felt about their sexual and reproductive bodies except in general terms. While it might be tempting to conclude from their silence that they simply did not think about such matters, a more likely explanation points to the power of social conventions that proscribed even a whisper about them.

# CHAPTER 3

# Placed Bodies

Physicians who claimed that country women lived healthier lives than those in the city for the most part did so as a means of explaining elite white women's apparent ill health. In spite of their racial superiority, physicians argued, such women suffered the consequences of their heedless adherence to the demands of fashionable civilization. However, as they watched sectional tensions escalate, southerners who found themselves more and more on the defensive in the political and intellectual life of the nation transformed their debate about the influence of urban civilization on bodies into the belief that bodies were shaped by the geographic location in which they were born and lived. During the 1850s, physicians developed the argument that bodies were defined not only by their race and sex, but also by the very region in which they were placed. Bodies were either northern or southern, African or American or European. The bodily consequences of being thus placed were seemingly just as profound as the differences created in them by race and sex.

Southern physicians who made such claims in the 1850s did so with full awareness of the sectional tensions shaking the nation. It is not difficult to argue that their voices were a crude effort to contribute to the rhetoric pulling the nation asunder. However, while some of their pronouncements were undoubtedly influenced by fire-eating politicians and the desire to set themselves apart from northerners, they were also influenced by their growing claims for the science of medicine. Determined to heal their patients' ills, physicians believed that attention to location could improve their diagnostic accuracy and therapeutic efficacy. The result was a curious mixture of regional distinctiveness and medical theory, which historian James O. Breeden called "states rights medicine."[1] Placed bodies required an explicitly southern understanding and an explicitly southern medical practice, encouraging physicians in the region to develop their own expertise as well as allowing them to refine the implications of race and sex differences.[2]

Awareness that some places were inherently unhealthy and that some people were more likely to get sick in them was part of the anecdotal medical lore that informed mid-nineteenth-century physicians' thinking about bodies as placed. They were similarly informed by the related notion that climate had a significant influence on the constitution and on diseases and their treatment. Like the miasmas that made certain places unhealthy, climate could influence the body's reaction to its environment; the South's heat (as perceived by whites) or cold (as experienced by blacks) was widely understood to be dangerous for the raced bodies that resided there. Not only were diseases experienced differently in different places and climates, so were their treatments different. Physicians recognized a growing responsibility to explore the implications of place for the bodies they sought to understand and whose illnesses they tried to cure. One stated plainly: "The moral or intellectual status of a race has a very intimate relation to its geographical location and physical conformation."[3] A Georgia physician noted: "Nature presents the same great features everywhere . . . saving those modifications usually attributed to climatic and social differences."[4] John Stainback Wilson noted that "there is more danger in heat and in sudden changes than in uniform cold." As a result, the southern climate, with "long hot summers and short variable winters, is very trying to the constitution," especially for women.[5]

Samuel K. Jennings, author of *A Compendium of Medical Science,* which he claimed was based on fifty years of experience, believed that "physical organization," habits, and "moral character and degree of sensibility" were all influenced by place. People who lived in "equatorial zones" were "almost constrained to prefer a careless and sedentary life" while their bodies "sink into effeminate weakness," leading to "a short life of pleasure." Those who inhabited northern climates were characterized by "hardihood, with little nervous irritability." Those who were from mountainous countries and who had to work hard to support themselves were "a strong vigorous and unconquerable race, always jealous of their liberties and ready to contend for or defend them." By contrast, those from fertile regions were "tame, indolent, and easily conquered" because "indolence and ease . . . produce effeminacy."[6]

Writers outside the South shared these beliefs. Textbook author Thomas Denman, writing about difficult labors, noted that women's experiences in childbirth differed depending on employment and climate. He argued that "though we retain and act upon the same principles, . . . the events . . . must be different in different places, and . . . the authority of the best writers must in some measure be local."[7] Physicians who believed in the individuality of suffering bodies also believed that where those bodies were from and where they were located shaped their medical experiences.

Although arguments defining bodies as placed were most thoroughly elaborated in the last decade before the Civil War, they were built upon familiar theories about the cause of disease. A traditional explanation for disease that was maintained throughout the middle part of the nineteenth century and beyond attributed it to miasmas, foul emanations from rotting organic matter often found in low-lying places. Malaria, not yet identified as a distinct disease as we understand it today, was a term derived from the Italian for bad air and used to label such poisons as well as the diseases they carried.[8] Nearly all fevers were believed to be the result of poisons arising from the earth in specific locations.[9] What would today be considered contagious diseases were also usually identified with place. For example, strangers' and travelers' fever were so named because their victims were most often travelers arriving in southern ports during the summer. Today, historians recognize that they could have fallen victim to an epidemic of yellow fever and the disproportionately low number of cases among the local population be ascribed to exposure or acquired immunity.[10]

Even in the earliest years of colonization, European immigrants recognized the often severe health consequences of what they called seasoning, the process of becoming accustomed to the environment of the New World. Historians partly attribute Virginia's turn away from indentured servitude toward slavery in the mid-seventeenth century to landowners' recognition that seasoning was more often fatal for the English than it was for Africans. Although the explanation would not be known for centuries, such observations were generally correct, especially in the eighteenth century.[11] Many West Africans carried in their blood the trait known as sickle cell. When inherited from both parents, this trait causes a painful and debilitating form of anemia. However, individuals with only one copy of the trait in their genetic code inherit "some protection" from one form of malaria, making them less vulnerable to the disease, especially in its acute form.[12] Seasoning, like malaria and other fevers, was primarily a southern phenomenon; relatively few complaints about its dangers were recorded in more northerly places, although malaria certainly existed elsewhere on the continent. These early notions about the importance of place would only become more highly developed as time passed, physicians' knowledge increased, and sectional tensions escalated.

As early as 1836, a Georgia physician, Edward Delony, warned that in Georgia, Alabama, or Louisiana, the treatment that would successfully cure a disease in the North would "not only prove unsuccessful, but, in all probability, dangerous to the life of the patient." He offered cholera, pleurisy, rheumatism, and typhus fever as examples. Delony criticized his southern colleagues for being "too much in the habit of looking to the north for medical light and knowledge," when in practice they would "have to avail themselves of their own resources." Instead, he noted, "their own judgment and experience soon teach them the fallacy of suffering themselves to be governed and guided by the views and opinions of those who can know nothing of the difficulties which we have to encounter in the management of the diseases which occur among us."[13]

Similar recognition of the need for a specifically southern medicine was offered the next year by S. M. Meek, an Alabama physician. Meek applauded the "thrilling interest" southern physicians took in female complaints. He claimed "it must be obvious to every close observer, that a southern climate and the constitution of females born and raised in the south, render them peculiarly subject" to uterine diseases and "impose on the medical profession the duty of attempting to afford them that relief which is not to be looked for from any other source."[14] Delony's and Meek's ideas about placed bodies were prescient in 1836 and 1837, but they would become much more common as sectional tensions intensified.

By 1850, with the nation convulsed by wrangling over the extension of slavery into the territories recently won from Mexico, southern physicians increasingly turned their attention to the consequences of place for the body, its functions, and its diseases. While only rarely couched in the language of sectional rivalry, their arguments emphasized instead a southern medical distinctiveness that marked the region as home to different diseases from the rest of the nation, or sometimes the same diseases in different forms, requiring different treatments. All of this was predicated on the existence of different bodies, more or less adapted to the South's climate. However, perhaps reflecting a sectional political agenda, they did not usually demarcate the boundaries within the South, in spite of growing social and economic distinctions between the upper and lower or old and new Souths, or in longer-settled areas and the frontier.

Southern physicians who sought to understand placed bodies vacillated between understanding them as having fixed constitutions and as subject to change. The constitutional consequences of race and sex were clearly fixed; no one could change from female to male or black to white at will. The constitutional implications of race and sex for an individual's experience of disease were seen as immutable as well. Physicians disagreed only on the details, not their existence. But the consequences of place were harder to understand because bodies could and did move from place to place: from the Old World to the New, from North to South, from the coast to the interior. Physicians asked themselves whether the constitutions of people born in particular places remained fixed or whether they could adapt to new surroundings, a process they termed *acclimation*. The answers were important. If placed bodies had fixed constitutions, then individuals who moved away from home were inviting trouble because they would be vulnerable to a new climate and the diseases associated with it. But if bodies could acclimate, that vulnerability would be reduced over time. No one could be sure which bodily characteristics were fixed and which subject to change or if the answers were the same for all categories of bodies.

The possibility of acclimation was fundamental to physicians' understanding of placed bodies. While this term still exists in popular explanations for how bodies adapt to changing environments, it no longer has a precise medical meaning. Today, physicians, epidemiologists, and public health workers distinguish between inherited and acquired immunity to explain differing degrees of resistance to disease. Roughly speaking, inherited immunity is passed along in the genetic code of an individual, although it is often supplemented by resistance supplied by the mother through the placenta or in breast milk. Acquired immunity results when an individual body successfully weathers a disease and thereby learns both to recognize and resist its causative agent. Each kind of immunity can be complete, rendering individuals impervious to the disease, or partial, leaving them susceptible to milder, less dangerous attacks than those with no immunity at all. Population groups that have remained relatively distinct for long periods of time develop characteristic patterns of immunity to diseases that they encounter frequently (such as malaria in West Africa) while remaining completely vulnerable to those with which they have had no experience. In addition, some diseases, including malaria, exist in both acute and chronic forms, with the latter state often the result of the body's immune system developing a kind of equilibrium with the infection. Without an understanding of genetics and the germ theory of disease, mid-nineteenth-century physicians could not begin to think in these terms. Even so, they were observant enough to recognize that demographic variables influenced relative susceptibility to disease and that race and place were chief among them.

The debate between constitution and acclimation, while never couched in such stark terms, was fraught with contradictions for southern physicians. Arguing that differences in the experience of disease were due to the fundamental constitutional differences of race and sex was a familiar position, easily justified by the assumptions of a slaveholding society. Yet significant numbers of physicians recognized that blacks and whites, men and women who lived in the same place, also shared disease experiences. Theories of acclimation helped them explain such similarities. At the same time, political rhetoric stressing regional differences made defense of a uniquely southern experience both desirable and expedient. For a host of reasons, then, acclimation offered physicians a way to understand the limits of constitutional difference even as it added another dimension to it. The constitutions of raced and sexed bodies could not change, but the constitutions of placed bodies could with time perhaps be modified, suggesting once again that southern physicians had a key role to play in understanding and treating the region's people and their illnesses.

The concept of acclimation, however, also encompassed possibilities that southern physicians found disquieting. If bodies could acclimate, if constitutions were flexible rather than fixed, then how could the bodily consequences of race and sex differences be as immutable as everyone assumed? Might the similarities between the various kinds of bodies be as significant as or even more significant than the differences? Such possibilities were too antithetical to antebellum understandings for serious exploration, but in their considerations of placed bodies, these physicians were addressing issues that would eventually lead to widespread acceptance of the implications of population genetics for understanding disease patterns.

## Climate, Disease, Acclimation, and Race

For nineteenth-century physicians seeking to understand the consequences of placed bodies, the South's climate seemed an obvious beginning point. With a population divided between people from tropical Africa and temperate Europe, the South seemed ill suited to either group. Physicians worried that the South was too hot for white bodies designed for a temperate environment, while it was too cold for Africans accustomed to heat. These physicians assumed that bodies placed in an inhospitable climate were prone to disease. Not surprisingly, they understood the influence of climate to operate differently on black and white bodies. For whites, the South's tropical climate was indeed harmful. A reviewer of Josiah Nott and George Gliddon's *Indigenous Races of the Earth* noted their belief that "the pure white man carried into the tropic, deteriotes [*sic*] both in mind and body; the average duration of his life is lessened; and, without fresh importations, his race would in time become extinct." The reviewer suggested that a Scandinavian who moved to the tropics became "tanned, emaciated, debilitated; his countenance, energy, everything undergoes a change." He considered this "not simply a healthful modification of the physical and intellectual man, but a positively *morbid degradation*."[15] White bodies were, in this view, not intended by nature to thrive outside the regions in which they had originated, which had more temperate climates than the South.

According to physician Erasmus Darwin Fenner, professor of the theory and practice of medicine at the New Orleans School of Medicine, acclimation was a dangerous process, especially for whites. He noted that soil and climate differences in the various regions of the earth were so great "that no race of animals is capable, at once, of enjoying equal health in them all." The gradual changes associated with "adaptation of the constitution" required "time and exposure." Few could accomplish them without danger. "There are but few individuals who can make a great change of residence with perfect impunity. With the great majority of people, it is done at the peril of their lives." Fenner noted that it was "universally admitted that all immigrants from more Northern regions to the South were very liable to suffer from the endemic fevers, for the first two or three years of their residence, but that after that period they obtain comparative immunity, and in the course of time may enjoy as good health here as they did where they came from, and some of them *much better*." He explained this by noting that they "become habituated to the climate and its diseases," but that this usually required "the endurance of one or more spells of the customary endemic fevers."[16] According to Fenner, acclimation was possible but not certain for white bodies, since some people would lose their lives while their bodies tried to adjust.

Some observers, less sanguine than Fenner, were convinced that acclimation compelled significant sacrifices from the white bodies attempting to undergo its rigors in the South, in part because it could never be successfully completed. Such bodies might survive in the southern climate, but they would never adapt to the point of thriving in it. According to Dr. Dawson, editor of the *Oglethorpe Medical and Surgical Journal,* published in Savannah, Georgia, the southern white man's mastery over the slaves provided him with "social advantage," yet "he fails to live out the length of his days. His life as compared with his own race, in the Northern States, is shortened." He believed that whites "attain their highest intellectual and physical development, and most perfect health," in more northerly latitudes. Dawson warned that even in healthy locations in the South, "the ruddy complexion of the New Englander fades, his muscles shrink, and a general languor takes possession of his body." Avoiding labor as much as possible would modify "the decay of the white race in the Southern States."[17] While partly intended as a warning to northern whites to stay out of the South, Dawson's comments were also an indication of his conviction that the region was dangerous for whites, whose bodies were not intended to thrive in its heat and could not be made to do so no matter how long they remained.

Physicians who worried about the harmful effects of the South's climate on white bodies and their apparent inability to acclimate successfully to it ran the risk of viewing white bodies as vulnerable and perhaps inadequate, a position they found racially unacceptable. At the same time, they recognized in it a potential justification for slavery. If whites were incapable of work in the South's heat, then slavery was necessary if the region were to remain inhabited and its economy to thrive. Yet physicians did not want to claim white bodies were in any sense inferior to black, even in their ability to adapt to new environments. As they struggled with these dilemmas, their conclusions on the implications of place for white bodies inspired similar investigations for black.

However devastating the South's hot climate was for whites, physicians believed that it was far too cold for the region's blacks. Dr. A. P. Merrill, in his essays exploring the consequences of race differences, noted that the "negro constitution" was "eminently adapted to the torrid region," which meant that "the climate in which we find him in our country, is much too far north for him." Exposed for much of the year to cold temperatures and unable to provide enough body heat to make up the difference because their bodies were less adapted "to the generation of animal heat," blacks needed to "be protected from the evil influences" of cold on their "animal functions."[18] He warned that only careful attention would keep them alive and able to work hard.

Like Merrill, most physicians agreed that blacks' removal from the African climate to which their bodies were best adapted rendered them exceedingly vulnerable to disease. At the same time, they wondered whether bodies brought from Africa to America would eventually adapt to new circumstances. The question was particularly important given the argument of many proslavery ideologues that the economy of the South and by extension the nation depended on slaves' ability to labor in the fields, since whites were not biologically suited for hard work under the hot sun. According to Dawson, differing reactions to the climate explained why "the white man has taken the relation, indeed, of master; the African that of a slave laborer."[19] Physicians were eager to avoid the contradiction of viewing black bodies as vulnerable to southern diseases because the climate was too cold for them and at the same time able to withstand grueling labor in what no one could deny was the South's summer heat. Therefore, they resorted to debating racial theories of acclimation; in particular, they wondered whether black bodies experienced the process of acclimation in less risky and more complete ways than did white. They also wondered whether viewing blacks' bodies as better able to withstand its rigors would mean that they were in some sense superior to whites, a position the physicians considered untenable.

A. P. Merrill, perhaps more moderate in his racial views than many of his colleagues yet who worked hard to distinguish black bodies from white, noted that in hot climates the races experienced disease differently from each other. He explained that "whatever diseases prevail among one race, may prevail, also, among the other, under similar conditions, affecting the negro race sometimes more and sometimes less severely and fatally." Only "very rarely in the southern states" did any disease exist "exclusively among the colored race, and to which the white race was not subject under the same circumstances of exposure to its cause." Yet Merrill was convinced that blacks suffered differently from whites, the result of their bodies' different adaptation to the South's climate. He noted that blacks were "fitted by nature for the enjoyment of health in a hot climate," the implication being that whites were not—and that the South was not quite hot enough for them.[20] At the same time, blacks' less resilient bodies left them vulnerable to the climate's damaging influence.

According to Merrill, Africans' ability to resist the continent's fevers and tropical heat made them ideally suited to live there, unlike whites, who "can scarcely manage to exist." However, Africans were still less able to survive in the South than in Africa, but not so much as to prevent them from being able to work. Instead, the key distinction was between those accustomed to the climate and newcomers. Blacks who had been in the South for a long time had adjusted and could not be sent home.[21]

Not all physicians agreed with Merrill's positive assessment of blacks' relative healthiness in the New World. At the end of a survey of the "diseases of the colored population" of Alabama, Mississippi, and Louisiana, pioneering medical geographer Daniel Drake remarked, "if half the colored population of a Southwestern plantation were sent to [Liberia], they and their descendants, in ten years, would number more than those left behind."[22] Joshua White believed that the South's climate was "a melancholy notoriety" for blacks, forming "a considerable drawback to their increase." He thought that "the constitution of the African Negroes is as unfit to guard against the effects of our climate in the cold months, as that of Europeans, and our northern brethren in the hot."[23] Slaves, like whites, were subject to the dangers of the South's difficult climate; neither thrived there to the same extent that they would in places to which their bodies were better suited.

Whether the South was too cold or too hot, both blacks and whites were widely understood to be vulnerable to its illnesses because their constitutions were inherently unsuited to its climate. Both races had to experience acclimation in order to survive and thrive. Physicians were uncertain, however, which category of body was able to do so more successfully. Merrill noted that "the color of the skin" and the "woolly covering" of the head protected blacks and qualified them "for enduring the heat of a tropical climate, and a vertical sun" and disqualified them "for a cold climate, and for great and sudden transitions of temperature from heat to cold."[24] Similarly, Josiah Nott remarked that "while the white man is darkened by the tropical sun, the negro is never blanched in the slightest by a residence in northern latitudes. . . . He is inevitably killed by cold; but it never changes his hair, complexion, skeleton, nor size and shape of brain."[25] He did not, however, think he needed to explain why this mattered. Most observers focused less on the permanent changes that climate might make on the appearance of the body and more on the ways in which it responded to specific diseases in new locations.

Observations about the relative health of blacks in Africa and America, and thus their relative ability to acclimate to the South's environment, were offered in the context of a debate among physicians regarding blacks' and whites' susceptibility to characteristically southern diseases, particularly yellow fever, malaria, and the various other fevers that plagued the region. As was so often the case, Josiah Nott enraged his fellow physicians by arguing that "there is no acclimation against the endemic fevers of our rural districts," particularly for white bodies. He noted that "those of the tenth generation" worried just as much as newcomers about moving from dangerous to salubrious locations during the summer. There was, he thought, "no acclimation against intermittent and bilious fevers, and other marsh diseases." Nott believed that blacks, "being originally natives of hot climates," did not need to become acclimated to the South's temperatures and thus were "less liable to the more inflammatory forms of malarial fevers, and suffer infinitely less than whites from yellow fever" as well as being less vulnerable to marsh poison.[26]

Nott was aware of many interior plantations where "negroes of the second and third generation continue to suffer from these malarial diseases, and where gangs of negroes do not increase." He contrasted these unhealthy slaves with "the negroes of the rice-field region [who] do undergo a higher degree of acclimation than those of the hilly lands of the interior." His view of the relative health of the rice-growing areas as compared with the interior is to modern eyes unconvincing; flooded rice fields were perfect breeding grounds for the mosquitoes that carried disease while the higher, better-drained interior was not, although no one at the time was aware of this explanation. Nott attributed his knowledge of these matters to his role as "examining physician" for life insurance companies, which had an obvious interest in questions of acclimation.[27] He asked whether there was "an experienced and observing physician at the South" who disagreed with him, presumably confident that none would.[28]

In this as in so much else, Nott's views generated controversy among the region's physicians, many of whom did disagree with him. E. D. Fenner considered himself one of "*thousands,* not only of physicians, but planters, too, who differ with him" on the question of acclimation against the South's endemic fevers. Fenner claimed that his experience as a physician and planter convinced him that "*but for the attainment of a greater or less degree of acclimation,* the extensive malarious region of the Southern and Southwestern States never could have reached its present state of population and improvement." He noted that "practical men" valued the "*acclimated* negro, horse, ox and milch cow," and that even "the dogs, turkeys and chickens have to undergo acclimation before they can do well here." In fact, he said, "an acclimated negro, horse or milch cow, commands a higher price than an unacclimated one." Disagreeing with both Nott and one of his reviewers, Fenner noted that there were "malarious *seasons* as well as malarious *regions,*" exposure to either of which would cause "the inherent conservative powers of the animal constitution" to "habituat[e] itself to the deleterious influence of deadly poisons." After calling on other experts to buttress his views of the "consanguinity between the types of fevers," he remarked that "persons who have lived long in Southern malarious district[s] suffer much less from yellow fever, when first exposed to it, than those from the North who have not been thus seasoned." In other words, not only did bodies become acclimated, their exposure to one type of fever could protect them from others since they were all related. Even so, Fenner noted, "malaria is certainly a *poison* to the negro as well as the white, but it is less deleterious to the former, and he more readily becomes seasoned to it."[29] His complex efforts to refute those who tried to distinguish between the South's endemic fevers as well as on their impact on different categories of bodies was a reflection of his conviction not only of the existence of acclimation, but of its importance as a prerequisite to good health in the South as well.

Daniel Drake also sought to distinguish those diseases that particularly afflicted the South's black population. He noted that "acute inflammation of the lungs . . . produced by changes of weather in winter and spring, occasions more deaths than any other" cause except various fevers. "Intermittent, and remittent fevers; simple, and malignant or congestive, are the greatest outlets of human life" among slaves. He observed that they were seasonal, "and one attack is no security against another." Drake was aware that diseases varied from place to place; his catalog of diseases of the Southwest noted that "further north, tetanus and autumnal fever get less, but consumption and inflammation of the lungs increase."[30]

Nott, Fenner, and Drake were not, in this instance, exclusively concerned with the racial implications of acclimation. Their dispute had more to do with whether it even existed and for which diseases. However, for other physicians, the relative vulnerability of the races was central to the discussion of acclimation. For

A. P. Merrill, a disease could have many causes, depending on circumstance and location. However, the fevers that were the most common diseases of slaves were "almost uniformly attributed to the influence of malarial exhalations" associated with "marsh lands" or "low alluvial soils, into which dead and decaying vegetable matter largely enters as a constituent part." Merrill noted that "our largest and most productive plantations are mostly situated upon just such soil as would seem best adapted . . . to the production of this class of diseases." He concluded that "experience alone is the safe guide" in explaining "the healthfulness of a particular location"; there could be no "*a priori* reasoning."[31] In Merrill's view, then, apparent racial differences in acclimation were better understood as the result of the location of the plantations on which blacks lived and worked.

Merrill's careful observations led him to recognize that even "contiguous" plantations could have different experiences of disease, without consistent patterns or apparent explanation. He recognized that living and working among decomposing cotton seed, sugarcane, and other "putrid effluvia" did not cause illness, but he could not say what did.[32] Even so, Merrill acknowledged the complex ways in which the races reacted to the diseases of particular locations. For example, he noted that "fever prevails and always has prevailed among the slave population of the southern States, to a remarkable extent." Nothing offered slaves any exemption from it, not "condition of life, occupation, exposure, or variety of location," nor sex, nor age. In their vulnerability to fevers, slaves were not unlike whites "occupying the same localities." He noted that "it is probably true of both races alike, that laborers in the open air, tillers of the soil, and all whose occupations subject them to constant out-door exposure, are more obnoxious to attacks of febrile disease, than those" who work indoors.[33]

In spite of his confused—and confusing—comments about race differences and acclimation, Merrill steadfastly argued that location was central for explaining variations in the incidence of some diseases. He argued that whites were more vulnerable to periodic fever than blacks because "the owner of slaves has generally chosen for himself and family the most insalubrious locality." Planters built their own homes on the higher ground, which they thought was healthier, while locating their slaves "upon the bottom lands" or on the shores of rivers and lakes. Planters recognized that such low areas were more dangerous, but they believed the "partial immunity of the race would preserve them from greater danger . . . hence there could be no moral wrong." But their assumptions turned out to be incorrect. Not only did such arrangements mean that whites were "more liable to fevers than the negro," but those slaves who worked in whites' homes "were more obnoxious to febrile influences than their more fortunate but less cherished compeers" laboring in the fields. Place, in this instance, was very local indeed, while race hardly seemed to matter. When "from choice or necessity" the two races lived in close proximity, "the difference in the susceptibility to attacks of febrile disease, has been less distinctly marked." Periodic fevers, at least, depended more on the place in which the bodies subjected to them were located than upon their race. Even so, "negroes' . . . exemption from the graver forms of periodic fever, consequent upon their peculiar adaptation to climates where these fevers most prevail, render[s] their attacks less serious and obstinate" than those of whites.[34]

Merrill believed that yellow fever was different; here, race mattered more than location, although that continued to be important. He noted that "it appeared to be generally conceded that negroes are much less liable to be attacked" by yellow fever than were whites. In tropical cities, they were considered exempt from the disease, while in the South they were liable "only to a moderate extent, and in its mildest form." Still farther north he believed "the negro race more liable to suffer from this form of fever," especially in epidemics. He attributed these geographic differences to the influence of "their adaptation to hot climates," which made them "among the most favored of climatized persons," and to their relative immunity to "gastric inflammation," apparently a factor in causing the disease.[35]

Merrill's confused and contradictory analysis of susceptibility to illness, the racially based possibility of acclimation, and the importance of place for explaining the incidence of disease suggests how little consensus southern physicians had achieved on these matters in the decade before the Civil War. Unable to explain the causes of disease adequately and thwarted by a racial logic that emphasized difference, physicians struggled to make sense of the locally and regionally distinct experiences of disease that they were sure existed. For Merrill, the physician who made the most concerted effort to come to grips with these matters, consistency could not have been a high priority as he proclaimed that sometimes acclimation was possible and sometimes it was not, for blacks and whites alike. For other physicians, perhaps even less scrupulous in their logic and certainly less committed to his habit of close observation, there could be little doubt that place was an important variable in defining bodies. For them, as for Merrill most of the time, the place in which a body lived and worked shaped its experience of illness as surely as did its race and sex. Even if they could not agree on the correct explanation, which they thought had something to do with race and acclimation, they knew that southern bodies were unique.

## Place and the Practice of Medicine

Uniquely southern bodies required a uniquely southern practice of medicine. Physicians might not have been consistent in their explanations for how and why bodies did or did not acclimate to place, but they were nearly unanimous in their conviction that medical treatments, both preventive and interventionist, had to be adapted to their environment. If the disease implications of acclimation and the dangers of misplaced bodies were to be overcome, people had to be encouraged to behave in ways that would enable their bodies to thrive. For whites, this typically meant leaving dangerous places during the sickliest months, usually from before the hottest part of the summer until the first killing frost. Those who could not leave their homes were at least encouraged to build them in healthy locations, which most authors defined as high ground, away from the miasmas that infected low, swampy places. Nott, for example, in arguing against the possibility of acclimation to the South's endemic diseases, noted that "all prudent persons, who can afford to do so, remove in the summer to some salu-brious locality, in the pine-lands or the mountains." In fact, far from becoming acclimated, those who remained "from generation to generation in malarious districts become thoroughly poisoned."[36] Few whites needed doctors to encour-age them to leave dangerous summer locations; the wealthy already had been doing so for generations.

For slaves, of course, such advice was not appropriate, since slaveholders deter-mined where they must live and work without regard for the slaves' preferences. However, physicians were not reluctant to offer planters suggestions for ways to improve the health of their slaves by minimizing the impact of place on their bodies. Once again, Merrill led the way. He warned planters that placing African bodies in a climate north of the tropics to which they were best suited and thus exposing them "to a temperature to which [they are] ill adapted" required that they be "protected from the evil influences upon [their] animal functions . . . by being better fed, and better clothed, and lodged, than in [their] native country." Without such "changes in [their] mode of living," the "natural result" would be "disease and an abridgment of the duration of life."[37]

Merrill was quite specific about what those changes should be. He warned planters that their practice of "afford[ing] their slaves less liberal supplies of meat" during the winter was dangerous; slaves required "more of fatty and hydro-car-bonaceous food in cold weather than in warm." Similarly, they should be allowed to sleep in a warm room, given blankets, and prevented from sleeping outdoors. Their lodgings should be supplied "with both ventilation and warmth," which Merrill thought could best be provided by warming them with "hot-air furnaces" most nights of the year. In addition, their homes should be provided with "glazed windows," fireplaces, and, again, furnished with "a plentiful supply of warm blan-kets." Not only did houses need to be carefully constructed and furnished, they also had to be placed in "a healthful locality," which he defined as one with fertile soil and "a luxuriant growth of vegetation of some kind."[38]

Merrill was equally insistent on the importance of clothing to overcome the dangers of the southern climate for slaves' bodies. He thought cotton clothing appropriate for seven months of the year, "but for the other five months it is safer, and good economy, to provide all who labor in the open air, and are subject to the vicissitudes of the weather, with woolen shirts." The "old and feeble" as well as those "in all sickly localities" should wear wool shirts and drawers year-round, "for it has been well ascertained, that the use of flannel next the skin all the year, affords the most certain protection against malarial diseases, of any means known" except daily quinine, a far more expensive and physically quite unpleasant proposition. He noted that it was "a rare thing . . . to meet with a violent case of fever, cholera, or other malarial affection, so called, in a negro who habitually wears flannel next the person, and particularly if he sleep with a woolen covering at night, and in a cabin properly warmed and ventilated."[39]

Merrill likewise warned of the dangers of allowing slaves to work in wet clothing and with an empty stomach, both of which could lead to "constitutional injury" or "disease, and often fatal disease." His prescriptions for slaves' clothing extended to overcoats, which he viewed as the article most "necessary to the health and comfort of field negroes," and he spoke of the importance of warm and dry clothing for those who labored in the dew or rain. He rejoiced in the "fortunate, if not providential fact" that the best foods for slaves, Indian corn and pork, were "produced in high perfection, and with moderate labor, in all that region of country where slaves are owned and worked." When carefully prepared, both were "of the most nutritious and wholesome character." The "fattest pork" was especially appropriate for slaves in a cold climate, where "such oleaginous food becomes as essential to his health, as is the blubber diet to the Esquimaux." Pork was the only meat upon which a slave could subsist "with any hope of returning to his owner such large profits of labor." Without it, "the negro not only cannot become an effective laborer in cold climates, but must necessarily suffer in his bodily and mental health, become short-lived, imbecile, and unprolific." Merrill recognized that slaves also required "milk, garden vegetable[s], ripe fruits, and sugar or molasses" as well as "liberal supplies of good vinegar."[40]

Merrill knew that his recommendations for keeping slaves healthy in a climate too cold for their bodies were costly. He urged them upon slaveholders as serving their self-interest, noting that "the time lost by negroes in unnecessary sickness, and the cost of medicines and medical aid saved by such arrangements, not to mention the increased average duration of life, would amply repay the expense." According to Merrill, such treatment was also a blessing to blacks, as was slavery itself. A slave left to his own devices in a cold climate, "too feeble-minded to compete with white men in his struggle for a livelihood, and too improvident to provide, in the heat of summer, for the requirements of winter, . . . is reduced to the necessity of subsisting upon unsuitable food, and often compelled to wear insufficient clothing." The "natural consequences" of blacks' improvidence would be "disease of body and mind, leading to early dissolution, and to deterioration in the bodily and mental vigor of his descendants."[41] Merrill believed that those of African descent in the United States required material conditions of life that suited their misplaced bodies, but even so they were more likely to thrive as slaves in the South than as free people farther north. Good treatment and acclimation could overcome some consequences of living in an unsuitable climate, but their inherent constitutional inferiority remained. Merrill was certainly more vehement than most physicians in his recommendations to slaveholders hoping to avoid the illnesses caused by requiring Africans to labor in the South. Others, however, certainly shared his conviction that slaves' misplaced bodies were liable to illness.

Merrill was not alone in advocating better material treatment for slaves in order to ensure their health. John Stainback Wilson warned that because of slaves' "feeble heat generating powers," planters should provide carefully for their diet, clothing, and housing. Like Merrill, he urged planters to provide "woollen outer garments" and overcoats, along with "long cotton aprons, well covered with paint" to protect them from getting wet. The cost of these "would be nothing when compared with the gain in time, health, and comfort" because the slaves "could continue to work regardless of the weather, without the risks arising from wet clothing."[42] He also advised that their houses be elevated off the ground and the surroundings raked yearly to remove "the accumulated filth of years, which lies festering about negro cabins," to protect them from "typhoid fever, and other fatal forms of disease."[43] Similarly, Joshua White of Georgia recognized that "interest and humanity both urge to a greater attention to their comfort; thus, not only to ameliorate the pains of slavery, but to guard against the disease; often the greatest foe to the planter's hopes."[44]

Physicians' daily practice sometimes reflected these concerns. Joseph A. S. Milligan wrote his fiancée about "a little sick negro" who "had been sick for about two weeks with fever, but had been entirely neglected." The child lived only a few hours, causing Milligan to call upon the legislature "to provide for the protection of slaves in such cases, and for the punishment of their pernicious [sic] owners, who for the sake of a few dollars allow their servants to die of neglect." He thought the "case . . . entirely within the reach of medicine," and had the owner been willing to pay "five or six dollars the life of the child might have been saved." Milligan lamented that "this votary of mammon loved his money more than the life of his negro" and wondered "can such a man have a conscience?"[45] Milligan of course never tried to answer his own question, nor did he address the legislature himself. To do so would have been far too challenging to the South's peculiar institution.

Physicians who noted slaves' geographic vulnerability also regularly noted that they required a different medical treatment; just as bodies and diseases were sensitive to place, so, too, were the treatments they required. Samuel Cartwright, the physician most convinced of racial differences in diseases, noted "that very learned physicians from Europe and the Northern States, on first coming South, have felt and acknowledged their incompetency to treat" blacks successfully because of their regional peculiarities. Those who were educated elsewhere "find no such class of persons as those whom they have mostly studied to treat."[46] Merrill agreed, noting that "the teachings of medical authors, whose study and practice have been confined to the white race in northern latitudes" were "inapplicable" in the South.[47] Instead, physicians agreed, southern physicians required a specifically southern medical education.

Attention to the importance of a separate medical education for the South began early. In 1825, James W. Taylor addressed the Charleston Medical Society of Emulation, arguing that any doctor educated in the North "of necessity is compelled to lay aside many of the principles there imbibed." Instead, he had to learn for himself how to treat "most of the affections incident to our climate." Taylor thought it could take a northern-educated doctor two or three years to obtain "sufficient practical knowledge, to enable him to treat with any degree of skill, the diseases arising from our peculiarity of situation." Taylor added that "other considerations press strongly upon us" in encouraging local knowledge of medicine, but he did not elaborate because "they more properly belong to our well-being, as considered in a *political* and *civil* point of view."[48]

Taylor's address was printed in the *Carolina Journal of Medicine, Science, and Agriculture,* whose editors only a short time before had alerted readers to their "mortification that so many of our citizens should go to the North to obtain that medical and surgical aid which they could obtain equally as well at home." The editors wanted southerners "to encourage the distinguished among ourselves."[49] Although the journal's editors were not yet prepared to make an entirely sectional argument about medicine, they were opening the possibility.

Only a decade later, Edward Deloney, a physician from Talbotton, Georgia, applauded the beginnings of the *Southern Medical and Surgical Journal,* based at the Medical College of Georgia and destined to become one of the South's premier medical journals. He argued that the "influence of climate, especially on the human constitution . . . and the consequent variation and peculiarity of symptoms which characterize disease" required southern doctors to practice medicine differently from their northern counterparts. Deloney welcomed the journal as "a medium through which we may kindly interchange our ideas, and present to each other our experience," rather than allowing doctors to continue "the fallacy of suffering themselves to be governed and guided by the views and opinions of those, who can know nothing of the difficulties which we have to encounter in the management of the diseases which occur among us." He urged southern physicians not to "neglect so favorable an opportunity for the improvement of medicine, and the mitigation of the sufferings of our fellow creatures" as the journal offered.[50]

These early advocates of sectional medicine did not base their enthusiasm on theories about uniquely southern bodies or diseases that differed from those in the North. Nor were their arguments yet contributions to the intensifying political animosity between the regions, as would be the case later. Instead, their comments formed a kind of regional boosterism, designed to inspire local physicians to the achievements of their neighbors. They wanted to attract wealthy clients, strengthen local institutions, and sell journal subscriptions, not fan political tensions.

It was only with the heightened political tension of the war with Mexico that doctors began to call for a specifically southern medical education in the context of understanding bodies in place. Samuel Cartwright was among the first to argue for the necessity of a southern medical education in terms of the bodies physicians would be treating when they began to practice medicine. As early as 1846, in an address to the Mississippi Medical Convention, he complained that much "of the practice of the physicians of our state is among a race almost unknown to medical books and schools." He supported a society "for learning the laws of those affections, and the remedies that each of us has found, by dear experience, to be the most successful in their treatment" and asked for help from the legislature.[51] In 1851, he noted that slaveholders "consider it safer, in most cases, to trust to the empiricism of overseers, rather than to the regular doctors who are new comers." Recently arrived young doctors were capable of treating slaves successfully, he thought, but only "if they were to study their diseases, their anatomy, physiology and pathology" as carefully as they did those of the white poor. The problem stemmed from the textbooks used in northern medical schools, which "contain not a syllable" concerning race differences.[52]

Cartwright believed that the problem could be solved by a medical education that stressed comparative anatomy. He criticized southern schools that used "the same text books and echo[ed] the same doctrines" as northern, urging them instead to "have their own text books, containing not only the anatomy, physiology and therapeutics applicable to the white race of people, but the anatomy, physiology and therapeutics of the black race also." Doing so would cause "the empire of medical learning" to come South and "give students better opportunities of acquiring knowledge." Students were not the only people in the region who would benefit. Physicians would "reclaim the practice among three millions of people that the overseers have mostly got." Medical men would no longer find themselves "superseded by overseers and empirical practitioners" because they had insufficient knowledge of local diseases; with such knowledge, "a Southern country physician [would] never want practice." Employing physicians would also "be for the interests of the planters," presumably because their slaves would be healthier.[53]

In spite of all of these anticipated advantages, Cartwright's claims did not go unchallenged. One anonymous reviewer noted that "medicine and politics are as incompatible as acids and alkalies, and he who mingles the two is no friend of either." While he endorsed the suggestion that southern schools establish "a chair on the special branch of diseases of negroes," he objected to Cartwright's "bitter denunciation of Northerners and Foreigners, because they choose to differ in opinion with the worthy professor." He worried that young medical graduates whose minds were "thus neutralized by such unwise teachings, will be totally unfit to treat the sick negro."[54] The reviewer warned that minds "biased by political prejudices cannot do justice to a medical subject," adding that truth must be "the sheet-anchor of medicine" or it would be "worse than a humbug." By implication, Cartwright was accused of mingling "medicine and politics" an "unholy contamination."[55]

The reviewer's ire was particularly directed at Cartwright's tirade against north-ern medical schools, which he described as "either the impotent effervescence of a mind distracted by political enthusiasm, or a wanton calumny which noth-ing can excuse." The author, a southerner by birth and rearing, was educated in the North, where he claimed his professors were "quite as well acquainted with the anatomy of the negro, as well as with the science of comparative anatomy" as Cartwright could wish. He similarly refuted the claim that planters trusted overseers to attend to sick slaves, noting that "the physician is always called in to attack any serious symptom." Cartwright's criticism of northern physicians and their textbooks was "all wrong"; his aspersions "illiberal, unprovoked, and unjust," the result of his "unconquerable prejudice against Northerners."[56] This anonymous reviewer, writing in 1852, did not share the growing sentiment for a uniquely southern medical education, but as time passed his point of view would become less and less often expressed.

Shortly after Josiah Nott was appointed professor of anatomy at the University of Louisiana in 1857, he, too, joined the discussion. Nott admitted that at one time he shared the prevailing prejudice against medical schools in southern cities be-cause of "the difficulty of pursuing dissections during our mild winters, for not only is the putrefaction of bodies disgusting and unwholesome, but it is inimical to the successful pursuit of minute dissection." Since "anatomy is the ground work of the science and art of medicine," this was a serious drawback. However, Nott reported that his "doubts are now entirely removed" because bodies could be perfectly preserved "in any weather, an indefinite period of time . . . by means of antiseptics." This opened the door for excellent medical instruction in New Orleans, for "no city . . . can at all compare . . . in point of abundance of material for the anatomical student." Nott was an eager booster of his new employer, boast-ing about its museum and the anatomical models the school had purchased.[57]

More than just the availability of cadavers gave "great weight to the value of southern schools" in Nott's eyes. They also allowed students "who are to practice in malarial districts" access to "professors who have been for twenty or thirty years treating daily the diseases of the south." Such professors "should certainly be more competent to instruct southern young men than teachers who have little or no experience with our diseases." It was "well known that the diseases of warm and cold climates differ as much as do their fauna and flora." Nott claimed that northern medical writers "knew nothing" about "remittent or yellow fever," while they would "laugh at the idea of a New Orleans physician attempting to teach [them] anything about pneumonia, so different is the type of the disease in the two latitudes."[58]

Nott claimed that he did not "desire to make invidious comparisons, or to say unkind or ungenerous things of other schools." He declared, "the field of science is a Republic equally open to all." New Orleans could "become one of the lead-ing seats of medical instruction in the United States" if the faculty lived up to the "energy, industry, and fidelity to the great trust reposed in them." Should the school fail, "it will be from the indolence, incompetence, and want of character of our teachers." Nott urged his peers to "learn useful lessons from some of our brethren of the North" who were "beacons to stimulate our exertions in the cause of science."[59] Nott did not remain long at the University of Louisiana, moving to help found the Medical College of Alabama in 1858.[60] Nott's views were simultaneously a reflection of his self-interest and part of his determination to enhance the prestige of southern science, medicine, and institutions.

By the end of the decade, southern medical schools regularly followed Nott's example and advertised their advantages as including a regional perspective that offered students the opportunity to study the diseases and treatments of southern bodies. Among the advantages of study at the University of Maryland was its location in Baltimore, "a Southern city . . . in a medical point of view, as regards the classes of persons who come under the supervision of her physicians, and the nature of the affections which they are called upon to treat." The school's proponent, a Baltimore physician, repeated the familiar notion that "no man who has received his education exclusively at a Northern school can be prepared to practice Medicine to advantage at the South." Such a physician would be unprepared to treat "that class of the population which is comparatively scarce at the North," namely slaves. This was an important disqualification because "all who have had experience in these matters know, that between the blacks and the whites there are vast differences, both as regards the course and character of the diseases which affect them, and their susceptibilities to the action of remedial agents." He noted that "Northern graduates have to learn all these things at the bedside . . . whereby . . . much time is lost to them, and perhaps a considerable amount of property destroyed for their patrons." By contrast, "Southern graduates begin the practice of medicine with these important facts well indoctrinated into them," so that "it must be palpable to all unprejudiced minds, that, so far as the treatment of negroes is concerned, they have a decided advantage over physicians from other localities."[61]

Among the advantages offered by the University of Maryland were the "black wards," which "furnish the most admirable opportunities for the study of such maladies as pertain to the negro race." They allowed its students to gain "that peculiar knowledge in regard to the predispositions, proclivities and susceptibilities of the two races, which can not be acquired save in a Southern school." A southern education would save "the life and property . . . which must, of necessity, be sacrificed whilst the lesson which should have been taught in the premises" was acquired by those trained elsewhere. The author warned that "those who are interested in this species of property . . . jeopardize their most essential interests, when they prefer the graduate of a Northern school to one who has acquired his degree" in the South.[62]

For this author, one of the chief advantages of a southern medical education was the understanding it offered of the nature of the diseases physicians there were called upon to treat. Those diseases were "modified by certain agencies which originate in the particular locality where they occur, and are peculiar to it." This was especially true of malaria, the result of a "certain subtle influence [that] is generated in particular sections." To think that it could be understood from textbooks or "the occasional cases which present themselves in northern latitudes . . . is perfectly absurd." Instead, "it must be carefully and continuously observed where its manifestations are most numerous, and its operations the most potent." Specifically, malaria "must be studied in a Southern institution, under the direction of Southern teachers, and on Southern soil, before it can be understood." A medical student who did not do so was "blind, not only to his own interests, but to those of his patrons."[63]

Perhaps appealing to those same self-interested patrons, the editors of the *Charleston Medical Journal and Review* endorsed the "commodious Hospital for slaves" recently built in that city. They recommended it not only for the skilled nursing it would provide and the qualifications of the physicians, but also to the students at the Medical College. Students would benefit from the hospital's "clinical opportunities," which offered them "an admirable field for acquainting themselves with the diseases peculiarly incident to a class from which the majority must expect to derive their largest number of patients." The hospital was the best place to study "the personal and race peculiarities of the African, as influenced by our climatic and industrial conditions."[64]

Placed bodies demanded a placed medical care, a position that inspired increasing acceptance as the North became ever more tainted with abolitionism. Only Cartwright accused all northern physicians of abolitionism and viewed the education provided in their schools as suspect because of it, but southerners' unease with northern teachings grew as sectional tensions escalated. Ideas about placed bodies had a firm footing in that the South did have both a different pattern of disease and a different population from the North, but these realities were heightened by the political storms sweeping the nation. How much of the physicians' rhetoric was influenced by politics and how much inspired by their attempts to understand the significance of their empirical observations can never be accurately determined; both factors clearly entered into their thinking. Those educated in northern medical schools, like Josiah Nott and Samuel Cartwright's anonymous reviewer, simultaneously defended their own training and their regional expertise. They were the most committed to eliminating the taint of politics from the debate about medical education, but even they recognized that placed and raced bodies demanded a specifically southern form of medical care.

Differences in medical education led to differences in medical practice as well. Physicians familiar with both regions were well aware that diseases and their treatments had a regional component. When William Peirce graduated from medical school in his native New York, he looked for a place to practice and found himself "strongly inclined from my knowledge of the prices which medical services demand in Virginia to the South." He established himself instead in

Mississippi, which he described to his sister as "very sickly." He reported "the diseases here are of a very different type from those of a more northern latitude they are rarely inflammatory but diseases of debility." Treatments differed from those at home as well: "[Q]uinine is here dealt out by the spoonful and Calomel and Blue Pill are prescribed with reckless carelessness." Peirce did not say what his neighbors and patients thought of him.[65] Similarly, in rejecting the position of another doctor regarding a specific treatment, Joseph Eve, professor of obstetrics and the diseases of women and children at the Medical College of Georgia, noted "most assuredly physicians of the great metropolis . . . must have much less repugnance" to using the speculum "unnecessarily, than physicians in this latitude, who are much more apt to neglect them when proper."[66] Doctors were becoming ever more sensitive to regional differences and thus advocated for a uniquely southern medicine.

The entrance of politics into physicians' efforts to understand the implications of placed bodies was as apparent in what they did not discuss as it was in what they did. Nearly all of their efforts to make sense of the bodily consequence of place were intertwined with their efforts to understand race, not sex. What made the South medically distinct as a place was the presence of large numbers of black bodies as well as white, while women were found in approximately equal numbers to men everywhere. As a result, the consequences of race and place were entangled in physicians' analysis, while sex rarely appeared. Even so, physicians who struggled to understand placed bodies also occasionally wrote about sex, specifically about white women. Their comments were not developed to anything like the same extent as those about race, but they were nevertheless quite telling. For the most part, southern physicians viewed the consequences of place for northern and southern white women's bodies as beneficial for the former and harmful for the latter.

For example, John Stainback Wilson thought that southern women's beauty was subject to "early decay," the result of "climate, constitutional weakness, and bad habits of living." Women's "sexual peculiarities . . . consist in a certain softness and laxness of all the fibres and tissues of the body, and an excitable, impressible state of the nervous system." While women everywhere shared those peculiarities, they were exacerbated in the South, where "a hot climate produces exactly these effects, and hence, Southern women are subjected to the combined and powerful action of a natural weakness and susceptibility, aggravated by the direct and concurrent effects of climate."[67] Alabama physician S. M. Meek noted that "the number and extent of female diseases [was] much greater in southern than in northern latitudes." In addition, he claimed, in the South "the precocity resulting from climates" led "females [to] arrive at puberty from two to six years earlier than in northern latitudes." It also "produc[ed] greater relaxation of the muscular fibre, and the parietes of the uterine and genital organs in general."[68] Together with early childbirth and "the delicacy felt by young, inexperienced females" that produced "delay in making application to the physician for the necessary assistance," these "contribute[d] largely to augment the sufferings of females in southern latitudes beyond what they suffer in colder climates."[69]

Even Thomas Denman, the English author of a widely used textbook on midwifery, wrote of the impact of climate on women's reproductive organs, although he disagreed with the southern doctors in thinking that cold was beneficial to women. In his view, climate influenced the timing of menarche as well as the experience of labor. He noted that "in hot climates, all natural labours are said to be more easy, than in those that are cold," a difference he explained "because the disposition to relax and dilate is sooner assumed, and more perfectly accomplished" in warm places. He fretted that "modes of treatment have been enjoined to women in childbed universally . . . without due regard to the heat or coldness of the climate, or the season of the year when the patient might be confined."[70] Like other physicians who thought childbirth easier in the South, he based his argument on the tendency of muscles to contract when cold, relax when hot, a pattern of moving from a specific circumstance to a general principle that reflects both their efforts at developing theory and the ease with which their conclusions could be in error.

Perhaps inspired by Denman, physicians providing gynecological and other forms of care to women sometimes took the weather into account when determining treatments. For example, when T. L. Ogier's white patient required an operation to remove a fibrous tumor from her uterus, "she did not readily consent." Ogier "did not insist upon its being immediately done" because the weather was "very warm at the time," which he was glad to avoid.[71] In treating a Savannah slave woman suffering from what he supposed was an extrauterine pregnancy, B. W. Harder noted that he did not attempt an operation because "we were satisfied that she must die, and that soon." The nearly sixty-year-old woman was "debilitated" and "the weather warm."[72] These physicians were not so much concerned with women's response to the South's heat as they were with the consequences of that heat for the female constitution, even though they were of different races. They very likely believed that women's bodily inferiority made them more fixed in place than were men, less able to adjust to changing conditions.

Physicians who sought to understand the effects of place on white women's bodies and minds sometimes turned their attention to their behavior rather than their illnesses. Place could influence how women acted as well as their health; here, the advantages were in favor of southern women. For example, the southern reviewer of a volume on prostitution by William Sanger noted his comment that "in all Southern cities the majority of prostitutes are from the North." The reviewer explained "this great disproportion, so much in favor of, and to the credit of the South," in terms of "the different condition of her Society, which imposes . . . greater personal responsibility for the actions and severer penalties for the offenses of its members, and in the dissimilarity of her institutions and pursuits."[73] He thought that white southern women did not become prostitutes, but he did not comment about white men's sexual exploitation of slave women. An editor of the *Oglethorpe Medical and Surgical Journal* noted a case of infanticide committed by a New York servant girl, which he thought was hardly isolated. He reflected on "the accursed situation of the poor white slaves of the North, and the dreadful doom which awaits them in the future" and wished they knew "the bright land of the cotton, the orange and cane, where the children of Japhet and Shem luxuriate in the happy freedom the Almighty ordained for them!" He, too, noted that "nearly all the unfortunates who crowd the brothels of both the North and the South, are Northern women," adding that "Negro maidens never kill their children" because they could count on them being provided for as slaves.[74] These differences, attributable to social circumstances and not to the characteristics of the female bodies inhabiting the two regions, nevertheless allowed southern physicians to reflect on the importance of place.

Physicians in the 1850s who sought to understand bodies and minds as placed as well as raced and sexed did so in the context of escalating sectional tensions that would shortly erupt into war. While couched in the language of science and medicine, their concerns could not help but reflect their political context. Although those who strayed too far over the line of politics were taken to task, southern physicians generally may well have recognized that a specifically southern medical practice enhanced their opportunities and their status. Physicians were determined to build their professional credibility, and their efforts to understand placed bodies served scientific, social, and political purposes.

Physicians who wrote about placed bodies did not attempt to juxtapose those factors they attributed to race or sex with those they attributed to place. In fact, physicians did not attempt to construct a typology in which each of a body's characteristics—race, sex, and place—was balanced against another in a systematic fashion. To do so would have required a rigor and a logic far beyond what was possible at the time, to say nothing of forcing them to confront the contradictions in their analysis. Still struggling with the tension between empiricism and system in medical thinking, they were too caught up in the difficulties of explaining the consequences of race, sex, and place for individual bodies and minds to try to consider their influence on one another in any but the simplest fashion. Their notions of what constituted an acceptable method of practicing medicine, particularly when that method required thinking statistically, were too crude to allow them to consider such matters. In addition, had they followed the consequences of their thinking about acclimation and placed bodies, they would have had to consider the possibility that the impact of other bodily characteristics was mutable, or perhaps not as dramatic as they believed, a position they could not admit. Still finding their way professionally, eager to gain credibility, they did not recognize the contradictions in their analyses, much less worry that these would be detected. Writing for one another in the relative obscurity of medical journals, their efforts to work toward a theory of disease causation that rested on the characteristics of individual bodies were imperfect at best, yet they were a reflection of the assumptions and confusions of the society in which they lived and worked.

## Laypeople Consider the Consequences of Place

Physicians were not alone in their efforts to understand placed bodies. Such think-ing had been part of common sense about health and illness for generations, although not couched in the more formal language of medicine. Laypeople, in their everyday communication with one another, routinely commented on the impact of climate and the weather on their bodies and minds and considered the health benefits of travel from one place to another. We still do this today, even though we recognize that germs rather than miasmas or bad weather cause ill-ness. To some extent, nineteenth-century physicians did little more than couch the assumptions of their society in formal, scientific language, notwithstanding their commitment to the search for explanations. Their success in defining bodies as placed and creating a southern medical practice depended in no small measure on the inherent familiarity of the idea.

Belief that the weather caused or contributed to ill health was widespread. There was, however, no consensus on what kind of weather was bad for the body. Unhealthy weather was variously described as cold, warm, hot, dry, damp, rainy, stormy, windy, wintry, out of season, unsettled, gloomy, and changing. For exam-ple, Lucila Agnes McCorkle noted one June that "the warm weather—& sudden changes are very trying to my constitution. My heart as well as body is languid & lifeless."[75] Mary Jeffreys Bethell of North Carolina remarked in summing up the year's events that "there was much sickness in our country this summer there was a long spell of hot and dry weather."[76] Another woman wrote her nephew that "it is very sickly with us, almost every negro on the plantation has been laid up with severe colds, the consequence I suppose of the very warm weather we had about Christmas."[77] Priscilla Beall McKaig of Maryland complained in her journal in 1858: "My health has been precarious all winter, suffering with colds, sickheadach and dyspepsia, owing I think in a great measure, to the house being open so much since they commenced the improvement . . . and I am exposed to every blast of wind, when ever I leave my room." On another occasion she noted that it had "rained 27 days in May. . . . The general health has been remarkably good, for a rain storm of such long duration."[78] Eliza DeRosset wrote one sister about another who had just left for home, noting "she had a slight touch of tooth-ache (caused I suppose by the damp weather.)"[79] Such comments were repeated endlessly in the letters and journals of the day.

Just as common as references to the weather being the cause of illness were those that attributed recuperation or death to it. Eleanor Douglass wrote that she knew her mother was "still very weak" and worried that "the very warm weather will will [*sic*] prevent your gaining strength."[80] Ellen Ewing wrote her aunt that she had "a hard lump in my left breast, from cold I suppose," as well as sore ears. She hoped "when the weather becomes settled that I will be better."[81] Eliza Clitherall thanked God, who had "by his great Mercy sent" the "gracious heavy frost" that would "check the Scourge with which our town has been visitted [*sic*]."[82] James Bryan noted a sickly season in which "not a single individual on my Lot escaped[;] . . . the County was never more sickly." He was relieved that "the weather is now very cold which I hope will be the means of restoring health."[83]

For many writers, good weather was cold weather, although the cold had its own dangers. Young Smith wrote: "Old Black Sam died of winter fever three or four weeks ago that disease has been verry [*sic*] prevalent this winter and numbers have dyed."[84] The climate itself could be dangerous. After his brother died of country fever, G. M. Wilkins wrote of the imprudence and "ardent anxious temperament" that left him "another example of confidence, fatal & fruitless, in the climate of Carolina."[85] However it was defined, good weather could bring a welcome end to illness, but southern whites nevertheless recognized its dangerous potential that could quickly and easily turn even the most apparently healthy individual into a corpse.

White southerners who feared the impact of the South's climate on their bodies likewise worried about the consequences of travel, especially when travel included the possibility of bad weather. Just as Wilkins's brother risked disease by venturing "into the country before a frost had made it safe," in spite of repeated warnings of the dangers, so did everyone have to fear the dangers of movement from one place to another for their bodies.[86] Wilkins's brother-in-law John Berkley Grimball noted in his diary that he was "suffering from a very severe cold—from wet feet when in town—and from traveling in the rain all Saturday."[87] Sophia Watson began to miss her husband almost from the moment he left their Alabama home in the spring of 1848 to settle his father's estate in the North, yet eager as she was to see him, in early August she wrote about "quite a conflict in my feelings with regards to your return. I fear to have you come back before October on account of sickness and it seems a long time to have to wait yet two months before seeing you. . . . Having spent the summer months at the north may render you more liable to the diseases of our climate."[88] Eliza Clitherall reminisced that it seemed odd to her to spend the winter on the plantation and the summer in the city, "but such are the pernicious effects of the country malaria, in a southern climate that a late sojourn upon a Plantation, or a visit by the planter to his estate, of more than two nights, inevitably produces sickness & often death."[89] Laypeople could never be sure which places caused sickness, which were healthy, or when it was safe to move between them. Tristrim Skinner attributed his mother-in-law's "sudden illness . . . to the sudden change from hot, musquito breeding, Norfolk, to the pure sea air of Hampton."[90] Just as physicians worried about the possibilities of acclimation for placed bodies, so laypeople tried to minimize the health dangers of their own movements from place to place.

Physicians and their patients who worried about the dangers of movement from place to place also recognized that travel could benefit the sick. While the benefits of spas and springs were well known and widely advertised,[91] so, too, were shorter trips that could provide the sick with a change of air. Leaving the city or the country, bathing at the coast, or seeing the sights in the North could all refresh and reinvigorate an ailing, weary body. Joseph Milligan advised Octavia Camfield that after "confinement in your bed & in your room for such a length of time you will need the country air to restore your strength and health," suggesting that it would "be best for you to go as soon as possible after your recovery."[92] Milligan wrote his wife about a "palpitation" that he attributed to "a piece of apple-pie which my stomach refused to digest" and hoped that "the change of air" would benefit him.[93] When John Berkley Grimball's mother suffered "from a violent cold," he sent her "to town, where she could have many comforts which the country can- not supply," including a doctor "in whose skill she has the utmost confidence." Grimball's mother was "extremely anxious to go."[94] Travel could aid more serious illnesses as well. Sophia Peck reported that a woman addicted to opium was "much better now than [when] she left Greensboro—the change seems to have been of great benefit to her" even though she was often "up all night and entirely crazy from the effects of it."[95] In a letter describing what he was learning in medical school in Philadelphia, a man noted that in cases of syphilis, "a change of air and sea bathing is recommend[ed] to all who are able to leave their homes."[96]

This student's warning limiting travel to those able to leave was typical. Many people who traveled for their own health or urged others to do so nevertheless worried that the fatigue and exposure would be harmful. During the Civil War, Mary Bethell noted in her diary that her daughter "has been sick and feeble, she was so fatigued from the long trip of 4 weeks."[97] Margaret Devereux wrote her sister that when their mother mentioned to her physician that she thought of going to Philadelphia, "he shook his head tho' and told Mother that so far from benefitting her—it would be the worst thing that she could do—for the fatigue would make her sick—and advised her by all means to stay at home and keep quiet and in a few months she would be quite well."[98] Arabella Bolton wrote that her mother's physician "has kept her a close prisoner and will only agree to her coming home upon condition it is mild weather and a close[d] carriage."[99] Travel had physical as well as emotional consequences, and its dangers could easily overcome its intended benefits.

Unlike physicians, who rarely considered the significance of sex when writ- ing about placed bodies, laypeople paid careful attention to the consequences of travel for white women, especially when they were pregnant. Travel could benefit pregnant women, as Penelope Warren noted in a letter to her husband after a visit during which she had not felt well but said she "hoped the country air would cure me—I think it has had the desired effect. I feel very well today."[100] Mary Jane Milligan wrote her husband that while the weather was pleasant "mother has been out visiting . . . when she can," since "she will have to stay home for the next three or four months."[101] It could also help those recovering from giving birth. In 1836, Henry Burns wrote of his anxiety about his wife's "feeble" health since her confinement, which made him want "to take her to some country place, where she might recruit her wasted strength by a change of air and diet."[102] Most of the time, however, pregnancy and childbirth limited women's opportunities to travel, as it was considered dangerous as well as immodest. Emily Rutherfoord noted that "Sallys *situation* is such that I think they will give out the trip to the west."[103] Martha Dupree Treadwell wrote her absent husband, who invited her to join him, that "it would be best for me to remain at home for the reason that I expect that I shall be confined in the course of a month or two & the fatigue and heat that I should have to under go in going out there would more than likely bring about abortion."[104]

The place white women chose to deliver their babies required careful deliberation. Many preferred to be near their mothers, sisters, or other female kin, which meant they had to return to their former homes well before the time or their kin had to travel to them. Some women chose to deliver near a trusted physician, which could also require travel. Maria Bryan suggested that her sister "go home and stay some there." She was "sure the journey, if conducted with proper prudence, would not hurt you, and Dr. Gilbert seems to be your best physician."[105] Meta Morris Grimball's pregnancies influenced her husband's travel plans as well. In November 1837, he noted that he "went into the country today—alone. The family will not move up until after Meta's confinement." Fourteen years later, another pregnancy also dictated the family's movements: "Meta expecting to be confined shortly made it necessary to leave the country earlier than our wont."[106] Pregnancy and childbirth were considered dangerous enough that unwonted travel could only make things worse; white women wanted to deliver in what they and their families considered the safest place.

Travel could have particularly intense consequences for children, positive and negative, and white parents eager to preserve or restore their health often considered undertaking it. Kate Meares wrote her mother that "the children have been poorly for some days & maybe the trip will do them good. . . . I hope they will be better for a change, particularly as it has fair to be a little cooler than it has been."[107] On another occasion, Meares's mother worried about her granddaughter and encouraged Kate to "carry her out of the City[.] I know that change would do her good, more than all the medicine she can take."[108] Cities could be especially dangerous places, and mothers were especially eager to travel with their children to avoid them. One woman told her sister that her daughter "wishes to leave town" for the summer "on account of the children."[109] Eliza Skinner was similarly eager to leave Baltimore because her son was teething.[110] Cities were not the only source of potential danger to children. Martha Dupree Treadwell's husband offered to bring her and their daughter to join him, but, she told him, "as much as I wish to be with you I cannot force my reason to believe that it would be right for me to take our darling there." She had been "told that the water is limestone & I do not think that it would agree with her at all."[111] Cities could also offer a refuge.

When several slave children became sick and two died on John Berkley Grimball's plantation, he "thought it prudent" to send his own children to town.[112]

Children could also make travel difficult, especially for white women caught between their own health requirements and the often conflicting demands of their husbands and children, as Frances Robertson found to her sorrow. Robertson worried in her diary whether to leave and what to do with her infant when her husband required her to join him at home where "whooping cough" prevailed. "The trials of this life" left her pillow "wet with tears," but "at length my better judgement overcame my feelings," and she joined her husband, leaving her son behind.[113] In the summer of 1833, Sarah Gayle considered her health "worse than it has ever been—habitually worse." While she had "no disease," she suffered "great debility, apathy, utter want of all energy." She thought "a trip to the Blount Springs might renew my life, but with my number of children, such a step is out of the question, unless there were undoubted necessity for it."[114] John Bryan wished his wife could "take a little trip—for she needs it & is anxious to do so—but what to do with all the children is the question."[115] Women who had to travel with children were to be pitied, as one woman noted about Charlotte Green, a minister's wife, who "looks very badly—and was very unwell during their stay here. she seems quite unfit for such a journey, with her six little children & one so young—only two months old."[116]

White men could find traveling for their health easier. Ann Pettigrew wrote her sister that their brother "appears to be in bad health," but it was "very fortunate for him he is not encumbered with a family he can now go about for his health, without any cares comparatively."[117] Some men, however, found that the pressures of work prevented them from leaving home just as children made it difficult for women. Meta Morris Grimball noted in her diary that Mrs. Barnwell was "very much concerned by the ill health of her husband." She reported that the doctor had told him "he ought to go away & take care of himself[.] [H]e said he could not leave his business, & now he looks very badly has the most painful symptoms."[118] Other men felt it necessary to travel to look after their pecuniary interests, in spite of the dangers. John Berkley Grimball noted in his diary the death of a friend who was "devoted to his planting interest." The man "suffered no considerations of danger to prevent his visiting his plantation at all seasons—necessarily exposed to miasma which long & melancholy experience has abundantly proved that it is impossible for a white person to inhale with impunity."[119]

Even slaves were sometimes allowed or required to travel for their health. John Berkley Grimball, who worried about the dangers of miasmas for whites, noted in his diary that he "Had January, who is threatened with Dropsey,[120] brought down here for change of air." Years later, Grimball's overseer wrote "that Robin my driver has been quite ill have replied that he be sent to town as soon as able to bear the fatigue for change of air."[121] Sophia Watson repeatedly brought sick slaves from the plantation to her home in town so that she could supervise their care.[122] Even so, travel by sick slaves was undoubtedly quite rare; when it did occur, it was more likely to be local.

Slaves themselves were well aware of the dangers of place for their bodies. Reuben Rosborough, who had been a slave in South Carolina, recalled that during slavery people believed "it was de miasma dat de devil bring 'round you from de swamp and settle 'round your face whilst you sleep, and soon he git you to snore you sniffed it to your liver, lights[123] and gall, then dat make bile, and then you was wid de chills a comin' every other day."[124] Awareness of the dangers of miasmas brought by the devil might well have been inspired by the West African belief reported by folklorist Newbell Niles Puckett in *Folk Beliefs of the Southern Negro.* According to Puckett, "because of sickness and deaths, the natives will change the location of their villages, running away from the malevolent spirits just as they would run from actual enemies."[125] At least some blacks believed that place had a range of consequences for the body. Another folklorist, Elsie Clews Parsons, was told by Jack Brown how a woman "learn to talk proper." A visiting doctor married her and "take her out travellin' an' change her woice. Dat's de reason, you go in differen' climate now, yer woice change."[126]

As southern whites sought to care for themselves, their children, and their slaves, their every thought and action was imbued with the notion that climate and place were central determinants of health. Bodies were embedded in a particular local context; only by paying careful attention to the consequences of that context could health be maintained or restored. White southerners wrote about such matters almost without thinking, for they were deeply ingrained in the culture, so much so as to be taken for granted as truisms. The South's laypeople, no less than the physicians they consulted when necessary, understood bodies as placed and fretted about the harm that could come to them if they lived in an insalubrious location or moved out of a familiar environment. What separated them from the physicians was the very ease with which they accepted such ideas; they were for the most part uncritical of the received wisdom about place that filled their letters and diaries. Unlike physicians, whose efforts to provide explanations caused them to try to develop an analysis of placed bodies and minds, laypeople simply took for granted that bodies were placed without wondering why or exploring the consequences.

That the South's physicians shared the assumptions of its lay white population should come as no surprise. Medical knowledge, like all knowledge, exists in a context that shapes its parameters. Nevertheless, the strong congruence between cultural truisms and physicians' efforts to develop a medical analysis suggests the importance of this particular set of beliefs. As southern whites, laypeople and physicians alike tried to keep themselves and their families healthy; as they tried to define their place in the nation, they could not help but consider their placed bodies as significant, different from bodies in other places.

# CHAPTER 4

# Ambiguous Bodies

Nineteenth-century Americans of all sorts assumed that the story the body told was easily read. At a glance, they believed, race, gender, class, and other identifying characteristics could be determined by the color of skin, shape of nose and lips, texture and style of hair, and cut, fabric, and style of clothing. At the same time, Americans recognized that the body could tell an ambiguous story. Surfaces did not always speak plainly. Clothing could hide a body that did not match what it claimed to represent. Unwilling to tolerate the threat of social disorder inherent in ambiguity for a host of social, political, and economic reasons, Americans in the middle third of the century were committed to an increasingly rigorous program of classifying bodies and eliding differences. This they thought necessary in order to protect themselves and their communities from the consequences of what they perceived as bodily incorrectness, such as marrying the wrong kind of person, identifying a "black" person as "white," or allowing a woman to vote. Often, they called on physicians for help.

Physicians were natural allies in the effort to fix categories of bodies. By virtue of their profession, they could claim both legitimate access to bodies and legitimacy over them. Their growing sense of themselves as scientific and objective led them to question the sureties of the appearance of the body's surface and its coverings; indeed, physicians were often eager to take on the role of arbiters. Especially in the South, physicians easily recognized the cultural power inherent in the role of defining bodies. Such a role allowed them to position themselves at the forefront of regional and national debates about race, sex, and place.

Physicians' willingness to take on the role of policing the boundaries of bodily categories was also a reflection of their growing interest in defining what was normal. By focusing on ambiguous bodies, they believed that they would gain a better understanding of the more ordinary bodies they encountered in daily practice. Studying what they considered the errors of ambiguous bodies allowed them to sharpen their ability to understand not just normal bodies, but also what happened when normal bodies became sick. Inspired by scientific curiosity, their desire to categorize and classify also offered a measure of prestige since only they could determine who was normal and who was not, who was healthy and who was sick.

Southern physicians brought to the debate a particularism that defined raced, sexed, and placed bodies as creating distinct patterns of health and illness. While they rarely agreed on the details, most shared the assumption that black (or African) bodies were fundamentally different from white (or European) ones; that women's reproductive organs influenced their bodies' and minds' experiences far beyond the obvious functions of menstruation, pregnancy, and lactation; and that the geographic location of a body influenced both the diseases to which it was subject and the course and treatment of those diseases. It was but a short step from attention to such particularities of the normal body to concern for bodies that appeared to slip between the categories, those that were mixed race ("mulatto" in the physicians' parlance), intersexed ("hermaphrodite" or "of doubtful sex"), or physically anomalous in some other visible fashion ("monsters"). The power of defining bodies allowed physicians not only to participate in establishing the categories, but also to police the boundaries by assigning classifications to individuals whose surfaces were not easily read or were otherwise ambiguous. The manner in which they did so allowed them to enhance their own authority even as they traversed the intersections of science and politics, biology and ideology.

Classifying the race or sex of bodies was especially important to midcentury physicians who were convinced that the characteristics of a particular body determined the illnesses to which it was subject. Believing as they did that the symptoms of many diseases as well as their treatment were dependent on the characteristics of the body in which disease was to be found, they could not help but concern themselves with proper placement of individuals into categories. The very nature of their work depended on doing so correctly. At the same time, their determination to understand the nature of disease inspired in them a good deal of curiosity about disease in those whose bodies were ambiguous. Were those of mixed racial background less healthy than those with either pure white or pure African blood? Were the constitutions of those with reproductive organs of both sexes dominated by their male or female parts? Were the minds of those with ambiguous bodies similarly ambiguous? Finding answers to such questions, physicians believed, would help them better understand disease itself, as well as the consequences of race and sex. Categorizing the suffering body was for them essential to the very understanding and practice of medicine.

Enhancing their understanding of bodily suffering was not the only reason southern physicians concerned themselves with understanding ambiguously raced and sexed bodies. For many physicians, the question of the fertility of such bodies was equally important. While the question of whether the intersexed could somehow impregnate themselves was largely theoretical, that of the fertility of mixed-race individuals was not. Southern physicians had special reasons to worry about fertility. As aspiring members of the elite, they worried about the region's ability to sustain its place in the nation, which in a majority-rule democratic society depended on the size of its population. Threatened by the increasing tide of foreign immigrants to the North, southern whites feared anything that would diminish the size of their own population, including the perceived inability of mixed-race bodies to reproduce. All southerners were familiar with the sterility of mules; slaveholders worried about the potential sterility of mulattoes. Additionally, slaves' ability to reproduce was one way in which calculating owners measured the return on their investment in slaves as property. While in the short run it was clear that those of mixed race could become parents, whether they did so as often as those with pure African blood, whether their children were as healthy, and whether those children would themselves be able to reproduce were questions of more than academic interest.

Slaveholders' political and economic interests as well as their concern for social order led them to express concern for other sorts of ambiguous bodies as well, especially those of women. Here, too, physicians were uniquely positioned to provide answers. One of their key concerns was to define the existence of pregnancy. Given the social, economic, and biological implications of pregnancy, determining whether a given woman was pregnant could easily become a requirement in a doctor's practice. Moreover, women who were unambiguously pregnant were often considered to be in a liminal state in relation to the fetus, a relationship that was expressed in terms of what one author called "transcendental anatomy": the mother's often inadvertent influence on the characteristics of her unborn child.[1]

The ambiguous body could take many forms. Both doctors and the general public had reason to be concerned about distinguishing between death and life, as well as the manner in which particular deaths occurred. While the latter was primarily a matter of medical jurisprudence for which doctors were called upon to provide expert witness, the former spoke to more primal fears of being buried alive.[2] Public health authorities in midcentury did not yet require birth and death certificates, nor was the cause of death recorded with any rigor, even in urban areas. Yet determining whether a baby was born dead or alive or when and how an unconscious person died demanded levels of expertise only physicians could provide.

In addition, physicians were frequently expected to distinguish between sickness and health, particularly in their slave patients. Slaveholders expected the physicians they employed to expose instances of shamming, which threatened both slaveholders' authority and physicians' credibility.[3] Physicians were also called upon to testify about the status of the bodies of slaves in court proceedings. As witnesses for buyers and sellers, owners and hirers, their expertise about the health and illness of disputed bodies was increasingly valuable and increasingly recognized.[4] In all of these instances, physicians were expected to define the ambiguous body, in the process categorizing it as black or white, male or female, pregnant or not, healthy or sick, alive or dead.

Physicians who understood the core of their practice to be the treatment of disease perhaps did not relish the responsibility of categorizing ambiguous bodies of any sort.[5] With the exception of shamming, few were called upon to do so. Most mixed-race children were born to slave mothers, and so their identity was rarely called into question. Most physicians undoubtedly never encountered an intersexed person in a lifetime of practice. Only a small number would find themselves called upon to adjudicate the race of a baby born to a white mother, the presence of a pregnancy, or the cause of death. Since determining the answers to such questions had the potential to alienate their clients and neighbors, most physicians were undoubtedly grateful. Even so, their growing scientific curiosity led the editors of medical journals to fill many pages with discussions of such matters. Physicians accepted the responsibility of categorizing even the most puzzling of bodies, even if they did not always welcome the practical consequences of doing so.

Physicians who wrote about ambiguous bodies did not do so with the confidence of those who discussed race, sex, and place. They rarely generalized about the significance of ambiguity or attempted to address philosophical perspectives. Instead, they presented the cases that had come before them. As a result, their writing is more anecdotal and less abstract, typically focusing on individual ambiguous bodies rather than any sort of ambiguity as a category.

## Physicians Consider Ambiguous Bodies

For southern physicians convinced of the fundamental distinctions between black and white bodies, those of mixed race posed a range of intellectual dilemmas. If blacks and whites were subject to different diseases, even, according to some, members of different species, how could bodies of mixed parentage best be understood? The question was of special importance because there was not a perfect overlap in the South between the categories of black and slave. While the law defined those with even small proportions of black blood as black and subjected them to all sorts of restrictions, the presence of free blacks as a social category, many of whom were in fact of mixed race, was troubling.[6] While defenders of slavery would have preferred that all blacks be enslaved, the presence of a liminal social and legal category within the southern body politic left them scrambling for ideological consistency. One solution was to turn to physicians for assistance. If mixed-race bodies could be shown to be infertile and thus doomed to extinction within a few generations, the separation of society into slave and free, black and white would automatically be preserved without the messiness of intermediate categories. In addition, freedom itself could be seen as medically dangerous for those with black blood circulating in their bodies. Once again, because of physicians' presumed ability to address such issues, they assumed an important role in the region's efforts to justify its institutions.

In fact, physician debate on the relative health of those of mixed race was extensive. Josiah Nott, the Alabama physician and ethnographer who claimed that blacks and whites were separately created and thus fundamentally different types of human beings, was convinced that mulattoes were "a degenerate *Hybrid race*, and subject to much greater mortality and lower average duration of life span than either whites or blacks."[7] Similarly, physician Samuel Cartwright, who had identified several diseases to which only blacks were subject, believed that "the blackest negroes were always the healthiest, and the thicker the lips and the flatter the nose, the sounder the constitution." Cartwright maintained "all negroes are not equally black—the blacker, the healthier and stronger; any deviation from the black color, in the pure race, is a mark of feebleness or ill health."[8]

Lesser-known and less-controversial physicians shared their conviction that mixing of the races led to decreased vitality and increased illness. Dr. A. P. Merrill, who had written so extensively about placed bodies and the treatment African bodies needed to survive in the South's cold climate, also believed that "amalgamation" of black and white blood (later referred to as miscegenation) tended "to impair the energy of the vital forces, predispose to adynamic diseases, and to shorten life." Amalgamation also tended to impair "the procreative powers, and thus to retard increase." He believed there could be no doubt that "the mixed race of all grades, is more liable to those diseased conditions, principally of the nervous system, and to those depressions of the vital energies" that caused tuberculosis and "neuralgic disease, . . . check[ed] their natural increase, and curtail[ed] the average duration of their lives."[9] Slaves themselves sometimes held similar beliefs. Sophie D. Belle, who had been a slave in Georgia, claimed that her mother was three-quarters Indian and that both her mother's father and her own were white men, making her "eight-ninths white race." In spite of marrying twice, Belle never had any children, which she explained by saying, "They tell me now if I had married dark men I would maybe had children. I married very light men both times."[10]

Physicians who believed that those of mixed race were inherently less healthy and less able to reproduce than those of either race whose blood was pure often relied on their understandings of heredity to justify their position. Since the propensity for disease was inherited, these physicians believed that those of mixed race were especially unhealthy because their vulnerabilities to illness came from both parents, each of whom had a different set of weaknesses. As a result, they were not likely to reproduce successfully for many generations. Dr. J. Dawson, an Ohio physician whose article was reprinted in the *Oglethorpe Medical and Surgical Journal,* noted that the offspring of parents of different races could be "prolific to a certain extent, but not to the extent of maintaining a permanent existence; or, like the parent races, of being able to perpetually reproduce itself."

He added that "Mulattoes . . . run out at the third, or, at the farthest, the fourth generation"; after that they become sterile.[11] A few physicians used this thinking to argue for the reopening of the international slave trade, claiming that "without fresh African blood" the fate of the race was "*fixed.*"[12] Drawing on their experience with the sterility of mules and their conviction that the mixture of blood from what some of them understood to be different species of mankind led to a "greater feebleness of constitution,"[13] at least some physicians feared that mixing the races would be fatal.

At the same time, race mixing could have some advantages, particularly for the minds of individuals, albeit advantages that were perhaps troubling. The same Dr. Merrill who believed that amalgamation shortened life noted that the more white blood and the "greater the remoteness of the hybrid from the original stock, [the more] the mental constitution . . . approaches . . . the superiority of the white race." Thus, he noted, the "hybrid race" when enslaved occupied "places of trust and responsibility, requiring the exercise of judgment and reflection, as well as tact and ingenuity." Those who were free "often become prosperous, trustworthy and skilful in their several occupations."[14] D. F. Nardin, a Thomsonian physician in Charleston, South Carolina, believed that "as the race becomes amalgamated with 'white blood,' you see comfort and industry in proportion to their approach to the European parent, with all the marks of a superior intellect."[15]

Only a few southern physicians were willing to challenge their colleagues' assumptions about the consequences of race mixing for bodies or minds. A reviewer of Samuel Cartwright's work worried about the consequences for physicians of defining ever-narrower gradations of humanity, suggesting that Cartwright's thinking would require different explanations for the physiology of every possible combination of blood. The reviewer warned that "henceforth, the first question of the practitioner at the bed-side of his patient, must be in relation to the purity of his or her blood." If that blood were mixed, he warned, the "case is more stubborn, of course, and black and white powders must be mixed according to the extent of the tincture."[16] His views, however, were not widely shared. Because so many of the justifications for slavery were built upon the assumed inherent inferiority of blacks, the emergence of large numbers of mixed-race bodies could only be perceived as threatening to the survival of the institution itself.

For many physicians, defining the characteristics of bodies of mixed race was a humanitarian effort: They saw themselves as providing a warning of the dangers of amalgamation. While such views were of course politically self-serving in that they reinforced the defense of slavery, they also offered physicians an indirect means of commenting on the morality of white men, since there could be little doubt that the origins of nearly all mixed-race bodies came from the sexual activities of white men with black women. While physicians were not often tactless (or foolish) enough to comment directly on the sexual behavior of other men like themselves, there was certainly a coded warning inherent in their remarks.

Mixed-race bodies were dangerous bodies, both because they were prone to ill-ness and impaired reproduction and because they contained some of the mental superiority of whites. Their very existence reminded white men of the dangerous bodily consequences of their own behavior.

Even more troubling than deciphering the bodily consequences of amalgama-tion was determining the racial categories of particular individuals, most notably when those individuals were the offspring of white mothers. Such cases presented a quite different form of threat to white male domination, a threat found in the pre- or extramarital and interracial sexual activities of white women.[17] There were few greater taboos in southern society, and physicians were occasionally called upon to arbitrate the results of their violation. For example, Dr. W. L. Sutton of Kentucky reported that town physicians were called upon by the "reputed father" of a baby and his rural physician to provide the child with medical attention and "to silence some neighborhood talk which had arisen on account of its color." While two doctors attributed the baby's dark color to an opening in his skull or "inflammation of the brain," the town physicians asked about the mother's complexion, which was "reported to be very dark," and also invited "moral testi-mony." Although the family physician "had unshaken faith in the chastity of the woman," she eventually "acknowledged that she had had occasional connection with two negro men in the neighborhood." Sutton reflected that the subject of telling a white child from a black one presented "knotty points": "the more it is studied, the more difficulties start up" and perceived the matter as one for medical jurisprudence.[18] It was also, apparently, a subject for neighborhood gossip, which demanded that physicians be even more careful in their pronouncements.

Sutton and the other *ten* doctors consulted about the race of this baby found themselves the arbiters of private morality, expected to pass judgment on the behavior of a white woman in a context that viewed white women as inherently passionless and the idea of their sexual contact with black men unspeakable. Even so, Sutton used the opportunity the baby presented to explore the "popular notion" that some children "tainted with African blood" have a dark scrotum and dark streak down the back along the spine, while others were reportedly spotted. He carefully considered the evidence for dark spots on the skin, con-cluding that they were "certainly rare" and that he did not "know to how much consideration they are entitled," while placing "no reliance" on the dark scrotum and spine because they were contradicted by his experience.[19] Clearly, Sutton recognized that deciding the race of the child was a matter worthy of serious consideration. There were serious consequences for mother and child alike, as well as for the physician's standing in his community, given the potential embar-rassment of an incorrect decision or even a correct one. The very care with which he and presumably the other doctors consulted considered the matter suggests the importance he attached to the moral integrity of racial categorization. Yet Sutton and his colleagues certainly encountered the mixed-race babies born to black women quite frequently, without examining them for spots and streaks or acknowledging them as ambiguous. The mixed-race babies born to white women contained within themselves the potential to disrupt the social order and so had to be classified as ambiguous, while the mixed-race babies born to black women did not and so were not considered to be in the same category.

Physicians' concerns with the too-dark babies of white mothers reflected their sense of moral order and social responsibility. Their concern for the twins of apparently different races born to white or black mothers reflected their scientific curiosity. In the absence of any convincing theory of genetics and with only a limited understanding of the finer biological details of reproduction, doctors intent upon defining the limits of the normal—as well as the possible—found the differently raced twins of the same mother and different fathers compelling evidence of human variation. A Georgia physician, A. F. Attaway, attended the birth of a white woman whose firstborn twin was very dark. "Not being willing to suggest a thing," he explained the baby's color by attributing it to cyanosis, meaning that insufficient oxygen in the blood had caused its skin to appear darker than normal. After the second twin was born, he noted "the great difference between the children" as of "peculiar interest." Later, he asked the mother for an explanation of the babies' conception, which she provided with some hesitation, admitting that she had once "cohabited with a negro man" as well as more often with "the father of her white child."[20] Similarly, Thomas Taylor, a Mississippi physician, reported on what he called a case of "mixed birth," in which a "negress" gave birth to twins, "one a mulatto, and the other a negro child." Taylor believed the woman's account that she had intercourse only once with a white man, three weeks "from the time she first felt she had conceived." He noted "at their birth the mulatto child bore marks of being at least three weeks younger than the negro."[21] For both Attaway and Taylor, the details of these women's conceptions offered the opportunity to learn more about reproduction as well as race. Oddly, physicians rarely addressed the possibility that a child of black or even mixed-race parents could be albino.[22]

Physicians concerned with establishing the racial identities of infants were intent on more than simply understanding the mechanics of conception and racial categorization. At the same time, they were claiming for themselves authority over the boundary between white and black, defining it as a medical issue as much as a legal and moral one. While the legal standard proclaiming that a child followed the status of the mother solved one of the fundamental problems of amalgamation, it did not speak to the more vexing if less common question of racial identity in all cases. No matter what their racial identity, slaves were by definition black, but the mixed-race offspring of white mothers had to be classified as such.

For some physicians, racial categorization was an especially difficult task because they believed the categories to be unstable even within an individual body. Dr. A. Harvey suggested that not only do "offspring exhibit, more or less distinctly, over and beyond the characters of the male by which they were begotten, the peculiarities, also, of a male by which their mother had at some former period been impregnated." While his most graphic evidence came from animals, he thought it would be simple to subject his ideas "to a pretty decisive test" in people by examining the "distinct breeds of the human family." It would only be necessary "to observe accurately, whether the children of European parents, where the woman has, in the first instance, had offspring by a negro, exhibit traces of the latter in the colour of the skin, the form of the features, &c." Similarly, Harvey asked "whether the children of negro parents, where the woman had, first of all, been impregnated by a European, exhibit the peculiarities of the latter." He thought the subsequent and apparently pure white children of white women who had first had a child by a black man would show the taint of race mixture. Furthermore, he thought that the father's influence on "each successive impregnation" would be increased, so that "the younger children begotten by him, rather than the elder, might be expected . . . to bear their father's image." Harvey considered the best explanation to be that of another physician, who claimed that "when a pure animal of any breed has been pregnant to an animal of a different breed, such pregnant animal is a cross ever after; *the purity of her blood being lost,* in consequence of her connection with the foreign animal," by which he meant the developing fetus. Harvey extended this analogy to human beings, concluding that "the blood and constitution generally of the mother may . . . become so imbued with the peculiarities of [the father], as to impart them to any offspring she may subsequently have by other males."[23] The obvious implication of his argument was that she, too, would become mixed race. Few southern physicians adopted his thinking, perhaps because so few white women were in this situation, yet the instability of racial categorization was clear.

Physicians were similarly concerned with defining the boundary between male and female bodies.[24] Believing, as the French author of a midwifery textbook put it, that a woman's body was "not only female in the peculiar disposition and arrangement of her genital organs . . . but in every other part," physicians understood personality and behavior to originate in "the well-marked designs of nature, for the propagation of the species."[25] According to F. Le Jau Parker, the house physician of Charleston's Roper Hospital, founded for the care of slaves and free blacks and associated with the Medical College of South Carolina, individuals ambiguously presenting physical characteristics of both men and women were "almost incomprehensible deviations from nature in her ordinary processes of formation." He described the autopsy he performed on one such individual, Jacob, a sixty-seven-year-old slave who had lived, married, and worked as a man, but about whose sex the owner was "uncertain" and so requested the examination. Jacob's owner was himself a free person of color, suggesting perhaps a personal interest in the social consequences of ambiguous status. Parker deliberately referred to Jacob as "she" throughout his report, since "she was found to be a woman."[26]

Parker described Jacob as having a "mild and gentle" temperament, in spite of "hesitat[ing] as to her proper sphere in life, and . . . vascillat[ing] between the two opinions." This unhappiness resulted from "her suspected deformity," which caused men to ridicule him and "the dissatisfaction or contempt of his wife."[27] Jacob's regular menstruation caused "great pain" and "confirmed the suspicions of her doubtful sex," leading Parker to conclude that "[she] was without doubt a female." The autopsy Parker performed offered even more confirmation, revealing "that most wonderful organ, the uterus," breasts, and an enlarged clitoris, along with a "well-developed scrotum."[28] Parker's uncertainty about the meaning of Jacob's bodily anomalies matched his discomfort with Jacob's inability to conform to the requirements of either the male or the female sphere. His only solution was to define Jacob as female.

Jacob was not the only intersexed slave to come to the attention of southern physicians. Ned, a slave in Virginia, likewise lived as a man. Although the physician who reported on him never explained why he came under examination, Dr. Harris noted his "strange and anomalous appearance," observing breasts, a "naturally formed" but "dwarfish-looking" penis, what resembled the "external labia of the female," and no testicles. In addition, he reported, "this singular creature has been regularly menstruating for three or four years *through the penis*," accompanied by a range of dramatic symptoms. Harris "naturally" wondered "to which of the sexes does this human being belong?" He answered that "the conclusion . . . is forced upon us, that the female organs predominate" and that Ned most likely had "a uterus with its appendages," thus making him female.[29] Harris attributed his conclusion to "those attributes, both moral and physical, which mark the presence of such an organ," even though Ned was sexually attracted to women. Harris viewed this behavior as the result of being "taught to look upon himself as a male" so that now, "in imitation of others, [he] deports himself as such to the other sex." This was as close as midcentury southern physicians could come to perceiving gendered behavior as learned, rather than rooted in the race and sex of the body. Harris did not know if Ned's "amorous advances to the dusky maidens around him has ever resulted in any practical display of virility." In spite of Ned's claim that his penis was "eminently endowed . . . with virile sensibility," Harris concluded that "no seminal discharge has, or ever will take place."[30] With a uterus and without semen, Ned could only be a woman.

Both Drs. Harris and Parker concluded that slaves who considered themselves to be male and were perceived as such by others were in fact female, a conclusion that may well reflect their sense of the inherent inferiority of black and female bodies. If women were by definition less than men, weak and imperfect, then Ned and Jacob's black and imperfect bodies were more easily seen as female than as male. And since slave women generally did the same kinds of work as slave men, there could be few overt consequences for defining them as such.

Physicians generally found the task of labeling sexual ambiguity more complex when the individual was white, perhaps because inferiority was harder to assume and sex roles even more rigidly defined. For Samuel D. Gross, professor of surgery at the Louisville Medical Institute in Kentucky, the three-year-old white child brought to him presented a "novel and interesting" case. The child had been pronounced female at birth, but "began to evince the tastes, disposition, and feelings of the other sex" at age two, rejecting dolls and becoming fond of sports. In this case, Gross was disturbed by the contradiction between the child's apparent sex and her behavior, believing that contradiction between mind and body to be a symptom of her medical condition. Gross carefully examined the child's external genitalia, discovering that she had "neither a penis nor a vagina," but did have testes. He considered surgically removing them, to prevent her from later experiencing sexual desire and marrying, since he was sure "impregnation could never occur."[31]

Given his concerns about the child's future, Gross consulted her parents and a colleague, all of whom agreed that depriving "her of an appendage of so useless a nature . . . [which might] ultimately lead to the ruin of her character and peace of mind" was "an act of kindness and of humanity to the poor child." In the three years since the operation, Gross reported, the child's "disposition and habits have materially changed, and are now those of a girl," including "great delight in sewing and housework." He offered this example "as a precedent in similar cases," because "defective organization of the external genitals . . . exerts so baneful an influence over his moral and social feelings" and nothing causes "such a sense of self-abasement and mental degradation" as being "forever debarred from the joys and pleasures of married life, an outcast from society, hated and despised, and reviled and persecuted by the world." However, the editors of the *Southern Medical and Surgical Journal* who reprinted Gross's article doubted that many readers would agree with his reasoning. While they did not explain their own thinking, it is likely that they did not consider even the child's surgically constructed female body a suitable candidate for marriage in the future, perhaps because it would never be capable of reproduction.[32]

Intersexed individuals like Jacob, Ned, and the unnamed child treated by Dr. Gross were of more than academic interest to many physicians. A Connecticut doctor was called upon to determine the sex of Levi Suydam, whose right to vote in a close election was challenged by the opposition party "on the ground that he was more a female than a male." Although two physicians declared he was entitled to vote, further information revealed that he menstruated regularly and had "a feminine figure" and "feminine propensities, such as a fondness for gay colors, for pieces of calico . . . and an aversion for bodily labor," causing the physicians to rethink their conclusions.[33] Medical testimony was also an issue when Paul Eve, professor of surgery at the Medical College of Georgia, was asked by a "gentleman" about "the condition of his wife," who, in eighteen months of marriage, had not conceived. The woman had never menstruated, but periodically she had "an efflorescence and mottled appearance on the skin" that caused her to suffer "great malaise." Eve's probing finger revealed that her vagina terminated in "a perfect *cul de sac*" but nothing resembling a womb. Suspecting that the uterus was absent, Eve asked "might not this marriage involve a question in medical jurisprudence?"[34] Both Gross and Eve were primarily concerned with the moral legitimacy of marriages with white intersexed individuals, an issue that was never raised for slaves, while the Connecticut doctors, along with the southern editors who reprinted the article, were worried about preserving the legitimacy of male suffrage. All saw themselves as uniquely positioned to determine such legitimacy, difficult as it might have been to do so.

In the apparent absence of a uterus, Eve in essence defined the person he examined as not-woman, although he certainly did not consider her to be male. As a general rule, physicians determined that the presence of a uterus or ovaries defined the woman, although the presence of a penis did not similarly define a body as male.[35] In their categorization of bodies, physicians considered the presence of female reproductive organs, most notably the uterus, as primary in determining sex, just as they defined individuals of mixed racial ancestry as black, even when the percentage of black blood was very small. In this, physicians reflected the assumptions of their society that female and black were themselves inferior categories, to which it made sense to assign those whose bodies were ambiguous.

Physicians involved in policing the boundaries between male and female, like those performing a similar function between black and white, believed that the evidence of the body could be read, but only by those with their training and expertise. Determined to classify the bodies they encountered in their everyday practices as well as to define the meanings of those classifications, they had little doubt of the importance of their work. Their commitment to a scientific understanding of human beings, normal as well as anomalous, was necessary not only for the effective practice of medicine, but also for the orderly functioning of society. Society functioned best when bodies knew their place, which of course required that they be placed correctly. Since individuals could not be trusted to identify themselves correctly within a hierarchical system, physicians claimed for themselves the authority to define that place for the individuals who came (or were put) before them.

Physicians determined to label bodies in the manner they considered correct assumed that race and sex were binary categories, with the many mixed-race bodies and the few intersexed ones they encountered as aberrant violations of the laws of nature and of humanity. Not only did they read the biological body in terms of the categories to which it should be assigned, they also expected an individual's mind and behavior to match that of the biological body. While the institution of slavery made it nearly impossible for many mixed-race individuals to pass as white, if only because they were born to slave mothers, southern whites were committed to viewing them as socially black and biologically inferior as well.

Doctors who claimed for themselves the power to define even the most ambiguous bodies enhanced the social authority of white men in the name of science.

In the process, they set themselves apart from other men as social arbiters and experts, with superior knowledge over bodies, able to name the unnameable, know the unknowable. By doing so, they helped avert the threat of social disorder inherent in the very presence of ambiguous bodies. Only by understanding ambiguity could they truly lay claim to policing the boundaries of what was normal. Science became for doctors the means to moral certainty and enhanced prestige, a way not only to help the suffering but to define them—and everyone else.

This commitment to classification was not limited to physicians; instead, their preoccupation reflected that of their society. Not only physicians but also the general public insisted on eradicating any hint of ambiguity, even at great personal cost. Ben, the slave sawyer discussed in the introduction whose injuries caused him to bleed from the urethra, imagined himself a woman as a result, while his owner and his community considered him insane. Similarly, a white man who "with a dull pocket-knife castrated himself, removing both testicles with a part of the scrotum" was considered mentally deranged. However, in this case the "act has cured him of his mental derangement, and he now repents most sincerely committing it." The physician reporting on this case noted that he did not know whether the man lived with his wife.[36] For laypeople as well as physicians, curiosity about anomalous bodies as well as the importance of the correct classification were paramount.

The commitment to sex and race classification inherent in the thinking of physicians and laypeople alike was part of a larger trend in American and European science in the middle decades of the nineteenth century. At that time, scientists were deepening their interest in classifications of all sorts as well as speculating about the divisions separating them. While the pioneers of natural history had already developed the schema by which living things are organized into categories (family, genus, species), scientists were eagerly attempting to expand their knowledge of those categories by collecting examples of all of the variations of life forms, such as plants and insects. Others were challenging that system and proposing alternatives. No one had as yet developed a comprehensive theory to explain the existence of variation, including what would become the fundamental concepts of genetics, hybridity, and mutation; Charles Darwin's *Origin of Species* would not be published until 1859. Yet even in the years before Darwin, scientists, including medical doctors, thought deeply about such matters and struggled to make sense of the ambiguities they observed around them. In many instances, their efforts to do so challenged their understanding of Christianity, which taught that God had created a world in which evil could exist, but not error. In their efforts to understand ambiguous bodies, physicians very likely wondered whether God or nature made mistakes. While few would have attempted theological answers, physicians' very insistence on binary classification of race and sex reflected the complexity of the moral issues presented by the existence of such bodies. For a science committed to classification, in which every form of life had its proper place and existed in proper relationship to every other form, ambiguous bodies not only suggested the dangers inherent in unknowable nature, but also represented a challenge to the fundamental principles of Christianity itself.

## Understanding Women's Ambiguous Bodies

Medical authority extended far beyond determining how best to label the doubtful racial and sexual identities of specific individuals. Physicians also claimed responsibility for understanding women's bodies. They were quite clear that women's bodies were fundamentally different from men's because of the pervasive influence of their reproductive organs. However, they also recognized women's bodies as inherently ambiguous, because the status of their reproductive organs was so difficult to determine with any degree of accuracy. The biological processes of menarche, menstruation, pregnancy, childbirth, lactation, and menopause all meant that women's bodies were in a permanent state of flux, permanently unstable. Female bodies' ambiguous status raised questions for physicians that they also considered themselves increasingly empowered to answer. They sought ways to determine whether women were virgins, whether they had been raped, whether they were pregnant, and whether they had aborted. Such questions arose with alarming frequency, reinforcing physicians' views of women's bodies as ambiguous. If ambiguously raced and sexed bodies were dangerous to the social order because they could not be easily categorized, women's permanently ambiguous bodies were threatening because of the very ordinariness of their ambiguity.

In their efforts to categorize women's ambiguous bodies, southern physicians were not fundamentally different from those in other parts of the nation. Doctors everywhere were eager to extend the range of their authority to women and their troubling reproductive functions. However, southern doctors may well have perceived themselves to have more at stake in this process, given the importance they attached to extending their control over racial categories. If they could establish legitimacy over the ambiguities of women's reproductive bodies, a goal they shared with other physicians, there could be little doubt of their right to define other categories of bodies as well. In addition, southern physicians may well have considered that their efforts to understand reproduction would enhance their ability to explain the similarities and differences between women of the two races. Southern physicians had professional and cultural reasons to want to categorize bodies and define the parameters of what they considered normal.

Every aspect of women's reproductive functions could present doctors with ambiguous signs and symptoms that emphasized their liminality. Among the most perplexing was menstrual blood that escaped the body from irregular places, including "the nose, lungs, stomach, bladder, nipples, or some other part of the body."[37] This was known as vicarious menstruation, an uncommon but nevertheless dangerous condition. According to Hugh Blair, professor of general and special anatomy at the Oglethorpe Medical College in Savannah, Georgia, in 1858, "when certain organs of the animal economy cease or fail to perform their proper functions, some other organ or organs take on an increased or vicarious function, and the system is rescued from oppression and disease." The most "deeply interesting" example "of perverted actions of organs" occurred in the uterus, which "at regular periods . . . requir[ed] prompt depletion." If those "efforts" were "foiled" or "arrested, and the circulation" redirected elsewhere, such as the lung, brain, nose, or ears, "the most violent symptoms ensue." Blair believed "these exceedingly distressing symptoms are relieved by '*vicarious menstruation*.'" He offered "the most decidedly unique case" of this in a fifteen-year-old white woman who was "about approaching puberty." Although she had never menstruated, three times at twenty-eight-day intervals she experienced "an almost insupportable pain" in her right eye. Blair considered this as "quite suspicious" after the second time; the "third time this young and tender plant had suffered from the blighting influence of this formidable malady was convincing proof, without the probability of a doubt, that this was a case of attempted vicarious menstruation." He treated her "by everting the eyelids, and freely scarifying them" to promote "the hemorrhage," bleeding her from the temples, and administering a variety of drugs. After more than a month of treatment, he claimed, "her eye was entirely restored, and her catamenial discharge had been regularly established."[38]

The eyes were not the only site for vicarious menstruation. Far more common were other parts of the body associated with reproduction. In 1847, E. C. Baker of South Carolina reported on another young white woman "who had been suffering for a length of time, from an affection of the breast, supposed to be 'cancer.'" In fact, it resembled an ulcer and felt like a tumor. According to the woman's mother, "about *every month* the *breast enlarged,* the *ulcer inflamed,* and a discharge of *sanious purulent matter*[39] took place." The woman herself remembered being stuck in the breast by the pointed edge of a palmetto royal leaf five or six years earlier, the sore from which "had never since been healed completely." Because of this history and her periodic suffering from "giddiness, severe pains in the lower portion of her abdomen, and sickness of stomach" at the same time that she bled from the breast, Baker "regarded it as a case of *vicarious menstruation.*" Like Blair, he prescribed a variety of treatments over a long period of time, which gradually resulted in increasing the quantity of menstrual discharge from her uterus, with "that from the ulcer diminishing in proportion."[40]

S. B. R. Finley reported on a similar case in a slave woman in Charleston. Since she was forty-four or forty-five years old, no one was alarmed when she stopped menstruating, but after a month, "at the next regular period, a discharge appeared from the nipples." She described the pain associated with this "as resembling in every respect, the pains she had formerly experienced in her menstrual efforts." After some doubts and consultations, Finley, too, diagnosed vicarious menstruation. Because of the woman's age, Finley decided only to keep "the patient constantly under my inspection, watch symptoms as they may arise, and if dangerous apply proper correctives."[41]

Other physicians reported cases of vicarious menstruation in a slave woman in whom for three years "*at every monthly period the menstrual fluid was discharged through the [umbilical] opening*";[42] in a married white woman with what at first appeared to be "a dangerous attack of hemorrhage from the stomach and bowels" who "vomit[ed] and purg[ed] what seemed to be decomposed [menstrual] blood"; and in a slave woman with "a slow oozing of blood" from an ulcer on her leg "so extensive and threatening" that it required amputation. After the woman's leg was removed, she formed "sacks" every month "around the stump of the amputated limb, [that] require[d] to be lanced." The appearance of these sacks was "so uniform . . . in their periodic character" that the woman kept a lancet herself, allowing her "thus *surgically* to perform the work of menstruation."[43]

Doctors who diagnosed vicarious menstruation rarely worried about the body's unusual discharge of blood, although they recognized it as abnormal and usually tried to restore the uterus to proper functioning. Gunning Bedford considered it beneficial, with the "compensating discharge acting as a waste-gate, and thus protecting the system measurably from harm."[44] Tomlinson Fort considered bleeding from the lungs "a most fearsome disease," but added "when it arises from suppressed menstruation, it is not considered dangerous, and sometimes appears for years to return, from month to month, and yet the patient suffers very little deterioration of health." He similarly thought "vomiting of blood" to be "an alarming—frequently, a dangerous disease," but recognized "the least dangerous of its forms, is that which occurs from suppressed menstruation" because the stomach "perform[s] the office of the uterus."[45]

In spite of these reassuring assessments, most southern physicians considered vicarious menstruation a sign of danger and a medical problem demanding treatment. Convinced that women's bodies were dangerously ambiguous sites seemingly liable to menstruate at any time from any orifice or surface, doctors were willing to see nearly any blood as menstrual blood. Controlled by an imperative to menstruate so strong that blood could flow from anywhere, women's bodies could only be seen as ambiguous, able to deviate from what was normal at any moment and in the process confuse the unwary physician about their very nature.

Physicians who were wary of women's ambiguous bodies also struggled to find ways to determine whether a particular woman was pregnant at any given moment. One anonymous author noted that "most practitioners think it a very easy matter to decide on the existence of pregnancy at almost any time" and that their decisions were "very often correct." However, he warned, "other causes than pregnancy" could be at the root of "nearly all of what are commonly considered evidences of this state," noting that in the first four months especially, for a physician to decide whether a woman was pregnant was "one of the most difficult problems in all the practice of his profession." Mistakes could let doctors treat a pregnant woman as if she suffered a disease, using drugs that "may have the power of *abortives*," which would be a "dangerous and criminal disaster." But the reverse could also be dangerous. If he "decide[d] in favor of pregnancy" because of a woman's "symptoms," he would be "lost to all other views both of causation and pathological condition." This could let the truth of her disease remain hidden "until the golden moment passes, beyond which there is no hope" to cure her.[46]

This author warned that women's accounts of their bodies could "not be depended on" because "they are often deceived by their own supersentiousness or by their desires or aversions; or they may have strong motives uncontroled by moral principle, which induce them to desire to deceive." He mentioned one white woman whose abdominal tumor led her to believe she was pregnant, even to believe "parturient pains had commenced." Another woman, similarly diagnosed with a tumor, eventually believed that she had "no less than seven children within her abdominal parietes," adding a new one every nine months. A third white woman, raped in the middle of the night by what she believed to be "a negro," was convinced that she had become pregnant and felt quickening, although the physician "could find nothing but her own fears to lead to the suspicion of pregnancy." Called to attend the birth, he "could not satisfy her" that there was no child, although afterward she "daily increased in health."[47] The truth about these women's bodies could not be read on the surface or even in the interior of the body, nor could it be subjectively experienced; instead, only the physicians' expertise could define the apparently anomalous body.

The confusion caused by one white woman's ambiguous body inspired her to consult Dr. Thomas L. Ogier of Charleston. According to his account, after the birth of her first child "the entrance to the vagina contracted more and more, until it was almost entirely obliterated," too small to admit even a fingertip. Mrs. C., as Ogier called her, was "somewhat depressed by her condition; she was under the impression that her pelvis was in some way deformed, so that she could never have a living child." In spite of her depression, she saw this as "an advantage, as a guarantee against her ever becoming again pregnant." She consulted Ogier when her menses were suppressed for three months. Ogier noted that "she was anxious to have the obstruction removed, if it caused the suppression; but yet she feared to have this done, on account of her then being liable to become pregnant." He found "the suppression . . . had been attended by many of the constitutional symptoms of pregnancy," which he thought caused them in spite of her belief that it was "out of the question" because "*physically impossible*." Ogier convinced her to have her vagina surgically dilated, which caused an abortion but facilitated her treatment. Some time later, she again became pregnant; Ogier delivered the baby using forceps because her vagina continued to be "perfectly firm and unyielding." Ogier considered forceps preferable to cutting the vagina in part because "my patient was exceedingly depressed, believing she would never get over it, and it was desirable to bring matters to a close as speedily as possible"; the forceps allowed the patient to be "at once relieved of her anxieties."[48] Determining which bodies could become pregnant as well as how those bodies should be treated was, for both Mrs. C. and Dr. Ogier, a medical matter in spite of her wish to use her ambiguous body as a form of contraception.

Cases of what one author called "spurious pregnancy" could occur for a variety of reasons. Ariel Hunton, a Vermont botanic physician whose article was reprinted in the *Southern Medical Reformer,* noted that the practicing physician would encounter "many novel, perplexing and unique cases" trying "to his skill and patience." He noted that "females frequently feign pregnancy for selfish or criminal purposes, and some who honestly think themselves in a state of gestation are deceived." He described several cases in which a woman believed herself to be pregnant and showed "all appearance of labor pains,—writhing, moaning, pulling at the hands of her attendants as in real labor—and all an imagination or an excitement of the mind." When he convinced these women that they were not pregnant, "immediately . . . their pain subsides, and they resume their domestic affairs." Hunton proclaimed himself "at a loss to account for such a transaction." He reported that the women's husbands were angered by these circumstances, noting that one was "offended, and manifested his boorish disposition by censuring his wife in rude terms for not knowing her situation," while another called the doctor "hard names" and a third suffered "disappointment and annoyance."[49]

Unlike Hunton, other physicians were able to explain, at least to their own satisfaction, why women who believed themselves to be pregnant were mistaken. Joseph Wright, author of a domestic medicine guide published in Georgia, offered menopause as one explanation. He suggested that "many women have such a dislike to age, that they would rather flatter themselves that they are with child than suppose that they are feeling any of the consequences of growing old."[50] Most cases of spurious pregnancy were not so easily dismissed. When Georgia physician George Smith was called to attend a white woman who believed herself to be four months pregnant with her second child, "having had the derangements of health usually attendant on gestation," he diagnosed her with "uterine hydatids" and "dropsical symptoms"[51] instead.[52] On another occasion, however, Smith was less certain. He consulted Joseph Eve, professor of obstetrics at the Medical College of Georgia, about a slave woman about forty years old who "supposed herself pregnant." Smith reported that he found the woman "apparently in labor, her pains, however, short and ineffectual." A day later, he noted that "her pains subsided, lactation supervened, but the abdominal enlargement remained unchanged"; two months later, she began menstruating again. Smith thought that she had an abdominal tumor and considered it a case of extrauterine pregnancy. He asked Eve's opinion because he was "deeply concerned," as were the woman's owners, who considered her "a valuable servant" and "feel great solicitude on her account, not knowing what may be the final result."[53]

Eve, who read Smith's description of the woman's circumstances but did not examine her, agreed with the diagnosis of extrauterine pregnancy as the cause of the abdominal tumor. He noted one case he had read about in which a woman who had experienced a similar abdominal tumor with signs of pregnancy and labor but no actual birth later delivered two children. After that woman's death, examination of her abdomen disclosed that "a male foetus was found entire with the exception of the bones of the cranium which were separated."[54] Abdominal tumors and extrauterine pregnancies were not always easy to distinguish from actual pregnancies, in spite of Eve's long-distance diagnosis. A Mississippi doctor called to attend "a light-colored, spare built mulatto woman" diagnosed "a hard tumor in the uterus," only to discover that she was pregnant when she delivered a child.[55]

Physicians who struggled to define pregnancy and distinguish it from other bodily states knew that their efforts to do so had both medical and social implications. Dr. G. Harrison of Georgia reported to his colleagues about a "servant girl of one of my patrons" whose symptoms indicated that she was "threatened with a miscarriage." He gave her laudanum, a preparation of opium, which stopped the pains. Two months later, she died and "a report was soon put in circulation that she had been killed as there had been a difficulty the day before between her and her mistress, who had stricken her several blows." The rumors gave rise to an autopsy, which revealed the fetus separated from the cord but no other injury, leading Harrison to find "an extra-uterine foetation of the ovarian class." This diagnosis presumably absolved the mistress of any responsibility for the slave woman's death. The circumstances were even more complex, however, as the woman's owner refused to pay the balance due for his recent purchase, "alleging that he had bought her and paid a high price for her, because of her pregnancy, and the future prospects of raising children from her." He claimed that "the woman was warranted to him sound . . . yet the seeds of death had been sown anterior to the purchase" and agreed to arbitration in the case. Harrison recounted the testimony given in the suit, which turned on questions of the signs and definition of pregnancy as well as whether the woman's stated claim to the doctor that she was pregnant could be considered. The court decided that the woman had been sound and pregnant, and so the new owner was obligated to pay the balance of her cost.[56] Determining whether a slave woman was pregnant or not was significant in part because her fertility added to her value. In addition, pregnant slaves could be given a stay of execution until they delivered the child, making the determination of pregnancy literally a life-or-death matter.[57]

Physicians like Harrison who were called upon to adjudicate pregnancy as well as treat women in apparent need of medical attention relied on the expertise of others even as they sought to develop their own. Textbook authors and medical educators were sensitive to this responsibility. Gunning Bedford, whose *Clinical Lectures on the Diseases of Women and Children* was widely read, wrote of a case of "concealed pregnancy in an unmarried woman." Bedford noted that "the question of the existence or non-existence of pregnancy is, under certain circumstances, one of the most embarrassing which . . . can be presented to the judgment of the physician." Bedford argued that physicians must "exercise a proper degree of vigilance," eliciting "the truth by all the means which are legitimately within reach." He impressed upon his students that they would "frequently be the sole arbitors, on whose decision must rest the honor of [their] patients, and on whose judgment must stand all that is sacred in life."[58]

Another textbook author, Robert Gooch, also wrote about the difficulties of determining whether a woman was pregnant. While women who relied on symptoms were right "in ninety-nine cases out of a hundred," he warned that "the symptoms are not infallible." His advice in doubtful cases was to "postpone giving a decisive opinion, till such time has elapsed as will enable you to ascertain" the causes of the woman's symptoms, specifically the seventh month. When dealing with unmarried women, Gooch advised prospective doctors not to give an opinion until six months from last menstruation, adding "do not believe one word they say. Listen to them as you would to a jockey praising his horse. . . . Never rely on the evidence of their tongues, but on that of their bellies."[59]

Both Bedford and Gooch urged young physicians to learn to read the evidence of the body in order to provide expert witness about its condition. Neither women's bodily perceptions nor their words could be trusted. Only they could decide whether a woman was pregnant, not pregnant, or suffered from an extrauterine pregnancy, tumor, or other anomalous state. Once again, the assumption of binary categories forced complex medical decision making about those apparently in between, decision making that as Gooch noted could easily have been avoided with the passage of time. In this case, women's ambiguous bodies contributed to the growing medicalization of pregnancy. If women could not be trusted to label their own status correctly without physicians' expertise, then pregnancy itself increasingly became defined as an illness requiring medical intervention.[60] By claiming authority over definitions of pregnancy, physicians also claimed authority over the course of that pregnancy, simultaneously enhancing their prestige and the number of their patients. While a few expressed a degree of anxiety about the responsibility imposed upon them by having to make decisions about pregnancy, most recognized that the right to make such decisions allowed them to define social order. Women's disorderly bodies might be confusing, but physicians viewed disciplining them into appropriate categories as part of their social responsibility as well as a sign of their medical expertise. Such distinctions were particularly important in the South, where a slave woman's value to her owner could easily depend on her ability to reproduce.

Women whose pregnancies were not in question could still present perplexing difficulties to doctors eager to make sense of their ambiguous bodies. Sometimes, the length and nature of gestation seemed to be questionable, as when North Carolina physician W. P. L. Jennings was called to attend a slave woman. She claimed to have "conceived some twelve months previous; and about the ninth month, according to her calculations, she felt some symptoms of labor, which soon vanished." Since she had five living children and "was a woman of unusual good sense for a negro," Jennings believed her at first, "but finally came to the conclusion that she had not given me a fair statement of her condition from conception to its terminus." His best guess was that she had experienced an extrauterine pregnancy. He remained puzzled until six years later when he was called to attend the woman for a violent attack of "cholic." At that time, he found two bones of an infant in her feces. After her death two years later, an autopsy revealed the infant "in a state of perfect preservation" in her uterus, except for "the bones passed by the bowels."[61] Another North Carolina doctor used elaborate calculations to "furnish conclusive evidence, that gestation may be prolonged to thirteen, if not sixteen, days beyond the usual period." In this case, he believed the woman, who was white and "of unexceptional character" and "above suspicion."[62] The range of normal human gestation could be either very rigid or quite flexible, depending on which of these two positions seemed most convincing.

In other instances, doctors struggled to make sense of women whose twins had different fates. Often, one twin died in utero while the other was born alive at full term, again making women's bodies rather confusing to doctors trying to define what was normal. A Georgia physician, S. N. Harris, reported attending a slave woman who gave birth to "a rather small, but healthy male child." When Harris removed the placenta, he found "enveloped in its membranes, a small foetus, of about the third month." The "blighted foetus" was "perfectly" preserved, "although compressed and distorted by the growth of the living child."[63] Dr. J. Douglass reported on a similar case, in which a white woman suffered an abortion of a three-month-old fetus, then six months later delivered "a fine, healthy child."[64]

The slave woman Elias Horlbeck attended in 1847 did not experience such a positive outcome. He reported that Maria was "ill with an alarming flooding which had been brought on from undue exertion" while she was "supposed to be about two months advanced in pregnancy." He assumed that she had miscarried, but nearly four months later Maria delivered both "a well grown foetus of between five and six months" and another "presumed from its development to be about six weeks old." He offered two theories to explain "their different degrees of development." One explanation was that the twins were "originally conceived" and that the smaller "was blighted or arrested in its growth and remained unchanged until both were discharged." Horlbeck's preferred explanation was that of "superfoetation"—that is, a second pregnancy separately conceived within a single uterus. He had read of approximately fifty cases of "superfoetation" in women with "a double uterus, having separate openings into the vagina." He knew that "no theory as yet advanced, is adequate to explain such a phenomenon in the normal condition [that is, a single uterus]; superfetation being opposed by material obstacles, insurmountable in the present state of the science." Even though no one knew how "fecondation of the ovule" occurred, Horlbeck thought "deviations from the regular order" were possible to explain Maria's experience.[65]

All of the physicians who tried to define the limits of a normal pregnancy sought in the process to define a normal woman's body. Recognizing the limits of their knowledge of reproduction, doctors nevertheless were sure that babies were normally born after nine months and did not remain preserved in the uterus; that the uterus was normally single, not double; and that twins were normally born or miscarried together. Their eagerness to report exceptions in medical journals is eloquent testimony once again to their willingness to probe women's bodies in order to classify them as normal and abnormal, enhancing their cultural right to define them in the process.

## Maternal Influence

Even when a woman's pregnancy could be assured and its status presumed to be normal, her body and mind existed in a complex and ambiguous relationship to the developing fetus. For many physicians, the debate centered around the nature of the mother's influence on the unborn child. While few physicians doubted that the health of the mother influenced that of her fetus, debate raged about the extent of such influence. For generations, folk wisdom claimed that the strong emotions a woman experienced during pregnancy would influence her child. Fear, shock, horror, surprise could all leave their mark, or so people believed.[66] Physicians entered this debate at midcentury with their usual mixture of claims to medical expertise and moral and social responsibility, urging on women a set of behaviors designed to ensure the health of their offspring. The language of their debate varied. Some wrote of prenatal influences, others of the inheritability of acquired characteristics. Unable or unwilling to view the pregnant woman and her developing child either as one body or as two, mid-nineteenth-century physicians struggled to make sense of the relationship between them. The debates shed light on their continuing confusion about how best to distinguish and to classify individual bodies.

Physicians who debated prenatal influences did so almost exclusively in terms of white women's bodies. Although their discussions rarely identified race except when presenting a specific case, the tenor of their writing suggests that they had only white women in mind. The possibility that any aspect of slavery could harm a developing fetus did not specifically occur to them. Even when pregnant slaves were forced to dig holes in which to lie to protect their swollen bellies while they were being beaten, or kicked or lashed into miscarriage,[67] physicians remained silent. Their silence perhaps reflects their conviction that black women's bodies were closer to those of animals than to white women's, and so less liable to the influence of the emotions. At the same time, the question of prenatal influence was particularly salient in the South, where white women's bodily vulnerability contrasted so vividly with slaves' presumed sturdiness. Physicians concerned about the health of white babies wanted to protect them from the harmful consequences of their mothers' experiences, while not simultaneously offering a justification for cossetting slaves.

Self-styled medical reformers were particularly sensitive to the operation of prenatal influences on white women's bodies, albeit without naming them as white. A Thomsonian physician noted that "much depends upon the health of the mother during utero-gestation." He warned prospective parents to avoid "a luxurious, effeminate or intemperate course of life."[68] Similarly, an anonymous author wrote of "a young female of some distinction" who corsetted herself so tightly that "she became hump-shouldered, and died in consumption." She "left an infant son, who, from the slenderness of his frame and the delicacy of his constitution, is threatened with his mother's complaint. He inherited her *corset-broken* constitution."[69] There were, however, limits to the reach of prenatal influence. One rather defensive Thomsonian physician felt compelled to refute the claim of a "professor of midwifery" who had "positively asserted that if the mother made use of our medicines during gestation, the fetus would be born without skin and scalped, as though it had been taken as an enemy by the Indians!" He noted that "such is not the fact, . . . and his prognostication was never verified by a single instance."[70]

Another botanic physician, Dr. J. R. Lasseter of Georgia, explained more fully the ways in which mothers could influence their offspring. He considered "the character of parents, both mental and corporeal" to be "entailed upon their offspring." If the mother had "a weak, delicate, and irritable body," her children were "apt to inherit the same." Lasseter attributed "many deformities and premature births" to the "unnatural condition of the mother." Such problems would be prevented, he suggested, if the mother would "avoid all emotional excitements of the mind; such as anger, fear, grief, &c., which exert a powerful and deleterious influence upon the bodily functions" as well as "all causes of a violent and of a mechanically injurious character." Lasseter was unusual in acknowledging that these prescriptions were "frequently difficult to maintain" because of life's difficulties and "the unusual anxiety that females feel while in this condition," which render them "more susceptible to the influence of exciting causes." Even so, he insisted, the "knowledge of the injury that results from a violation of these rules" should inspire them to "control their feelings."[71]

Lasseter believed that mothers also influenced their offspring during lactation, although not as strongly as during pregnancy. He claimed that the same emotional excitements that could harm the fetus "will alter or modify the secretion of milk . . . and impart to it a property that will cause disease and death." Women who became excited in spite of their best efforts should not nurse in that state, "but wait until it subsides and nature has time either to modify or free the secretion of its poison." Lasseter believed that "the peace and happiness" of children and parents depended upon the woman's ability to control her passions and "maintain that health of body and state of mind most desirable for her offspring."[72] Like the other physicians who wrote about maternal influences, Lasseter did not discuss the dangers babies faced from slave mothers who often had no choice but to nurse hurriedly and when overheated from work.[73]

Dr. Turck, who like Lasseter published in the *Southern Medical Reformer,* wrote of the way the "'longings' of pregnant females, accords to the mind a remarkable and sometimes fatal influence upon their yet unborn offspring." While he recognized that some physicians rejected this belief in spite of its widespread popular support, he considered that "at the present day . . . the popular view is considered as being more in harmony with the facts." He explained this influence in terms of the "nervous or electrical action of the mother upon her offspring" and urged acceptance of these views "to prevent the formation of monsters as far as possible." In addition, he thought that children would benefit from properly directing the mother's imagination and urged "commenc[ing] education with conception."[74]

A regular physician, Thomas L. Ogier, also recognized the importance of prenatal influences on the developing child's intellectual abilities. He noted that "the offspring most generally resembles the father, yet it often bears a strong likeness to the mother" and offered examples of this from both animals and human beings. Committed to "the improvement of mankind," Ogier used ideas of hereditary predisposition to justify his belief "that females should be well educated, that their good qualities may be transmitted to their offspring."[75]

Ogier was not alone among regular physicians in expressing his belief in the importance of hereditary predisposition, although few followed his lead in advocating women's education for this reason. As early as 1838, Milton Antony, professor of obstetrics at the Medical College of Georgia, considered the question posed to him by the Medical Society of Augusta concerning whether a woman's mental or physical state could "exercise any important influence on the foetus in utero." He considered the possibility of the mother's physical influence to be "settled beyond the reach of controversy," claiming that she could pass along both physical characteristics and diseases such as smallpox, measles, and syphilis.[76]

Antony considered the question of "transcendental anatomy" to be more complex, dividing it into the categories of "monsters by excess," "monsters by default," and "monsters without excess or default, but with peculiarity of structure or function." After distinguishing these categories and struggling with the nature of cause and effect, predisposing and remote influences, and the like, he concluded that the mind could have "ultimate physical effects" on the fetus. Not only were the facts "too common and too well characterized to leave a doubt" that maternal impressions could produce "anomalous appearances," but "women of the best intelligence and observation . . . confirmed the fact of the *sequence* of the phenomena" so accurately that it could not be disputed.[77] The fact that his view, like that of Turck, reinforced popular opinion rather than challenging it suggests how tentative scientific claims to legitimacy still were in American society and how thoroughly imbued with popular understanding supposedly objective observers could be.

William Hauser, professor of physiology and pathology at the Oglethorpe Medical College in Georgia, was likewise convinced of the importance of prenatal influences, drawing upon history rather than popular opinion for evidence. He noted that in ancient Greece, pregnant women kept "statues of the gods and goddesses in their bed-rooms, that they might worship them, and look long, lovingly, and frequently upon forms so perfect in all that was beautiful, noble, and divine, that their future offspring might receive the full impress of these divinities." He considered this practice "the reason why the ancient Greeks were born heroes and heroines" and their forms and faces seen as "the most perfect of any the world has ever seen." He thought that children born to mothers "who live in peace, plenty, and in social and religious enjoyment during the period of maternity" would be markedly different from those whose mothers spent their pregnancies "vexed, grieved, tortured . . . and . . . always unhappy." In spite of the "scoffings" of well-known obstetricians, Hauser was convinced that "in all ages, mankind has been forced to recognize mother marks on children."[78]

Physicians often reported in medical journals on the births of children they considered to have been marked prenatally by their mothers' experiences. In 1826, Dr. Charles Atkins wrote of a fourteen-year-old "mulatto girl" who since infancy was "incapacitated from discharging the ordinary avocations of life, from a defect of intellect and want of control over the muscles of volition." He reported that her mother saw "a similar object in the latter months of her pregnancy with this child."[79] Over twenty years later, Dr. Francis Peyre Porcher, a respected and erudite Charleston physician, wrote about a young white woman with eight toes on one foot and nine on the other as well as six fingers on her right hand and noted "the deformity was anticipated by the mother before the birth of her child." The mother, "naturally of a nervous temperament," had seen an elephant at the zoo, which "produced an exaggerated impression." The mother's "attention being particularly attracted to the size of the feet, the dread of some similar monstrosity formed the constant object of her thoughts during her waking moments, both day and night." Porcher noted that "frequent verifications" had "forced physiologists to look with more respect upon the effects produced by the mind, volition, thought and ceaseless anxiety upon the development of the fetus—once only ridiculed as the foreboding of superstitious old women or sensitive females."[80]

Physicians who were aware of these debates and skeptical of conventional wisdom nevertheless struggled to make sense of the anomalous births that they witnessed. Dr. E. V. Culver noted the "difference of opinion among the members of the medical profession for centuries, as to the cause of *monstrosities,* or irregular births." He considered it would "be presumption in me to offer an opinion upon such a subject," yet "without even presuming to form any conclusion in a matter so mysterious," offered information about a white woman's pregnancy with her thirteenth child. After a difficult labor, she gave birth to a stillborn child "with no part I could call a head" and only a quarter of a face. Culver noted that "the lady is unable to call to mind any instance in which she has been much alarmed," adding "the only thing of any note that has a bearing upon the case" was "pain and uneasiness on the right side" while horseback riding. "She says she has no doubt from her sensation, that the back part of the head of the foetus was firmly united to the right side near the stomach, and that she knew when it separated."[81]

Other physicians were more skeptical. When one reported the birth of a child with no right hand after the mother "was badly frightened by what she supposed to be one of her children cutting off the hand of another," the editor of the journal to which he wrote labeled it "doubtless a case of spontaneous intrauterine amputation, caused by the cord being wound around the wrist." The editor similarly attributed the birth of a "child with a deformed nose, which was in exact resemblance to that of an unfortunate girl's who lived next door, who had cancer of the nose" to "a case of incomplete development, which occasionally occurs as freaks of nature." He added wryly that he hoped "our women are not going to reproduce all the deformities they see."[82]

The births of other children with anomalously formed bodies raised equally perplexing issues. Two physicians from Savannah, Alexander Nicoll and Richard Arnold, reported to the Medical Society of Georgia that they were called on "to examine a female negro child" born a month premature, "to give our opinions whether violence had been used or not, which in consequence of the singular appearance it presented, was supposed by those who attended at the delivery." A "superficial examination" allowed them to pronounce "that no violence had been used to destroy the child, but that it was a monster of an interesting character." An autopsy revealed that the child had no brain. They noted that "the history of the mother affords no clue in this case," with "nothing pecul[i]ar during this pregnancy" or delivery. After studying the body in detail and comparing it with other such "monsters," the physicians concluded that embryos with "imperfect formation" are "*in all cases, primarily of the female sex,*" although they could not explain why.[83] Their conclusion perhaps paralleled those of doctors called upon to classify intersexed bodies, who regularly labeled them female, especially when the body in question was also black.

H. V. M. Miller, professor of physiology and pathological anatomy at the Medical College of Georgia, offered an "account of a case of double monstrosity," two-year-old conjoined twin girls born to a slave woman. Miller noted that "in the olden time each monstrosity was considered as the presage of some public or private misfortune, an example of Divine vengeance, the effect of witchcraft or the result of diabolical or beastly intercourse." However, he added, "in more enlightened modern times . . . the origin of monstrous births is still enveloped in great mystery," but now physicians look "to some original malformation in the germ from which they spring" or subsequent development, rather than "supposing sexual intercourse with the devil, copulation with beasts or with menstruating women."[84]

Miller knew that older explanations for the birth of what he called monsters could not be valid, but he was unable to offer a convincing alternative. Like many other physicians, he was reasonably sure that something in the mother's experience could be said to have an influence on the developing child, but what that something was or how to understand it was not clear. This uncertainty about the origins of bodily anomalies, like that about other forms of ambiguous bodies, reflects the era's confused thinking about reproduction and about what we now term genetics. For physicians determined to offer the best advice that they could to pregnant women, hedging their bets seemed the best solution to the problem of prenatal influences, especially since public opinion was so convinced of their existence. Physicians unable to offer a satisfactory alternate explanation had little choice but to accede to the popular view and at the same time maintain their credibility. As a result, while continuing to search for a better explanation, most were willing to concede that the frightening sights and strong emotions a woman felt during gestation could harm her developing child. Like the Boston doctors whose debates on the subject they read about in the *Charleston Medical Journal and Review,* they remained uncertain about the impact of prenatal influences.[85]

That uncertainty led authors of domestic medicine to warn women to avoid situations that would be dangerous to their offspring. W. H. Coffin, the unfortunately named author of a medical advice book published in Virginia, stated that "no pregnant woman should witness scenes of suffering or distress; the death throes of a friend, the convulsions of children, or the gaping and bloody wounds of accidental or other causes." In addition, he warned, "they should not be present where others are in labor, . . . nor witness disgusting objects of any kind."[86] John Stainback Wilson told readers that "the mental hygiene of pregnant women is not less important than the physical," adding "violent mental emotions may arrest the proper growth of the child, and cause deformity" or death. He thought "the mind and morals of the future . . . depend greatly on the state of mind and the feelings of the mother during pregnancy."[87] While these authors may well have been hedging their bets, they clearly accepted prenatal influences as legitimate concerns for white women. They did not urge similar protections or warnings for black women.

If physicians struggled to develop a rationale for prenatal influences and to account for the birth of monsters, popular understanding was unequivocal. Few laypeople doubted that a woman's experiences and emotions could influence her unborn child, as frequent comments in their personal papers make clear. For example, when James Campbell wrote to his brother to announce the birth of another child, he noted that "the little fellow came into the world under unfavorable circumstances. His mother a few weeks before, had heard of the death of her brother by a blow on the head & it is a little remarkable that he groaned for 24 hours after his birth, precisely like a person, under the effects of a wound on the head." Campbell warned his brother not to allude to "the supposed cause of the child's indisposition, as it appears to wound my wife's feelings, . . . so much so, that she would not even name it to the attending physician."[88] Carolyn Clitherall's foot slipped as she stepped from a boat to the wharf, causing her to fall backward.

As she was "stunned" and pregnant, she spent a day quietly, then resumed her travels. A few days later, she gave birth prematurely to "a beautiful little girl" who had "a *deep indenture* in the back of its head," who subsequently died.[89] Meta Morris Grimball noted a bit of parish gossip in her diary. The woman, a doctor's wife, "drank" and used "stimulants," then died young. Grimball remarked that the woman "left 7 children inheriters of her habit, for I believe intemperance is inherited,—just as much as gout or scrofulous consumption."[90] Peninnah Minnir wrote her sister about another relative who had recently given birth but was close to death from consumption. The infant was also failing, suffering from "something alike the croup and has shrunk down to nothing" and sleeping all the time. Minnir added "it was a sweet little creature but I think the disease come in the world with it."[91]

Black medical care providers shared the perspectives of many of their white colleagues. Easter Sudie Campbell, who was born shortly after slavery ended and worked as a midwife for forty years, warned that "mothers oughter be more careful while carrying dar chilluns not ter git scared of enthing foh dey will sho mark dar babies wid turrible ugly things. I knows once a young wooman war expecting en she goes black-berry hunting en er bull cow wid long horns got after her en she was so scairt dat she threw her hands ober her head en wen dat baby boy war born he hed to nubs on his head jes like horns beginning ter grow." Campbell also delivered a white woman who "like hot chocolate en she alays wanted more she neber hed nuff of dat stuff en one day she spills sum on her laig en it jes splotched en burned her en wen dat gal war born she hed a big brown spot on her laig jes like her Mammy's scar frum de burn." Campbell added, "Now you see I noes yer ken mark de babies." She offered additional examples, including a "colored woman" given a hog liver by her employer even though "hit made her feel creepy all ober en dat night her baby war born a gal child en de print of er big hog-liver war standing out all ober one side of her face."[92]

Former slaves also believed that babies could be born with marks from their mothers and from the whites who beat them. Henrietta King, who had been born a slave in 1843 in Virginia, reported that Lucy, a slave on the next plantation, was beaten for refusing to go to work in the fields when she was in labor, because "dey thought dat huh time was way off an' dat she was jes' stallin' so as tuh git outa wukkin." King reported that the overseer "laid huh 'cross uh big tebaccy barrell an' he tuk his rawhide an' whupt huh somepin terrible." The next day, her daughter was born. King said that she saw with her own eyes that "dat chile's back was streaked wid raid marks all criss-cross lak" and added that Lucy died the next day.[93] Here, the mother's experience was visited upon the child not because of her own lack of control over her emotions, but rather over her body.

White physicians who had to compromise on the explanations they offered for prenatal influences in order to accommodate popular opinion were willing to use their expertise to avoid anomalies in the first place. For botanic physicians in particular, that could best be accomplished by avoiding potentially incompatible marriages. One noted that partners should be close in age, not related by blood, in good health, and adapted in mental qualities.[94] As late as 1859, another botanic physician defined a set of physiological laws derived from Galen's classification of human temperaments into "Sanguine, Bilious, Lymphatic and Melancholic." He noted that "when both of the parties to a sexual alliance are physiologically the same, there will be no progeny" and warned that incompatible combinations could result in unhealthy offspring.[95] More reputable physicians expressed similar views, including Milton Antony of the Medical College of Georgia. He, too, speculated on the impact of mixing the temperaments of the parents on their offspring. The temperaments were so different, "not calculated to harmonize in running along the stream of life, . . . that they are perfectly unfit to be joined in matrimony." Were people of different temperaments to marry, he suggested, there would undoubtedly be an impact on the nervous system of the fetus through "the physical operations of the organism."[96]

Only a few doctors sought to understand the impact of both parents' bodies on their children. A developing embryo's sex "is determined by the vigour and predominance of the male or female contribution," according to one medical student. The newly married, "ardent in their attachments," were more likely to have female offspring because the man was "extravagant in his enjoyments to so great a degree as never to allow himself to be in a vigorous state." The result was that "his contributions to the formation of a similar being [were] not so consentrated, abundant or vigorous, & of course, not so able to stamp, by its predominance over that of the female, his own sex in the tender embryo." However, "in more advanced life[,] the male seeks only to gratify his venerial appitite when forced by the presence of a more considerable and more energetic quantity of semen" and thus was "more apt to stamp, or impress, his own sex on his offspring."[97] Physicians eager to avoid having their patients give birth to monsters—or daughters—were seldom reluctant to offer advice on how to accomplish their goals. They were, however, quite reluctant to address similar issues of compatibility between parents when it came to their slave patients. To do so would have raised the question of slave breeding, a politically dangerous topic in an era of abolitionist scrutiny and one that could easily have undermined their efforts at professional credibility.

Physicians' efforts to understand reproduction and the female bodies that accomplished it simultaneously reinforced their understanding of the importance of the differences between men and women and extended their control over the latter group. By defining women's very bodies as permanently ambiguous, they categorized them as problematic, fit subjects of medical authority. Physicians saw women as vulnerable, as subject to physical disorder, and yet as powerful, because they had so much influence over the unborn. Women's vulnerability as well as their power over the next generation allowed physicians to consider themselves responsible for understanding women's bodily state. In the process, doctors blamed women for the errors of their bodies and minds while rejecting the possibility of women's subjective understanding of them.

Physicians who wrote about women's ambiguous bodies wrote most frequently about white women, for whom the possibility of bodily subjectivity stemmed from the fact of their whiteness. However, in the physicians' views, their ambiguity defined their subjectivity, placing them between white men (whose bodily subjectivity was not in question) and slaves (who had no right even to bodily integrity, much less subjectivity). Physicians who understood women's bodies in this way were not so much concerned with distinguishing women's bodies from one another across racial differences as they were with emphasizing their differences from men, defining them as both different and lesser in the process. Ambiguous female bodies were inferior bodies that did not fit neatly into categories and whose place in society had to be defined, restricted, and reinforced by medical expertise.

Physicians concerned about ambiguous bodies of all sorts, whether mixed race, mixed sex, or female, were engaged in the process of establishing categories and fixing individuals within them. Their efforts reinforced their authority as physicians as well as their influence on southern ideologies of race and sex. While their thinking reflects a degree of intellectual integrity, if only because they were willing to raise such issues in the first place, it was also self-serving since doctors were claiming the role of biological arbiters for themselves. As a result, physicians could function as moral and social arbiters as well, defining the very nature of bodies and establishing normative categories. By seeking to eliminate ambiguity, or at least to confine it, they sought to eliminate the possibility of social disorder, a goal especially valued in a society facing external threats and fearing internal chaos. Devoted to developing their understanding of scientific truth, their biology nevertheless existed in the service of the ideology necessary to a slaveholding society predicated on underscoring race and sex differences. By claiming the responsibility to define and to treat nonconforming bodies and minds, physicians reinforced the importance of conformity to the very categories they had helped create.

# CHAPTER 5

# The Examined Body

For antebellum southern physicians and laypeople alike, no matter what their race or sex, defining the characteristics of the physical body, even a normal one, was insufficient for a complete understanding of its function and experience. Everyone recognized that bodies were influenced by the minds that were encased within them just as those minds were influenced by the bodies they inhabited, although they would have used different language. As a result, they believed the relationship between mind and body influenced every aspect of experience, whether physical or emotional. Yet minds were not just minds in the abstract; like the bodies surrounding them, they were raced, sexed, and placed. As a result, physicians and laypeople of all sorts in the South were intent on understanding the ways in which body influenced mind and mind influenced body in their particular social, political, and economic context. Such an understanding offered a way of thinking about a variety of perplexing problems and solutions to some of the dilemmas facing them in a racially and sexually bifurcated society.[1] Only by examining their patients' bodies and their minds in the context of their race, sex, and place could physicians hope to cure their ills.

By the mid-nineteenth century, doctors increasingly relied on direct examination of their patients' bodies in order to diagnose their ailments and determine proper treatment. While some physicians were still willing to offer advice long distance, to people whose bodies they never saw or touched but whose symptoms were described in letters, more and more often they recognized that direct contact with the suffering individual was necessary. Although few doctors as yet relied on instruments to measure any part of the body or enhance their own sensations of its functioning, they wished to touch the actual body, to feel the pulse and see the tongue. Such examinations also allowed them to observe the patient's behavior, helping them evaluate mind as well as body. The examined body was one whose mind and flesh were exposed to medical inquiry and subject to medical judgment.

Exploring connections between mind and body offered physicians in particular a mechanism for understanding the individual nature of disease as well as their own role in diagnosing and curing it. If individual bodies suffered individually, according to their specific characteristics, then understanding the connection between mind and body could help explain that particularity. Physicians in all parts of the country struggled to come to terms with these matters. They sought to understand the ways in which individuals' beliefs about illness and their bodies influenced the nature and course of their experience. They tried to make sense of the ways in which belief in the efficacy of a cure and the skill of a physician could shape the outcome, what we would today call the placebo effect. They sought to understand the influence they had as physicians to shape the experience of illness as well as the limits of that influence, grappling with such complex matters as modesty and when and how to examine patients, particularly women suffering from gynecological complaints; what and how much to tell patients afflicted with incurable diseases; and when to believe patients' accounts of illness as opposed to the evidence of their own examinations. Such questions were particularly difficult when the patient was a white woman, since physicians believed that women could rarely be trusted to provide accurate accounts of their own bodily experiences. But the questions took an even more troubling turn in the South, where so many of the physicians' patients were slaves and so, according to the racial assumptions of whites, could not be trusted at all.

Physicians throughout the nation were committed to untangling the connections between mind and body in part because they believed that those connections influenced the course and outcome of disease. They accepted the prevailing assumptions that health was linked to happiness, that soundness of mind and body were connected. But they also knew that as physicians, determining the exact nature of those connections was central to their mission. Successful practice, they believed, depended upon manipulating the connection between mind and body to enhance their own authority in the sickroom, which would then help their patients become well. Even more important was their commitment to understanding the ways in which patients' beliefs about the body contributed to their experience of illness. While few physicians were willing to argue that such beliefs were the sole or even necessarily the primary determinant of what happened during illness, they were certainly convinced that belief mattered and that, as physicians, they had a responsibility to consider and shape that belief. As was evident in the discussion of prenatal influences in chapter 4, they sought to characterize and understand that connection; few were willing to challenge its existence altogether. According to an anonymous writer in the *Charleston Medical Journal and Review,* the "nature of man" was composed of body, mind, and moral principle, which "are so inseparably interwoven, that we must study each, in order to understand the working of the whole." He added, "From the relation and dependence of these three parts in health, derangements in one must affect the others, so that medicine must extend its jurisdiction over the whole nature of man; and from no other source can human nature derive more aid in its approaches towards perfection."[2] Yet physicians also knew that such connections had limits and that the body sometimes operated independently of the mind. One noted that "the workings of a strongly excited mind may produce very great changes in the body, either immediate or remote," but he added that "this power of the mind is circumscribed within a limited circle." He wondered, "[W]ho, by an effort of his mind, could place another hair on his head, or add a cubit to his stature?"[3] Physicians believed that part of their responsibility was in mapping the limits of that circle.

Physicians' commonplace understandings of the connections between mind and body led many of them to define an expanded role for themselves as mediators of health. Convinced that they knew best how to define healthy living and cultivate the happiness it could bring, they increasingly took on the task of telling people how to behave. They did so in part because of their determination to professionalize medicine and enhance their own authority as well as that of the science they were convinced supported their claims. But they also did so because of their belief that mind influenced body, that people who controlled not only their behavior but also their emotions would lead healthier and happier lives. Physicians saw themselves as uniquely positioned to impart this wisdom to their patients, whose illnesses were obvious proof that their minds and bodies were not functioning properly. In the antebellum South, the advice they offered was filtered through their assumptions about the ways in which mind and body interacted with each other as well as proper behavior for men and women, white and black. As a result, the health advice they offered was tailored to the race and sex of their patients as well as their individual characteristics of mind and body. Physicians took seriously their roles as mediators of their patients' health, becoming ever more thoroughly convinced that they alone possessed the information necessary to construct the ideal life for everyone.

The mediating role adopted by antebellum physicians could clash sharply with the assumptions of their patients, who were often reluctant and sometimes unable to follow the advice they were offered; slave patients rarely got to decide without interference from their masters. Patients were not accustomed to having doctors diagnose their ailments as influenced by their emotions, even though common parlance loosely identified such causes. As a result, they behaved often enough in ways that today's physicians would term noncompliant and that provoked frustration among those of their own day. However, given the presence of competing medical sects, mid-nineteenth-century patients had even less commitment than people do today to accept the dictates of physicians whose assumptions about the origins of their illnesses they found unconvincing. Physicians were sometimes forced to negotiate both the diagnosis of the problem and the nature of its treatment with their patients, recognizing that patients who were told that their illness was under the influence of their minds were not likely to accept their doctors' conclusions. As a result of such negotiation, which if unsatisfactory could lead to patients in effect taking their business elsewhere, physicians had to frame their conclusions about the nature of individual illness with great care. As a general rule, they were far less tentative, far more successful in making their claims about the influence of mind on body and body on mind when the bodies in question were black, female, or both. As the most vulnerable members of society, already deemed weaker in mind and body than white men, these groups frequently found themselves subject to physicians' efforts to mediate their activities and unable to negotiate with them about diagnosis or treatment from a position of strength.

Throughout the antebellum years, physicians' acceptance of old categorizations of healthy bodies as balanced among the four humors (black bile, yellow bile, phlegm, and blood) was waning almost to extinction. Nevertheless, physicians were loath to abandon the connection between those humors and the four temperaments with which they were associated (melancholic, choleric, phlegmatic, and sanguine). These notions, particularly the ways in which the temperaments influenced the diagnosis and prognosis of disease, were still widely current among practicing physicians, who used them to explain the ways in which the mind influenced the body. Patients who were melancholic in temperament, for example, were subject to characteristic illnesses that were best treated by the use of tonics and other mechanisms for strengthening the liver. Persons of phlegmatic temperament likewise needed treatments appropriate to purging the body of excess phlegm and other forms of congestion.[4] Such assumptions are widely seen in the case reports physicians submitted to medical journals.

Even more directly, physicians believed that the weaker bodies of white women and people of African descent were more likely to be influenced by their emotions than were those of white men. White men, by virtue of their race and sex, were assumed to be more able to control their emotions than the other categories of people in the population and thus their bodies were less liable to the negative influence of their minds. For white women and all blacks, however, mental weakness led to bodily susceptibility just as the body's vulnerabilities caused them to be weak-minded and weak-willed. As usual, however, physicians considered these problems in racial terms first. They wrote about the ways in which women's bodies and minds influenced each other primarily in terms of white women, while the shortcomings of blacks were considered in less overtly gendered terms than those of whites. White women's racially superior minds nevertheless could be a source of harm for the bodies surrounding them, while black women's inferior minds helped protect them from disease. In this as in so many other aspects of their practice, southern physicians created complex intellectual dilemmas that forced them to work hard to avoid inconsistency even as they allowed them to reinforce the region's race and sex hierarchies.

Just as physicians sought to understand the ways in which mind and body influenced each other physiologically, they simultaneously tried to explain the ways in which illnesses (affections or derangements, in their parlance) in individual organs of the body influenced other organs not directly connected. Physicians believed that the concept of sympathy governed all bodies. In fact, they sometimes considered the mutual influences of body and mind as simply a special case of sympathy, between a specific organ and the brain. For example, they believed that sympathy between the stomach and brain meant that they directly influenced each other, so that dyspepsia[5] was aggravated as much by one's personality, habits, and emotions as by what one ate. Samuel Jennings listed as its causes "indolence, intense study, grief, anxiety of mind, diarrhoea, abuse of alcoholic drinks, excessive use of strong tea, coffee, &c. chewing or smoking tobacco, and in delicate persons insufficient clothing, or a residence in the basement story of a house or other damp situation."[6] However, in active practice, doctors were convinced that the concept of sympathy was most readily apparent in the ways women's reproductive organs, especially the uterus and to a lesser extent the ovaries, influenced and were influenced by their brains. That sympathy was most apparent in white women and during menarche, menstruation, pregnancy, childbirth, lactation, and menopause, although it could occur at any time.

Not only did physicians often consider each of the reproductive functions illnesses in themselves, they also were convinced that they could cause illness in other parts of the body, including mental illness. At the same time, they believed that women's feelings, attitudes, and emotions during the workings of these functions shaped their experience of them. As a result, doctors both attributed many kinds of illness located in various parts of the body to women's reproductive organs and warned women that their thoughts could quite literally make them (or their offspring) sick.

As usual, physicians writing about women meant white women unless they specified otherwise. The extent to which black women's reproductive organs existed in sympathy with their brains, and their reproductive functions influenced and were influenced by their emotions, was considered similar but not identical to those relationships in white women's bodies. For physicians determined to understand the links between mind and body and equally committed to curing the diseases of their (white) women patients, no matter what the disease might be or where it was located, reproductive organs and functions were the obvious place to start.

## Body, Mind, and Reproduction

Women's minds and bodies were first considered susceptible to the reciprocal influences of sympathy at menarche and during menstruation.[7] A Montgomery physician, H. R. Easterling, noted in the *Charleston Medical Journal and Review* that "many of the causes of a derangement" of menstruation "can be readily traced to the influence of the passions," which in turn caused "excruciating, and almost insupportable suffering to the patient."[8] This problem could easily be seen in accounts of individual patients. James Green, a Macon, Georgia, physician, recognized it in his twenty-four-year-old white patient E. T., whose good health was destroyed by "an act of imprudence" at age fifteen, when she waded into a pond up to her hips. As a result, "her first menstrual flow . . . was suppressed, and she was seized the same night with convulsions—of a hysterical character I suppose—and has had them frequently since."[9] At least some southern physicians were willing to attribute black women's sufferings from menstrual irregularities to the same interrelated emotional and physical causes as they did white. South Carolina physician John Douglass wrote about a thirty-year-old slave patient whose "menstrual irregularity, or other utero-ovarian derangement" he attributed to "her dissipated habits," even though he also felt a tumor in her ovary.[10] Douglass was not the only physician who believed that a woman's emotions or behavior caused the physical difficulties she experienced, even when biological explanations were simultaneously present. Such comments were commonly made in the case histories presented in the medical journals.

Imprudent behavior and dissipated habits were not the only ways in which mind and body interacted during menstruation. Fear also played a role. According to Milton Antony, an eminent Georgia physician and professor of midwifery and diseases of women and children at the Medical College of Georgia, "the severe influence of fear" was one cause of obstructed menstruation,[11] although he did not specify the nature of that fear.[12] Another Georgia physician, J. A. Hamilton, was willing to define the nature of at least one woman's fear. He wrote of a young white woman who suffered "extreme and alarming distress" as a result of prolonged dysmenorrhea,[13] a distress so great that it caused "great apprehension of death."[14] Yet another Georgia physician, writing nearly twenty years after Antony and Hamilton, noted that the "quantity of the menstrual discharge" is affected by "the emotions and passions of the mind." He noted that women should avoid "every kind of mental or corporeal agitation, or the process may be impeded, or hysterical or other unpleasant affections be excited."[15] Those affections could be unpleasant indeed. A Virginia physician attributed a young woman's "epileptic convulsions . . . of the most violent character" to four months of "amenorrhoeal[16] suffering."[17]

Many physicians agreed with the assumption that menstruation was closely linked to hysteria, epilepsy, and other illnesses that blurred the line between mind and body and voiced their warnings to women quite directly.[18] The author of one manual of domestic medicine told women that suspended menstruation of long standing could cause "hysterical symptoms," while another noted that it was caused by "passions of the mind" and could in turn cause "various hysteric . . . symptoms."[19] A third attributed it to "mental shock" and claimed it could cause "fever, headache, thirst, and sick stomach" and even "acute inflammation of the womb, or some of the vital organs."[20] Menstruation that was not suppressed was equally dangerous, according to J. Hume Simons, also the author of a domestic medicine manual. He warned that "the monthly courses" could cause "craziness, fits, and a loss, for a time, of motion or feeling" as well as inflammation of the brain.[21] Likewise, Joseph Wright wanted the female readers of his book to know that "a dull disposition" at menarche could lead to "vapors and hysterics." Even after menstruation was well established, "the greatest attention ought likewise to be paid to the mind" because "anger, fear, grief and other affections of the mind often occasion obstruction of the menstrual flow which prove absolutely incurable." Suppressed menstruation was itself most frequently caused by "violent passions of the mind" and could lead to "violent hysterical affections." Wright suggested that "every method should be taken to amuse and divert the patient" along with "a soothing, and kind, affable behaviour to females in this situation," but he also prescribed a variety of medicines.[22]

Both menstruation itself and its irregularities influenced and were influenced by women's minds. The sympathy between brain and uterus meant that every aspect of women's bodies as well as their emotions, personalities, and behavior were subject to their interactions. As a result, even when menstruating women tried to subject their bodies to their conscious control, they were unlikely to be successful. As often as not, doctors believed, women's unruly menstruating bodies made it difficult for them even to try.

The close connection between women's bodies and minds and the circular reasoning of physicians regarding their ailments did not manifest themselves only in discussions of problematic menstruation. Pregnancy, too, demonstrated the ways in which mind and body could interact. According to one doctor, "the brain is especially the seat of disturbance in pregnant women, principally by sympathy directly with the uterus."[23] The consequences could be devastating for mother and child. Medical and lay debates about the ways in which women's frightening experiences and terrifying dreams could be transmitted to their children before birth have already been discussed, but this was by no means the only mechanism for mind and body to interact during pregnancy. In addition, miscarriage, tubal (ectopic) pregnancies, and convulsions could also be caused by a pregnant woman's mental state, just as they could cause her to become hysterical or insane. James Green, who blamed one patient's long-term hysterical convulsions on suppressed menstruation from wading in a pond, believed another's three miscarriages were "hastened by a fright or a severe exertion."[24] Writing about tubal pregnancies, Charleston, South Carolina, physician W. C. Horlbeck noted that they could be caused by "a powerful impression made on the mind," including "emotions or passions, such as sudden fear, great terror, [or] indignation."[25] Joseph Wright attributed convulsions during pregnancy to "increased irritability . . . communicated by sympathy from the womb to the brain" or "violent passions of the mind," among other possibilities.[26]

Even women with seemingly normal pregnancies could show the dangerous effects of interactions between mind and body. Milton Antony noted that "mental causes are often antecedent to the physical phenomena [of pregnancy], and indeed exert decided influence on the physical organization to the end of producing physical effects."[27] John Stainback Wilson emphasized the "mental hygiene of pregnant women," suggesting that "mental emotion" could cause heart palpitations, fainting fits, difficulty breathing, sleeplessness, headache, miscarriage, and gloomy forebodings that could cause them to "die of madness and convulsions." Their emotions could also influence the developing child by arresting its growth or causing deformity; he was sure "the mind and morals of the future . . . depend greatly on the state of mind and the feelings of the mother during pregnancy."[28] Botanic physicians held similar views. According to J. H. Lasseter of Georgia, a woman who had "her anger aroused frequently, or even occasionally during the term of her gestation" would reasonably find that "the same passions would be so completely interwoven in the delicate fiber of the foetus, as to manifest itself in a proportionate degree in active life." A woman who remained "calm, tranquil and humorous" throughout pregnancy would find "these happy impressions would be made upon the foetus, and become prominent traits in its character."[29] Not only did a woman's emotions influence her own body, they shaped the character of the child developing within it.

If a woman's emotions influenced the physical experience of her pregnancy, so, too, did they shape parturition. When James Mims's patient suffered swelling and difficulty breathing shortly before parturition, she was convinced she would never leave her bed. Mims "told her of everything I could favorable in her case, and seemed as cheerful as I possibly could," including telling her that "she would soon be through, and with judicious management would ultimately recover." He said "a merry heart doth good like a medicine, sayeth the sacred historian," and proclaimed:

> The power of words,
> And soothing sounds, appease
> The raging pain,
> And lessen the disease.

Mims's fearful patient survived the birth (and his poetry), although the child did not.[30]

Physicians believed that emotions could cause quite dramatic changes in a laboring woman's body, even though they recognized it as a natural process not directly under her conscious control. For example, the *Medical Journal of North Carolina* published an article by Tyler Smith in which he claimed that "a very powerful influence may be exerted upon the uterus by emotion. A fright, or any violent mental disturbance, may bring on labour prematurely, or produce abortion." He noted that "the different effects of hope or despair on the commencement, progress, and termination of labour, have frequently been remarked," adding that the very entrance of the physician into "the lying-in room may arrest the pains of labour for a time, through the influence of emotion."[31] T. Gaillard Thomas agreed, claiming that "*mental emotion* is a well known cause of suspension of uterine action, during the parturient process," so that sometimes if "a strange physician[,] a nurse who was not expected, or an unwelcome guest, enters the room, pains previously vigorous and frequent, vanish entirely."[32]

Women's inability to control their emotions during childbirth could have disastrous consequences. Samuel D. Gamble, a Georgia physician, believed that "difficult and protracted parturition is occasionally fatal" due to the intensity of pain. This could be the case even in more ordinary labors with an otherwise successful outcome because the woman "never rallied, either in strength or spirit."[33] Milton Antony described such a case, in which his patient D. B. died after a delivery marked by "great fright, agitation, and fatigue."[34] Joseph Eve likewise argued that "pain is a great source of danger, as it may destroy life directly, or indirectly, by inducing convulsions or other fatal affections." He noted that "it is a difficult question to determine how much pain is strictly physiological, or essential to parturition, and how much is the result of the unnatural and injurious habits and customs of civilized life." Eve used his concern about the dangerous consequences of pain to advocate for the use of chloroform during delivery.[35]

J. J. Robertson, also from Georgia, similarly encouraged the use of chloroform, claiming that it prevented one of his patients from experiencing what she usually did after childbirth: "an unusual degree of prostration which generally continued for several days, and on one occasion was quite alarming,—what is usually termed the 'nervous shock,' amounting to almost fatal syncope."[36] Robertson considered her "unusual prostration" to be "the legitimate result of severe pain" and the "great exhaustion of the nervous system" it caused. Robertson described another woman whose recovery from confinement was similarly "slow and protracted, owing to the shock given to the nervous system, and complete prostration by pain," who was also helped by chloroform. She had suffered from "a functional derangement" and hysterical convulsions during pregnancy, which made chloroform in his view "peculiarly applicable" because it "would not only exempt her from pain during labor, but also arrest those unpleasant symptoms, which it most effectually did."[37] Protheroe Smith, yet another advocate of painless childbirth, via ether, noted that with its use, "a case of puerperal mania was immediately and permanently relieved; and several cases of dysmenorrhoea have been recorded, in which this agent has acted like magic." He was aware that "the pain of labour (incomparably the greatest which human nature is called upon to bear)" was so intense that "its severity is very greatly dreaded, and the depression caused by the anticipation of its inevitable occurrence, preying for months upon the spirits, has been known to produce very injurious effects."[38] Only John Stainback Wilson thought "women can be delivered with very little pain," for when bodies were healthy and "organs perform their functions properly, every natural act is attended with pleasure." He offered as proof "the pleasurable sensations experienced in emptying the bowels and bladder, when all is right."[39] Few women were likely to experience this ideal; perhaps even fewer would have appreciated his analogy.

Fear of physical pain was not the only mechanism by which emotions and the body's processes influenced one another during childbirth. According to Jesse Beck, a botanic physician, a patient who was a slave experienced "considerable difficulty" during the delivery of her first child, "the difficulty probably being much enhanced by, if not entirely dependent upon deep grief on account of the supposition that she had lost her husband a few days previous to her confinement."[40] A difficult delivery could also cause insanity, as a Georgia botanic physician reported in the case of a woman who suffered convulsions and was unconscious even before her child was born dead. He reported that she "slowly regained her mind and health" after "becoming frantic at times" and appearing for "two or three days . . . to be bordering upon insanity." He thought her debility was the result of recalling "to mind that she had been pregnant" and being "informed that the child was born dead." The same doctor reported a case of "temporary mania" in a woman who "became wild and raving during the labor . . . but became rational as soon as the birth occurred." He thought "her mental perceptions . . . improved as her pains increased in force and frequency."[41] An allopathic physician believed that pregnancy itself, especially a woman's first, could be a source of insanity, because it caused "a highly excitable state of the nervous system," especially in "individuals of delicate constitutions, and predominant nervous temperament."[42] It is not surprising that these physicians appeared to blur the line between cause and effect in their discussion of the ways in which childbirth and a woman's emotional state influenced each other. For them, there was no line because cause and effect were fundamentally the same.

Understanding the cause and treatment of what physicians termed puerperal insanity or mania could be difficult. Samuel Jennings attributed it to the debility caused by the fetus's "mechanical pressure" on the viscera and recommended emetics "to improve the state of the nerves [and] to agitate and resuscitate the torpid viscera."[43] William B. Atkinson believed the disease was caused by "irritation . . . acting upon the brain, and general system of nerves of a subject, hereditarily disposed to insanity, or of an extremely sensitive and impressionable temperament." Or, he added, it could be "dependent on moral emotion." He did not doubt that "the disease is evidently one of irritation, implicating especially the brain and reproductive system." Atkinson recommended the use of opiates to encourage sleep, after which "the patient . . . is found much more tranquil and manageable." Since patients suffering from the disease showed "prominent and distressing" symptoms, including "delirium, incoherent talk, perverted sensations, and extreme despondency," finding an effective treatment was urgent. Otherwise, "the general nervous system" could become "greatly disordered and . . . hysterical."[44] Birthing women's reproductive organs could cause devastating illness, even death, and women's efforts at self-control seemed to doctors feeble in the face of their organs' powerful influence on the body.

The immediate postpartum period was also fraught with physical danger for women unable to control their emotions. T. Gaillard Thomas, who worried about the consequences of unexpected visitors to the lying-in room, also warned about "the advent of zealous but injudicious friends, just after labor, whose congratulations serve but to harass and excite the already exhausted woman." He thought this could cause her to hemorrhage. He urged his medical colleagues to "*enjoin perfect rest and exclusion of visitors*" if they wished to prevent "evil [to] the already hyperaesthetic nervous system of your patient, and produce a corresponding depression of nerve power." Rest and the exclusion of visitors would "avoid many chances of mental emotions of various kinds, which could only exert a deleterious influence upon your patient."[45] Alfred Folger, author of a manual of domestic medicine published in Charleston, was also quite concerned about the influence of visitors on the emotional and physical health of birthing women, noting, "Women in childbed, are often seriously injured by a great many females collecting in the room, and each one relating some dreadful circumstance, that had occurred to females in labor and afterwards." He added that "such imprudence as this, should always be avoided."[46] The author of another domestic medicine manual, J. Hume Simons, warned more directly that if a woman who had recently given birth "talks much," she was apt "to have fever."[47] All of these practitioners believed that there was a seamless correlation between a woman's behavior, her emotions, and the physical state of her body during pregnancy, childbirth, and beyond, with each influencing the other in ways that underscored women's physical and emotional vulnerability. Women's diseases themselves were sometimes granted agency in doctors' writings, as was "this cruel disease" puerperal fever,[48] which sometimes "pursued its course obstinately to a fatal termination, defying medical interposition, seeming only determined to sever the tenderest ties of the dearest of human associations."[49]

Those correlations and vulnerabilities extended to the body of her infant as well. Medical men of all sorts believed that a nursing woman's body was influenced by all of her emotions, not just those regarding the child, and the baby was in turn shaped not just by the nourishment she provided at the breast, but also by the state of her emotional life. A woman's very emotions, they believed, modified her milk in ways that could easily be deleterious to her child. A botanic medical journal noted that "imprudence, neglect, or anxiety on the part of the mother" induced "irritation and suffering in the child." The author warned of the dangers of "ordinary bad temper, especially near or during the time of sucking." He offered the example of a healthy infant who "became restless, panted, and sunk dead on its mother's bosom" moments after nursing, because she had just before "trembled from fear and terror" and then nursed the child in a "state of strong excitement."[50]

In the context of a discussion of the question "ought a physician to tell a patient that he is going to die," to which the general answer was no, T. Bullard remarked on the "wonderful connection and mutual dependence" of the nervous system on "all the functions of the organism." He offered as one example "the milk of the nursling mother, [which was] so changed by sudden anger or deadly fear as to produce convulsions, and death even, in the before perfectly healthy infant."[51] Milton Antony asked whether any physician who attended nursing women "has not observed the injurious effects of that milk on the child which was elaborated during fits of violent anger?" He recommended regard for "the temper . . . in selecting a wet nurse."[52] A. G. Goodlett also implicitly urged white women to use wet nurses, claiming that women with "delicate constitutions, subject to hysteric fits, or other nervous affections, make very bad nurses; and these complaints are now so common, that it is rare to find a woman of fashion free from them. Such women, therefore, supposing them willing, are really unable to suckle their own children."[53] While Goodlett worried about women of fashion, few physicians appeared to be concerned for the nursing infants of slave mothers, who were routinely sent back to the fields a few weeks after giving birth. Their overheated, ill-nourished, and often exhausted bodies certainly could prove injurious to their offspring, but physicians focused on white women's emotions tended not to notice.[54]

White women who were unable to control their emotions properly were a danger not only to their offspring but to themselves as well. Gunning Bedford, author of a widely read text on the diseases of women and children, offered the example of a woman whose youngest child was six months old, who had "headache, vertigo, extreme restlessness, and her mind rendered morbid by this general disturbance of the nervous system." He diagnosed her as suffering from "the disturbing influences of *undue lactation*," which "has seriously involved her nervous system." He warned that this malady could cause mania along with "functional and organic disease of the uterus, together with various nervous disturbances, such as hysteria, epilepsy, &c."[55] Robert Gooch, author of a similar text, believed that women "debilitated by nursing" were vulnerable to "mental derangement," which he diagnosed as melancholia rather than mania. He distinguished between the two by noting that in melancholia, "there was an incipient stage in which the mind was wrong, yet right enough to recognize that it was wrong."[56] What that meant in terms of the best practice for women caught between warnings of the dangers of nursing their own children and advice that they should do so he did not specify. In spite of the dangers nursing posed to women's and babies' health, both authors informed women that nursing was best for mother and child if performed under the correct circumstances, even as they lamented the weaknesses that kept so many women from conforming to them.

Even white women's sexuality was linked to dangerous conditions of mind and body. The author of a long list of "aphorisms on the hygiene & nursing of infants" included among them the suggestion that "a nurse should abstain from sexual intercourse, if she experiences great excitement," although he did not specify what the consequences of violating this rule would be for child or mother.[57]

More often, physicians' warnings concerned the dangerous physiological and emotional effects of unrestrained sexuality on the woman's body, whether or not she was nursing. One author concerned about what he called subacute ovaritis suggested that its predisposing causes included "marriage, by the repeated excitement to which it gives rise," and "indiscriminate sexual intercourse, as in the case of prostitutes." However, too little sexual activity was as dangerous as too much; another cause was "the privation of sexual congress in women whose carnal appetite is strong, or its sudden denial, as in young widows," or "marriage late in life." In addition, women with "nervous, irritable, hysterical and scrofulous constitutions are most liable." Whether women afflicted with subacute ovaritis experienced too much or too little sexual activity was evidently the result of circumstance or the wishes of their husbands; its sufferers repeatedly reported "the utmost aversion to the approach of the husband, whilst previously they had derived a great amount of pleasurable excitement from coitus." The treatments were as variable as the causes. Women who suffered from "the want of the appropriate stimulus to the ovaries" should be encouraged to marry, to prevent "their becoming the seat of morbid affections." On the other hand, if the disease were caused by coitus, "the husband should be forbidden the marital bed until the disease shall have been subdued."[58] There is, unfortunately, no way to know how his colleagues reacted to his seemingly contradictory advice or how actual men and women reacted to this diagnosis or recommended treatment. However, this physician's willingness to enter into the intimacy of the suffering woman's bedroom suggests the extent to which he accepted the role of mediator of appropriate behavior.

Paul Eve, professor of surgery at the Medical College of Georgia, similarly displayed ambivalence regarding the consequences of sexuality for women. In an essay urging his colleagues to abandon use of the pessary[59] for prolapsed uterus, he listed among the reasons both that "they interrupt sexual intercourse" and that "their use may lead to immorality."[60] Twenty years later, Joseph Eve, professor of obstetrics and diseases of women and children at the same institution, advocated the use of caustics (cauterization) in the treatment of uterine diseases. Among other advantages, cauterization made it "unnecessary to interfere with 'family affairs,'" since the couple "if sensible, . . . will at least be temperate, and if otherwise, injunctions would not avail." He added that "moderate indulgence does not appear to exercise an injurious influence, unless it excites pain or causes hemorrhage, which would be apt to result soon after cauterization, and which thus itself becomes, to some extent, a barrier to excess."[61]

Physicians were genuinely troubled by the dangerous consequences of excessive sexuality for the minds and bodies of their white female patients. While Joseph Eve seemed to consider sexual activity appropriate, although without specifying whether for women, men, or both, Joseph Wright considered at least "excessive venery" one cause of menorrhagia, or excess menstruation, and Robert Gooch considered it a specific disease with specific remedies. According to Gooch, "furor uterinus" paralleled "the frequent excitement of the sexual organs by onanism" in men and led to "the same disordered and debilitated state of health in the female."[62] John Stainback Wilson warned that women who suffered "itching of the privates" could find that "through sympathy . . . the sexual feeling is sometimes so much excited as to render seclusion necessary, while the unfortunate sufferer is tormented in a way that is revolting to modesty."[63] He evidently feared that discomfort would tempt women to scratch themselves in a way that paralleled masturbation.

If excessive sexuality could be dangerous, masturbation could have truly debilitating causes and consequences for mind and body. In 1825, the *Carolina Journal of Medicine, Science, and Agriculture* reported on a German girl who "had existed in a state of complete idiotism from a very early age," whose physicians believed was the victim of "corporeal disease" and thus "susceptible of cure." At fifteen, it "became necessary to confine her arms in bed, to prevent her from committing incessant masturbation." Because she had shown some mental improvement, "it became a matter of considerable importance to put an effectual stop to the vice, which would so certainly have been the cause of her remaining in a state of mental hebitude." Since other methods failed, the physicians resorted to "extirpation of the clitoris," and "her libidinous propensities gradually decreased. From this time her mental powers slowly improved" until eventually she could write and communicate. The doctors concluded "that idiotism is curable, if it is not dependent upon some congenital malformation" and "that onanism, particularly when caried [*sic*] to excess, will confirm a state of idiotism." Even so, they acknowledged that "the disgusting practice of masterbation [*sic*] undoubtedly confirmed the mental imbecility of the patient" but was not necessarily the primary cause, since "self-pollution could hardly have taken place at a very early age."[64] The confusion inherent in this analysis, like that evidenced by later medical authorities, suggests the difficulty physicians faced when trying to sort out the ways in which sexualized minds and bodies influenced each other.

Men could also harm their bodies through uncontrolled sexuality, although doctors were far less likely to suspect them of doing so than they were white women, even though women were assumed to be passionless. A Tennessee physician, J. A. Long, wrote of the difficulty he had diagnosing the disease from which "a young man . . . of rather delicate constitution" was suffering. First Long thought his patient was suffering an attack of "chill and fever," then "spinal *meningitis*" and "*nephralgia*." None of the medicines Long offered seemed to help, including large amounts of opium, so that "death seemed to be his inevitable doom." Finally, the patient himself asked about "*self-pollution*," which "immediately unriddled the mystery of the case." Long prescribed "a more nourishing diet," tonics, quinine, and iron, and "directed as much cheerfulness as possible on the part of the attendants," which led to immediate but slow and gradual improvement. Long reported that this was "the first case of the kind" he had encountered in eight years of practice. "By way of excusing himself," Long's patient told him of "another, equally guilty with himself, who had abandoned the practice on account of a severe spell of chronic *rheumatism*." Both men appeared the same: "downcast countenance, old look in the face, dejected spirits." Long considered the problem to be "of rare occurrence," presenting it because he "thought it would be instructive, especially to the junior readers of the journal." Even white men's bodies could occasionally fall victim to the passions of their minds, so doctors had to be told to look for the possibility. When questioned, Long's patient made "a full acknowledgement of the baneful practice," suggesting that he knew that he was harming himself.[65] Few doctors would have believed that women could share the same degree of self-awareness.

Even men who did not masturbate could be harmed by the uncontrolled interactions of their minds and bodies, although here, too, doctors had to be warned to look for the problem. According to Professor Trousseau of Charleston, impotence could cause in men "an entire loss of health for years, and even death," while physicians struggled with either "cruel misapprehension or . . . the complete cure of a disease apparently unconquerable." Trousseau defined impotence as "an involuntary flow of semen, a passing out of sperm without any erotic provocation, or at least without *sufficient* erotic provocation." Trousseau noted that "patients affected by seminal loss have a sad and morose disposition; they suffer from headaches, vertigo, weakness of sight, and often fall into a habitual state of hypochondriacal melancholy." As if that were not enough, they could also suffer "paralysis . . . and various nervous disorders." In order to cure the disease, he developed a plug to be inserted into the rectum to put pressure on the prostate, which "very often suffices, after a week or two, to check involuntary spermatic discharges, to restore to an impotent man his former virile aptitudes, and to prevent uncomfortable accidents to the moral and intellectual faculties." However, he warned fellow practitioners to "be on your guard against those patients who are very rapidly cured, who set up too soon the cry of victory" because men who once suffered from the disease "always run great risks, and if they are not careful, sooner or later may come the renewal of the infirmaties [*sic*]."[66]

As a medical student, R. T. Dismukes was also warned of the dangers of onanism, "a vice, to which a great many youth are addicted" that was "very destructive to mind and body." He was taught that "it is a much greater crime to commit onanism than to have connexion with women, for a person destroys both soul & body in one, & in the other the soul only." Doctors should "prescribe prudent sexual intercourse . . . for Philosophical reasons" to any patient "who commits the crime in his sleep," along with "the highest diet & least stimulating food." He did not specify who their sexual partners should be. In addition, "if not a married man, he by all means awt to get married."[67] Men who masturbated might harm their bodies by their failure to have sufficient control over their minds, but men who suffered from involuntary impotence, as Trousseau defined it, were to be pitied because they could not even control their bodies. It was little wonder that they were melancholy; their disease left both body and mind vulnerable to the influence of the other in spite of their best efforts. Men's sexual and reproductive bodies were not as troubling as women's, but only when men were able to maintain control. Doctors were convinced that most white men, most of the time, did so successfully.

Masturbation and impotence aside, none of these physicians considered the physical or emotional consequences of differences between the sexual desires and social circumstances of white men and women. Nor did they consider the ways in which the possibility of becoming or actually being pregnant might influence women's feelings about sexual intercourse. Instead, they implicitly assumed that women should be sexually available to their husbands and at the same time assigned to women the responsibility for maintaining the appropriate frequency of intercourse—whatever that might mean. Physicians recognized one goal of their therapeutic interventions was to ensure that women's sexual and reproductive organs were in optimum condition for intercourse and reproduction. The treatments they offered clearly kept those goals in mind. They believed that restoring diseased women to bodily health would ensure appropriate sexual behavior, if only because the correct functioning of their reproductive organs would dominate their entire beings.

For all of these physicians, white women's reproductive bodies and minds were so intimately connected that no separation was possible. They warned women repeatedly that controlling their emotions was necessary for healthy bodily functioning. Yet their warnings had something of a hollow sound to them, for at heart most physicians were convinced that women's reproductive organs ruled their emotions, in spite of what they hoped would be their best conscious efforts to control them. White women's inherent weaknesses of mind and body, their inability to control themselves either mentally or physically, led them to be vulnerable to states of ill health of all sorts. White men were rarely so vulnerable, for their superior minds and bodies allowed them to exercise the admirable self-control so necessary for their position of mastery over themselves and others. Physicians who held such views did not often consider the influence of mind and body on the reproductive functions of black men and women. Living simpler lives in a more natural state, their bodies and minds were more likely than those of whites to exert a harmonious influence on each other, or so physicians assumed. They were unwilling to define blacks' sexual behavior as a form of illness of either mind or body, which might have called into question their ability to labor—and, in the case of women, their sexual availability to white men.

## Nervous Diseases and the Body

Physicians who believed that white women's minds influenced the normal reproductive functions of their bodies were even more adamant in their conviction that their interactions caused disease, particularly gynecological ones. One authority called them a "very troublesome class of affections" with a "rebellious nature" that was difficult to relieve or even control.[68] Inherent in his description of women's diseases was a view of women's bodies and minds as similarly rebellious and troublesome, because they were not immediately amenable to male authority. L. A. Dugas thought it unfortunate that "the influence upon the mind of any kind of uterine disease, real or imaginary, is such as frequently to amount to a monomania."[69] If women's minds, their so-called mental emotions, influenced their bodies even in a healthy state, the disorder they could cause during illness was dangerous indeed.

Many physicians believed that sympathy between reproductive organs and the brain rendered gynecological disorders particularly troubling. Columbia, South Carolina, physician J. McF. Gaston categorized some cases of ovarian disease as "nervous irritation." He confessed that these were "very slow in relieving" and that he found himself "heartily tired before I got them relieved." He described something of an epidemic of "cases of this nervous irritation of the ovaries, among whites and blacks, in Chester district" in the summer of 1850, which caused him to be "apprehensive of inflammation" and perhaps somewhat frustrated as well. Gaston reported that he "used every means to obviate such a tendency, but with little or no effect towards controlling the disease," which satisfied him "of the neuralgic nature of the affection." He treated women with this ovarian disease by "the introduction of anodynes, in the form of a pessary or in solution, to the vagina" because "a sympathy of a peculiar and very strong nature exists between" vagina and ovaries. The anodyne he used was opium in large amounts, or occasionally morphine.[70] Both diagnosis and treatment suggest the complex nature of Gaston's view of women's bodies and minds as well as his own emotional response to the difficulties they could present as patients.

Gaston's use of the term *nervous irritation* to describe a specific kind of uterine disease was particularly revealing. For midcentury physicians, irritation referred both to a physiological state, related to inflammation and other forms of tissue disturbance, and an emotional or psychological state of extreme sensitivity. As both a description of a symptom and as a diagnostic category, the concept of irritation did not require physicians to distinguish between afflictions of the mind and body. Physicians were particularly likely to use the term to describe white women's reproductive organs, which they considered especially vulnerable to its ravages, and to the emotional states such ravages induced. They also sometimes used it to describe disorders of the stomach, although that vocabulary usually took the form of more distinctly named illnesses such as dyspepsia. While never exclusively gendered as a female and reproductive complaint, as a description of illness the term *irritation* was used far more often to describe white women's ailments than it was used about men or slaves of either sex.

The word *nervous* was also indicative of physicians' way of thinking about disorders specific to white women. While the term referred directly to the nerves or the nervous system, it also described a pattern of behavior. Thompson McGown defined nervous as "pertaining to the nerves or nervous system. Also weak, irritable" in the glossary he included in his domestic medicine manual.[71] People who were nervous, like those who were irritable, were not in control of their emotions. They were subject to flights of fancy and were likely to imagine themselves sick, both in the sense of thinking that they were diseased when they were not and in the sense of making themselves sick by the actions of their minds. White men were generally assumed to be enough in control of their nerves to avoid such dangers, while the imagined illnesses of slaves were addressed in very different language. Instead, both nervousness and irritation, like the nervous diseases they caused, were closely associated with white women, whose weak minds and reproductive organs left them vulnerable to their ravages.

Alexander Stevens, a New York physician whose paper "On the Diagnosis of Nervous Diseases" was reprinted in the *Southern Medical and Surgical Journal,* argued that "nervous diseases present the far larger portion of strange, out-of-the-way symptoms, not to be embraced within the nosological definitions of other maladies." He offered a class-based analysis of such diseases, claiming that "when a case presented itself" he asked himself "did I ever see such a case in the hospital, or among dispensary patients, or among the poor in any of the walks of life?" When the answer was no, he "began to discover that generally it was a case of nervous disease that I had to deal with." Stevens believed that nervous diseases were subject to "*fashion*" and "adopted either in revenge of some misfortune, or in despair from some blighted hope." As "imaginary diseases," they required "more than any thing else, moral treatment."[72] He suggested that "the physician should endeavour to penetrate into the innermost recesses of his patient's heart, that he may fulfil the great indication, which is, *to present a powerful motive for recovery; and he should never suffer his patient to doubt for one moment that such a recovery will take place.*"[73] Stevens did not doubt that the discomfort his patients felt was real, but he thought that it had its origins in a complex mix of their emotions, their brains, and their nerves, as well as in the specific body part they believed to be diseased.

Other physicians used similar language when discussing gynecological diseases. The author of a review of *On Diseases Peculiar to Women* in the *Medical Journal of North Carolina* noted that the book discussed "the neurotic states of the uterus and its appendages," including those relating "to diseases of irritation or of exalted and deranged irritability or susceptibility."[74] Nearly every form of gynecological disorder could cause women to experience emotional symptoms, as numerous case reports demonstrate. According to North Carolina physician William King, a woman "of nervous temperament" who suffered "pain and other distressing sensations in the uterine region" some months after the birth of her eighth child also experienced "great mental depression, sleeplessness, palpitations, and many other symptoms of the hysteric disorder, all of which were greatly aggravated at each catamenial period." He diagnosed her as suffering from a "prolapsed and anteverted" womb and a "highly inflamed and engorged cervix." The anteverted, or tipped, uterus was of particular concern to him, since "the most distressing hysterical symptoms ensue, over which nothing in the long list of anodyne anti-spasmodics has any control." However, "every symptom of pain, spasm and mental disturbance can, as if by magic, be dispelled" by restoring the "womb to its natural position."[75] Simon Saunders reported more simply that one of his patients suffering from a prolapsed uterus and vaginal discharge was likewise rendered "exceedingly unhappy and distressed in mind."[76]

Curing the physical prolapse could cure the emotional problems it caused, according to South Carolina physician John Lake, who noted the case of a white woman whose prolapsed uterus had rendered her ill for twelve years and kept her confined to bed for six of them. The woman, her friends, and her physicians believed that "she could not long survive"; indeed, she thought death "was her best friend." After operating on her, Lake reported that "her general health began to improve, . . . and all the train of nervous affections attendant upon an aggravated case of prolapsus, was soon gone." He performed the same operation on "a negro woman, who had been confined to bed for the space [of] at least five years" without finding any treatment "which offered her sufficient relief to enable her to follow any kind of business." Rather than commenting on the emotional consequences of her affliction, as he had for his white patient, Lake noted only that "she was regarded by her owner as a nuisance." After the operation, she enjoyed "the like happy consequences" as the white woman, by which he presumably meant the reversal of the prolapse. Unlike the white woman, whose story ended with her able to visit friends in Alabama, Lake ended his account of the slave woman's case by noting that she was "returned home and placed in the kitchen as a cook for a large family."[77] Lake's comments suggest that the emotional impact of disease was different for black and white women, if only in the way it influenced their ability to perform the different roles expected of them in society.

In spite of such race-based assumptions, physicians believed the consequences of prolapsed uterus could touch all aspects of both black and white women's bodies. Milton Antony reported on the case of a black woman whose "recto-vaginal openings"[78] and prolapse were caused by "a fall down the stairway." Although he successfully cured her, the prolapse and fistulae returned and she became "extremely emaciated and desponding" and died "of mortification." As in the case of nervous irritation, the language here is telling. Antony's use of the term *mortification* blurred the line between a state of extreme tissue inflammation or infection and the woman's embarrassed discomfort with her condition. In the view of mid-nineteenth-century practitioners, both could have contributed to her death.[79]

Antony also reported on a white woman who suffered from similar dysfunctions, which caused "a regular recurrence of epilepsy every month, followed by great insensibility, and indeed entire loss of consciousness for many hours and sometimes for a day or two." She also experienced epilepsy "on the appearance of colic pains or headache." She, too, died after ceasing to menstruate and suffering "an obstinate and increasingly violent and harassing cough . . . and pulmonary ulceration," which Antony believed to be "merely metastases" of the original prolapsed uterus. A third patient enjoyed a better outcome of her prolapsed uterus and consequent menstrual obstruction after the birth of a child. After "labouring under chronic derangement of intellect" for many months, she was treated, and "her intellect improved and the distress of head . . . mitigated." Antony noted that "her powers of speech, of which she was entirely deprived, began to return, and she is now able to use a number of words very distinctly and accurately."[80] All three women's suffering demonstrated the absence of any real distinction between what he would call derangements of body and mind.

Antony's two patients were not the only women whose deaths were attributed to the mental and physical consequences of uterine disease. Joseph Eve believed that uterine disease often led to involvement of the nervous system, "as evinced in the development of various nervous affections such as the different forms of hysteria, chorea, and eventually epilepsy." He offered the case of a married white woman whose inflammation of the cervix was neglected "until her nervous system became very seriously affected." What began as "slight nervous seizures with very transient abolition of mind . . . gradually became more intense, amounting to decided epileptic convulsions." Although treated with "every remedy that promised the slightest hope of benefit . . . her disease constantly increased in intensity, until death kindly released her from a condition most pitiable and deplorable—her mind a wreck and her once comely person sadly changed and disfigured by disease." Eve thought that if the woman's cervical inflammation had "been treated before the nervous system had become involved, she would doubtless have avoided the epileptic affection altogether, and lived long to enjoy life and make others happy." He claimed to be able to present other cases "to prove that, after the nervous system has become gravely affected, although the uterine disease may be perfectly and permanently cured, the nervous affection will continue."[81] Joseph Wright agreed, warning his readers that when prolapsed uterus continued "for some length of time . . . the patient becomes hysterical, [and] emaciation and great debility are induced."[82]

Hysteria was hardly new in the antebellum years. It had been diagnosed and named for the wandering uterus believed to cause it by the ancient Greeks. However, as a disease, it was undergoing a gradual transformation that marked a shift in medical understandings of the ways in which women's bodies and minds interacted with each other, which would become increasingly proscriptive of women's behavior in the decades after the Civil War. Warnings of the dangers of hysteria would become the primary mechanism by which physicians sought to control women's lives, arguing, for example, that the mental rigors of education and careers would damage their reproductive organs, and so for their own good as well as that of the nation, women should be excluded from participating in them.[83] For the majority of antebellum physicians, however, hysteria was a dramatic and poorly understood symptom as much as it was a distinct disease, which could require behavioral changes but that was also subject to medical care. John Stainback Wilson pronounced it "as *real a disease* as small-pox or measles," whose "unfortunate subjects ... should receive our tenderest care and sympathy." He listed among its causes "a nervous temperament, idleness, effeminacy, menstrual disorders, ... sexual abuses, mental excitement, as fear, anger, disappointment, &c; and particularly that kind of excitement caused by reading lascivious books, and witnessing licentious scenes." To this already long list he added "excessive eating and sleeping, the use of opium and tobacco; stimulating drinks, as spirits, tea, and coffee; [and] the abuse of purgatives."[84] Such a disease with so many causes could easily mystify physicians and their patients.

For example, Virginia physician and author of a domestic medicine manual, W. H. Coffin included among the diseases "peculiar to the sex" what he termed "nervous state," which he said was "caused by a variety of the disorders to which the womb is liable." Its signs included "tremblings, shivering, palpitation, shortness of breath, pain in the left side, giddiness, fainting, loss of recollection, depression of spirits, and a variety of imaginings, which makes her always apprehensive of approaching evils." He distinguished nervous state from hysteria "by the absence of hysteric fits" but noted that some women also experienced "hysterical paroxysms" along with the other symptoms, without clarifying the difference. Nervous state, which he also called nervous irritation, could "terminate in complete mania"; it was treated with tonics, diet, fresh air, and exercise along with drugs, including digitalis, hyoscyamus, and morphine.[85]

W. Camps discussed hysteria in the context of insanity, noting that it was "in the moral state and motives, which not unfrequently attend or accompany the severer forms of hysteria, that we may recognise without difficulty the approximation of this disease to some of the forms of mental disease." He also noted that "insanity is far more a bodily disease than has hitherto been considered; and in cases of this malady there is mostly, if not always, impairment of the proper healthy cerebral structure." Because "the nervous system" was involved, "the proper functions of the brain often become deeply affected."[86] For both physicians and many of their colleagues as well, hysteria was caused by the interplay of disordered bodies and minds, the place where biology and what would later be called psychology merged in the sympathetic actions of uterus and brain.

Many physicians discussed hysteria as both cause and consequence of uterine disease. As early as 1838, an author in the *Southern Medical and Surgical Journal* noted the case of a nineteen-year-old unmarried white woman who suffered from "a violent fit of hysteria, which was characterised by incessant and violent fits of laughter of many hours duration." Examination led to the discovery that her uterus was distended to the point of contact with her hymen. Because "the paroxysm depended on irritation of the uterus from its monthly plethora," she was treated for the prolapse, after which "the laughing effort entirely ceased and the menstrual flux appeared."[87] Twenty years later, the same journal reported the case of a fifteen-year-old, also white and unmarried, who likewise was subject "at each menstrual period, to most distressing paroxysms of hysteria, attended with convulsions and temporary mental derangement." Her disease was attributed to uterine inflammation; she, too, was treated for it and "never had a paroxysm after the treatment was commenced."[88] Albert Henley diagnosed the "moans and shrieks," "state of syncope or coma," convulsions, and "violent fit of laughter" of a seventeen-year-old white woman as "hysteria or hysterical paralysis." After questioning the family, he attributed her behavior to "deranged menstrual secretion, and mental emotions from witnessing the delivery of her sister." When the woman suffered another attack after "she had assisted in shrouding a little girl," Henley attributed it to "irregular menstruation" and advised his patient "to avoid depressing passions, or mental emotions of any kind."[89] Women's bodies could be betrayed by their minds at the other end of their reproductive lives as well. One physician thought the hysteria of a woman in her fifties was "mainly connected with the cessation of the menstrual function."[90]

Other reproductive organs or their disturbances could also be the source of hysteria. An anonymous author observed that women's "hysterical and epileptoid attacks only came on at first menstruation and at the decline of life; and at each menstrual period, the nervous symptoms disappeared." He considered the source of the problem to be inflammation of the ovaries, "not the uterus, as the older authors supposed," and offered as evidence "the fact that in persons who have died while laboring under hysteria, the sub-inflammatory state of the ovaries was the only lesion observed." As explanation, he said, "inasmuch as the expulsion of the ripened fruit is frequently attended by nervous phenomena, puerperal convulsions, epilepsy, [and] mania, we can readily comprehend how the parturition of the ovum, by the ovary, may be attended by similar re-actions, or, though less intense, by the cognate, hysteria."[91] In other words, both childbirth and ovulation, functions in which the body expelled a part of itself, could cause a cluster of nervous disorders, including hysteria.

So, too, could menstruation, according to John P. Miller, a botanic physician. He discussed a derangement of menstruation called fluor albus, commonly called the whites,[92] whose symptoms included "general debility, irritable state of the nerves, palpitations and hysteric affections, . . . low spirits, [and] disturbed and unrefreshing sleep." He attributed it to "causes evidently productive of general exhaustion of the system," including "the vile habit of solitary vice, which is one of the prime causes in the unmarried female, and in the married, immoderate coition." In spite of its sometimes behavioral causes, Miller claimed it could be cured by cleanliness and vaginal douches, along with various medicines.[93] Likewise, Thompson McGown, author of a book on diseases of the South, believed that the whites could cause "various forms of nervous affections; as, hysterics, palpitations of the heart, faintness, . . . or other forms of neuralgia." However, unlike Miller, he attributed these "morbid affections of the uterus" to "want of proper attention in parturition" by "*ignorant or unqualified 'midwives'*" and urged "southern ladies to . . . employ competent physicians."[94] Both Miller and McGown mingled cause and effect so thoroughly that distinguishing them was nearly impossible, although they clearly linked menstruation, hysteria, unacceptable behavior, and the whites.

Other forms of sexual behavior also manifested themselves physiologically and psychologically as hysteria, leading physicians to explore the significance of a variety of anomalous cases of the disease in women. Joseph Eve hoped a "delicate and nervous" white woman's "nervous affection," which he considered "doubtless hysterical," would "disappear after marriage," a sign that he considered it related to the absence of sexual activity. Eve was sure this belief would have been validated, "had her married life been all calm and sunshine." However, "it was sadly overshadowed—the paroxysms became more intense and frequent, assuming a decided epileptic character." He did not make clear whether an unhappy marriage caused her disease to worsen or whether worsening disease rendered her marriage unhappy. When she became pregnant, the woman's "fits became more and more frequent," nor did they disappear afterward. Instead, her convulsions "have assumed a very serious character, uncontrolled, uninfluenced by every plan of treatment to which she has been subjected." Although Eve considered hers an "anomalous" case, he clearly understood the cause of her disease to be rooted in her reproductive organs, her circumstances, and her temperament.[95] Both Eve and Miller believed that sexual activity could be both cause and cure of women's emotional and physical distress.

Another anomalous case linking reproductive organs, the nervous system, and bodily experience and reported by an Alabama physician, E. Y. Harris, was that of a slave woman who went into labor during her seventh month. The night before, he learned, "a man had visited her for *carnal purposes;* that she had resisted him, at which he became incensed and struck her with his fist two or three times in the left side, when she cried out so loudly that he became alarmed and left." Harris bled her and gave her an opiate and was reassured the next day when she claimed to feel better and "said she felt the child move." However, he was called back six days later to find that she "seemed to be in a very deep sleep, from which she could not be roused." After two more days, he examined her again and found that the child had been stillborn, showing signs of having been killed by the blows the mother had received; a few days later, the mother died. Harris asked whether "this condition of the nervous system [was] brought on by the injury?" and wondered "would the same have produced similar nervous disturbance if she had not been pregnant?" While his questions remained unanswered and unanswerable, he noted that "here was a strange condition of the nervous system, brought on probably by the injury she received from the wretch."[96] Harris did not attribute the death of mother or fetus to the rape itself or to the blows the woman received, but rather to the "nervous disturbance" resulting from them, suggesting the complexity of the connection between the woman's awareness of rape and fetal movement and her body's experience of them.

A third anomalous case was reported by Francis Peyre Porcher, a prominent Charleston physician. Porcher described a sixteen-year-old Irish girl with extra digits on both feet and one hand, whose "deformity" he believed to be the result of her mother's reaction to seeing an elephant while pregnant.[97] However, the prenatal influence and the extra digits it caused were the least of the young woman's problems. Porcher diagnosed her with chorea, or Saint Vitus's dance, which he said was "generally brought on by anger, jealousy, . . . irritation, amenorrhoea and more frequently by fright." The disease caused her to be "inclined to imbecility, evinced by fatuous expression of countenance, impaired memory, and liability to causeless emotion," and to suffer "general irritability and mobility of the nervous system," what another physician termed "insanity of the muscles." Porcher attributed her case to "misery of mind produced by the deformity" because "her playmates . . . laughed at her a great deal." He also noted that she suffered "general constitutional debility" and had never menstruated. Porcher treated her for those ailments as well as for "a species of psoriasis" and for "very bad teeth," including the extraction of four milk teeth, which marked "the beginning of her recovery." Here, Porcher's description suggests not only his conviction of the mother's prenatal influence on the daughter, but also the extent to which her bodily anomalies of delayed menstruation, extra digits, and "delayed dentition" influenced her muscles and her mind.[98] His concept of cause and effect as well as his assessment of the ways in which her mind and body influenced each other suggest the complexity of those connections in his medical understanding. Chorea, like hysteria, was in his view both the physical manifestation of emotional distress and the emotional consequence of physical deformity.

For midcentury physicians, hysteria was not sharply distinguished from epilepsy, convulsions, chorea, or other ailments associated with women's reproductive organs, especially at reproductively liminal moments. Such beliefs were so widespread that Joseph Eve, professor of obstetrics at the Medical College of Georgia, felt compelled to inform his younger colleagues that not every case of convulsions was due to hysteria.[99] In spite of Eve's warning, a diagnosis of hysteria was common among the white women of the antebellum South. For physicians accustomed to viewing their white women patients as physiologically and psychologically vulnerable to the influence of their reproductive organs, the only surprise was that it was not more frequent. It was also a disease that served their professional interests well. Dramatic in its symptoms and difficult of cure, hysteria could not easily be attended using the advice of domestic medicine manuals, nor were lay practitioners particularly effective at curing it. Instead, hysteria, by conflating brain and uterus, required all of the skill and expertise and all of the trappings of scientific authority that physicians could bring to the bedside.

However, not all physicians were willing to attribute every perplexing symptom to hysteria and uterine disease. Instead, like several physicians treating slaves, Tomlinson Fort cataloged a new disease, which he named hyperaesthesis or excessive sensibility, in three of his female patients, one of whom was a slave. Careful to explain that none of them had ever suffered "any hysterical disorder," Fort described the women as at first disinclined "to submit to examination by the touch." As the disease progressed, their aversion grew, until the shock of being touched "produced more pain and alarm, than the thrust of two daggers," and caused "the most violent convulsions." The women perceived an approaching hand from two or more feet away, "and, as it approached, [would] recoil, or spring from it with horror"; this happened even when they were sleeping. One woman could not bear even the touch of her own hand. Fort likened "the shocks and excitement" these women experienced when touched, even with a feather, to "the operation of electricity" and wrote about their violent reactions to thunderstorms. He treated them with a variety of medicines but discovered that the remedies "usually beneficial in hysterical disorders" offered no benefit, so resorted to opium. All three women gradually recovered.[100]

## Race, Sex, and Hysteria

The vast majority of patients in whom physicians diagnosed hysteria were white women, whose overly civilized bodies, ways of thinking, and habits of life doctors believed left them vulnerable to such complaints. Southern physicians wondered whether slave men and women or white men could also suffer from the disease, a question with significant implications for their practice of medicine. The general answer was that they did not, or at least not very often. While black women shared the same reproductive organs as white women, their simpler lives and less vulnerable nerves offered them a good deal of protection from it. White men were even less likely to succumb to the disease; their masculine strength of body and character prevented them from losing control.

At the same time, physicians eager to explore the parameters of normal bodies and behavior were intensely curious not only about the causes of hysteria in white women, but also about its incidence in blacks of both sexes and white men. A South Carolina physician, E. Miller, acknowledged that "hysteria is by no means an uncommon malady in females," without specifying which race, adding that "its symptoms are those simulating almost every other disease" and that it "is often mistaken for other diseases." He described the case of "a negro girl, past the middle of life," who "had not enjoyed good health for some years, being very irregular in the appearance of the menses." He was called to treat her for "intense spasm of the abdominal muscles, fists clenched, and in short all the symptoms of labor, carotids throbbing violently, with a kind of hissing scream, indicative of the most intense agony; the spasm would return as often as every minute; she could not be restrained by three strong persons." She also suffered from "obstinate constipation," for which he decided to treat her first and then "departed till evening to await the action of the medicine." When he returned, he "found two more [slave] girls prostrate in the same condition," whom he also treated. The next day he "found still another added to my list, but with more of apoplectic symptoms, she could not be roused or made to speak, even pinching had no effect." He treated her like the others, with "the treatment commonly given in hysteria."[101]

Miller suspected from the start that all of these women suffered from hysteria, because he was called to see the first patient "after a negro meeting and preaching, with great noise and excitement." His request for "perfect quietude" was ignored by the overseer, who "gave permission to hold another such assembly, which was followed next day with a case in a small girl, eight years of age, and also in a boy of fourteen years." Although eventually the overseer stopped the meetings, the adult women "were subject to sudden returns of the fits, for three months more." One of them sometimes would be "taken all of a sudden when laboring in the field, and have to be carried home." Miller gave no indication that he suspected this woman or any of these slave patients of shamming.[102]

More interesting than Miller's frustration with the overseer's noncompliance with his orders was his reaction to the two children, in whom he "was scarcely prepared to expect hysteria" and so requested a consultation with a colleague. Miller's perplexity about the children led him to wonder whether "hysteria is a contagious disease? and is it dependent on some morbid condition of the uterus entirely?" He considered the cases he encountered to be "vivid pictures of epidemic disease," since "those who were taken displayed all the symptoms of contagious hysteria, . . . a kind of moral contagion." He noted that the first woman to be afflicted had "a nervous susceptibility, and the fanatic tone of religious frenzy, which is peculiar in the revivals of negroes, added a note of higher exultation to the excitement, and when the first case occurred, it was easy for the moral contagion to lay hold on others." Still, Miller was puzzled by the children. He wondered why, if hysteria "is dependent on uterine disease," the eight-year-old girl suffered from it "before the organs of generation were called into play for any purpose?" Likewise, he wondered how the boy, "who was well formed, and had well formed and well developed sexual apparatus," could have developed hysteria. His conclusion was to "admit it is commonly dependent on a morbid uterus, but not invariably." He also concluded that hysteria was contagious and warned that "once institute this condition among a number of females, and rigorous measures must be taken to put a stop to it." Miller recommended "free and pitiless drenching with cold water." Even so, he noted that "some of the cases were very obstinate, when the overseer becoming impatient gave them a severe flogging, and put a quietus on the noisy revivals, which was more effectual than any medicine in quelling the disease." Nevertheless, he added, the first woman "is now entering the confines of insanity, and with very little hope for a more favorable change" in spite of his continuing "the cold douche every morning."[103] While shamming never entered his discussion, Miller thought that unpleasant treatment could sometimes play a role in curing the disease.

Miller's description of these cases is important for several reasons. By raising questions about the possibility of hysteria in prepubescent girls and in boys as well as linking it to the religious practices of slaves, his analysis points to both the gendered and raced nature of the connections between mind and body. Hysteria was a disease caused by uterine derangements, yet it could exist in the absence of a functioning uterus, indeed in the absence of a uterus at all. Note Miller's careful insistence on the boy's "well formed and well developed sexual apparatus," which suggests that his first thought to account for the boy's suffering from hysteria had been that he was intersexed.[104] However, Miller's confusion was mitigated somewhat by the presence of the disease in slaves, whose uncontrolled religious excitement was more than their brains or bodies could handle. In this instance, the disease threatened to become epidemic because the overseer did not follow the physician's advice and instead allowed the slaves to continue their meetings; it only ended when he both stopped the "noisy revivals" and beat the slaves. Blacks' mental and physical weakness led them to emotional displays of religious fervor that had disastrous consequences for their health. Once again, black minds and bodies influenced each other in ways similar to those of white women, thus reinforcing inferiority on the basis of both race and sex.

Just as Miller wondered whether hysteria was contagious and could become epidemic among male and female slaves, James Green wondered whether it could be inherited by the women in a family, although not the men. He described his experiences with a young white woman suffering from a variety of menstrual disturbances and "frequent hysterical attacks, a striking phenomenon of which was severe erratic pains over the whole body but particularly the joints." He noted that "all the female members of this lady's family have been troubled in a similar way," including a younger sister with "the same train of symptoms" and "the same kind of hysterical paroxysms with flying pains in the limbs, joints, fingers, toes, &c." The woman's older sister suffered similar distress, as did their mother, who reported "that the hysterical phenomena and erratic pains are common to the whole of them as well as herself." Green concluded that "probably hereditary tendencies to this kind of disease are as easily transmitted as any other."[105] He did not, however, consider the women's common vulnerability to hysteria and other illnesses to be the result of contagion or epidemic, as Miller had for the slaves he treated.

While physicians could never be counted on to agree with one another's explanations, Miller and Green's difference of opinion may well have been the result of their differing assessments of the ways in which white and black women's bodies responded to the influences of their minds. Inheritance was a more neutral force shaping the health of Green's family of white women than was the epidemic of moral contagion that caused hysteria for Miller's slave patients. The two physicians reflected southern physicians' need to view white women's minds and bodies as more vulnerable than white men's, but at the same time superior to those of blacks.

Physicians experienced similar dilemmas in their quest to understand whether white men could become victims of hysteria. While they recognized that men could sometimes suffer from these diseases, they diagnosed them, especially in white men, only rarely and with a degree of intellectual struggle. For example, in a review of Charles Meigs's *Females and Their Diseases* published in the *Charleston Medical Journal and Review,* the anonymous author noted without comment that Meigs regarded hysteria "as originating in what he calls the sixth sense, the aphrodisiac influence; modifications of the vitality of the reproductive organs being the root of the evil in all cases of hysteria, which he admits in the male, as well as in the female."[106] Most of the time, doctors assumed, men's reason and their control over their emotions protected them from its ravages.

The problem of hysteria in white men was not solved by Meigs's cavalier statement that it could arise from the aphrodisiac influence of men's reproductive organs as well as women's. Gunning Bedford, who was professor of obstetrics, the diseases of women and children, and clinical midwifery at the University of New York, could not "conceive why sexual irritation in the male should not, as in the female," cause hysteria. While he acknowledged that it was "comparatively rare," he had "no doubt" that it existed and offered the case of a sixteen-year-old boy who "had fallen a victim to that most dangerous vice—*onanism*" as proof.[107] Ralph Schenck, the Virginia author of a domestic medicine manual, explained that "the hysteric disease appears most commonly in females; and the hypochondriac disease in males," although he acknowledged that the distinction was not perfect. Like those physicians who wrote about hysteria in women, his unstated assumption was that the males under consideration were white. Schenck characterized those suffering from "hypochondriac disease, commonly called Vapours, or Low Spirits," as having "a state of mind distinguished by . . . a langour, listlessness, or want of resolution and activity with respect to all undertakings; a disposition to seriousness, sadness, and timidity, as to all future events, an apprehension of the worst or most unhappy state of them; and therefore, often upon slight grounds, an apprehensive of great evil." Sufferers were also "particularly attentive to the state of their own health, to the smallest change of feeling in their bodies," which caused them to "apprehend great danger, and even death itself" and made it difficult to dissuade them from "the most obstinate belief and persuasion."[108] Yet Samuel Jennings warned that obtaining the truth from patients was difficult; even men were "strongly inclined to disguise the true origin of their complaints, and present circumstances and symptoms which have no relation to the case in hand."[109]

Schenck treated men's hypochondriac disease by diverting "the mind of the patient, to other objects than his own feelings," by encouraging him to attend to "the occupations of business" and by amusements, including sports and hunting, games and company, horse-back riding and driving. He acknowledged that "the firm persuasion that generally prevails in such patients, does not allow their feelings to be treated as imaginary," which meant that they were "not to be treated either by raillery or by reasoning." The masculine qualities of the activities suggested for the cure, as well as the language in which Schenck discussed his patients, suggests that hypochondria was indeed a disease of men and not women. Those who suffered from it were of "a melancholy temperament, and of a firm and rigid habit," while "the hysteric disease attacks persons of a sanguine temperament, and of a lax and flaccid habit."[110] The latter terms were not likely to be applied to white men under any circumstances.

A South Carolina physician, J. Y. DuPre, developed more elaborate explanations of the gendered nature of hysteria, rather than relying on the existence of a separate disease for white men. DuPre believed hysteria to be a symptom, "the consequence of diseased action in some portion of the system" that was "universally admitted to be a nervous affection" and "*partial* to the female." He added: "[I]ts *exclusiveness* to that sex, however, has been satisfactorily confuted by frequently repeated observations of its occurrence in the male," even though cases in men were "curious, and become exceptions to a general rule." DuPre described one such exceptional case, in a fifty-year-old "gentleman in this community." DuPre was called when the man suffered an "'attack of spasms'" that "simulat[ed] . . . an epileptic fit," of a sort "to which he had been subject during the last twenty years of his life." The "stout and plethoric" patient had been treating himself during those years with "ardent spirits," including "nearly a pint of brandy" on the occasion for which DuPre was called.[111]

Unlike any of the women whose hysterical fits were described by their physicians, DuPre's patient "was conscious of his situation, sensible of his suffering," and made "frequent efforts to speak." Also unlike female hysteria patients, "during the remissions of the paroxysms . . . he would relate very intelligently the history of his sufferings and distress *during a paroxysm*" and could "converse rationally." Yet DuPre diagnosed hysteria, because of "the previous history of the patient [and] the presence of consciousness during the attacks." He was able to stop the convulsions and quiet the patient with drugs and "the removal of his distressed family from his bedside." Further examination revealed him to be "a *dyspeptic,* in addition to his being afflicted with chronic hepatitis," although DuPre was "unable to say" which of the man's many symptoms were the result of which disease. DuPre explained his diagnosis by suggesting that it could "account for those strange irregularities in the nervous system constituting hysteria." He asked, "[I]f a diseased uterus may produce such, why may not the liver and stomach?" DuPre treated the man's liver and stomach disorders and "so far strengthened and invigorated his almost shattered nervous system, by imparting tone to the digestive organs and richness to the blood, that he has had but *one* paroxysm in the last five months." Afterward, the patient enjoyed "comparatively good health" and seldom felt "that sadness and gloom, the offspring of dyspepsia and liver complaint." In this case, the man's hysteria was aggravated by "the remedy which he usually resorted to," alcohol, which "was fast hurrying him to the grave."[112]

Like white women and blacks, DuPre's white male patient suffered from hysteria at least in part because he was unable or unwilling to control his body, instead consuming alcohol in what DuPre considered injudicious amounts. Combined with his plethoric constitution and diseased organs, the man's behavior left him vulnerable to hysteria in much the same way as those with weaker bodies and minds. His case was exceptional primarily because most white men, lacking uterus and ovaries, were not so vulnerable. Instead, their superior control over mind and body allowed them to avoid hysteria and enjoy good health, which white women and slaves could not duplicate. According to one physician attending a "feeble" woman who was "subject to spasms, affecting the extremities; frequent attacks of palpitation of the heart; difficulty of breathing, and many other disagreeable symptoms," she suffered because "*the mind is the main thing with her; I think if her mind was satisfied, she mout [sic] soon be up.*" This physician reportedly claimed "that there was but little the matter, except dejection of mind."[113] White men, with their vigorous constitutions and active minds, were rarely so dejected.

Midcentury physicians' efforts to understand the implications of the reciprocal influences of body and mind were informed by the unspoken assumptions of the society in which they lived. The race and sex of particular minds and bodies influenced the ways in which they interacted with each other. Physicians who took the oppositional binary categories of their society (male and female, black and white, slave and free) for granted created a medical science that reflected those categories; they literally could not imagine any other way of thinking. As a result, physicians concerned with the influences of mind on body and body on mind also took for granted the raced and gendered characteristics of those influences, viewing white women's and all blacks' weaker bodies and minds as appropriate for the social circumstances in which they lived, just as white men's stronger minds and bodies explained their dominant roles. In other words, medical science both reflected and reinforced the assumptions of southern society about the superiority of white male minds and bodies and the inferiority of everyone else's. Their relative lack of attention to the minds and bodies of black men and women was a sign that they saw them as relatively simple and so not likely to have significant health consequences. Black people's simplemindedness rendered them unlikely to fall prey to their emotions as did white women, and certainly incapable of the kind of emotional control doctors attributed to white men.

In contrast to their lack of attention to blacks, physicians developed complex theories about the influence of white women's reproductive organs on their minds, thus reinforcing their inferiority to white men. Women's reproductive bodies were at the center of their being, physically and emotionally, leaving them incapable of the kind of self-control doctors believed necessary to ensure good health. Instead, doctors were convinced that white women needed their advice in order to thrive and their care during the all too frequent periods when they were sick. For physicians determined to define bodies and minds within the context of southern society, medical and scientific explanations of their interactions reinforced the social hierarchy, defining white women's bodies and minds as subordinate to men's just as blacks' were to whites'. In the process, physicians enhanced the status of white men along with their own cultural authority; only they could be dispassionate enough to enjoy good health and help others who were not. Doctors' explanations of the interactions of mind and body allowed them to view white men as in control of their emotions while white women were vulnerable and blacks of both sexes relatively impervious to the influence of theirs. The consequences, they believed, could be seen in the patterns of health and sickness common to each race and sex.

# CHAPTER 6

# The Unexamined Body

Like physicians, lay southerners had their own ways of thinking about the connections between mind and body that helped them understand health and sickness, although their views were rarely in accord with those of doctors.[1] Views of mind and body enabled people of both races and sexes to explain their own illnesses as well as those of one another. Because theories about what caused disease and how to be healthy were in flux even among physicians, who did not yet command the level of cultural authority to which they aspired, laypeople considered themselves not only capable but entitled to define the causes and cures of illness according to their own views of how bodies and minds worked. They did so in ways that reflected the South's political and social institutions as understood and experienced by men and women, black and white.

Race, sex, and place were central to lay views of the connections between mind and body, just as they were for physicians. Not only did each race and sex have its own views about its members' experiences, so, too, did each understand the ways in which mind and body interacted to be different for different categories of people. Reinforcing the importance of race and sex differences, people's beliefs about mind and body interactions followed the assumptions of their society about slavery, subordination, and appropriate behavior, as well as health and illness.

Laypeople had no reason to articulate the kind of complex theories that physicians found necessary; they did not even attempt logical consistency. Instead, lay southerners of both races and sexes voiced their everyday understandings of the connections between mind and body informally, in a wide range of off-the-cuff comments that survive primarily in letters and diaries in the case of slaveholders and in folklore and oral history in the case of slaves. No matter how they were expressed, lay understandings of mind and body reflected assumptions of men and women, black and white, that were so much a part of the culture that they appeared to be common sense, so obvious that they rarely required articulation, never mind reflection. Yet what appeared to be common sense in fact masked a complex and often contradictory set of beliefs. Their unexamined ideas contrasted sharply with the carefully examined if not always consistent ideas of physicians. If physicians examined bodies in order to explain their workings to themselves and their patients, laypeople did not examine what they took to be the truth about those same bodies or even examine the bodies themselves. Yet they relied on unexamined assumptions to give meaning to their experiences of health and illness.

Lay views of mind and body derived from an unsystematic amalgam of what was considered common wisdom by members of particular groups in society, along with sometimes garbled versions of the views of various medical sects. They contained bits of received lore passed down through the generations; information from sermons, domestic medicine manuals, and other guides to correct living; and gleanings from such random sources as popular culture, advice books for travelers, and even advertisements for commercial nostrums.

Common sense coexisted in most lay southerners' minds with religious beliefs that sometimes contradicted its tenets. Many believed that whatever happened to the individual body and mind was God's will, not subject to intervention, much less free will. Yet most Christians also recognized that human agency was a real force shaping individual lives. They thought that people had a responsibility to live in a manner that would allow them to realize God's plan for them most effectively even as they reconciled themselves to their ultimate inability to determine every aspect of their lives, including health and sickness. Common sense taught the limits of human agency. The result was a blurred line between submission to God's will and active intervention in determining one's own fate by following the tenets of common sense. Lay explanations for health and illness often fell along that blurred line. Christians of both races believed that the state of one's body and mind—good health or illness, contentment or dissatisfaction, happiness or melancholy—was both a product of everyday belief and behavior and a result of the workings of God.

Since the meanings of life and death as well as illness seemed eternal mysteries that could only be explained by religion, most southerners turned to it to explain crises in both bodily and emotional experience. However, while most Christians believed in a personal God, their sense of God's workings in their everyday lives was sometimes remote. Ideas about God could provide comfort, and many white Christians offered platitudes about God's will when trying to reconcile themselves to loss and misfortune, but few people saw God as an immediate enough presence to explain every aspect of mind and body, especially when they tried to describe everyday experiences. Instead, they turned to the received wisdom of their cultures to provide themselves with answers. In most laypeople's thinking, religion and common sense reinforced one another to provide a web of answers to questions about health and disease.

For lay southerners, of course, the situation was made more complex because race and sex were always central in their lives and society. Christianity could be

a particularly potent force in shaping lay understandings of the connections between mind and body for the black and white men and women who subscribed
to its teachings because it assumed so many different meanings within southern
culture. Not only did its practice differentiate between categories of people based
on race and sex, its teachings were used by whites to justify the subordination
of some minds and bodies to others. Christianity did not simply ask believers
to submit to God's will; it also asked them to accept a set of conventions that
defined a social hierarchy of experience. White southerners found meaning in a
Christianity that validated their dominant roles, while slaves sought solace and
the possibility of redemption. Many of the former slaves interviewed by Fisk
University used the language of sickness and death to describe their conversion
experiences. They said that they were suffering with a sickness that brought them
close to death until Doctor Jesus came and healed them. Such language made no
distinction between mind, body, and soul.

Although the vast majority of both races considered themselves to be Christians, Christianity was flexible enough to admit varying interpretations and could
coexist with other beliefs. As a result, while many white and some black people
understood illness to be a warning or a punishment from God, most black people
who considered themselves Christians also saw it as the result of their lives as
slaves. Some also considered it a manifestation of another person's deliberate
efforts to inflict harm. Those blacks who rejected Christianity entirely in favor
of the set of beliefs commonly called conjure or voodoo were the least likely to
share the dominant view of the connections between mind and body. Instead,
they developed their own understandings of how mind and body influenced each
other in the production of disease. While by the antebellum period most slaves
accepted Christianity, those who did not exerted a disproportionate influence on
the black population as a whole, inspiring a continuum of beliefs about health and
sickness. Even those who claimed not to believe in conjure were usually wary of
its powers and respectful of its practitioners; this was part of the slaves' version
of common sense.

White southerners' views of common sense did not differ appreciably from
those of other native-born whites in the United States. However, white southerners were perhaps more restricted than those in other regions in their ability to
defy its tenets. Other parts of the nation offered individuals greater opportunities to diverge from prevailing ideas about health and illness, especially through
participation in what historians sometimes call the popular health movement.
This movement, encompassing such alternative ways of thinking and behaving
as dress reform, the Graham diet, water cure, spiritualism, and the like, had particular appeal to women but few adherents in the South. Its followers were too
closely associated with abolitionism and other reform activities to be considered
acceptable. Medical sects were common throughout the nation, and many white
southerners preferred the advice of Thomsonian and other botanic physicians,

homeopaths, and others who earned the contempt of allopaths. But few southerners could completely reject conventional assumptions about the body, and few deviations from prevailing notions of common sense were tolerated.

This was particularly true of the white women of the South. While women elsewhere could imagine competing ways of thinking about their bodies, if only to reject them, white southern women could not. Viewing their bodies according to competing versions of common sense would have brought them into conflict with too much else in their culture. In a society committed to reinforcing strict bodily categories and threatened by internal and external challenges to its prevailing ideology, such behavior on the part of white women could not be tolerated. Instead, white southern women were taught to see themselves as responsible for upholding cultural norms, including definitions of common sense. Challenging those norms by supporting any aspect of the popular health movement, seeking an education or a career, choosing to remain unmarried, supporting woman's rights, or otherwise rejecting definitions of appropriate behavior for women was possible outside the South but not within it. As a result, white southern women's beliefs about their bodies and minds adhered quite closely to what their culture defined as common sense.

For most white southerners, commonsense ideas about mind and body and their relationship in the sick person centered on the role of emotions. Common sense recognized that Christian faith influenced the mind, so both helped people stay healthy and cope when they fell ill, but faith was only one of the emotions that operated on the body. Whites believed not only that all sorts of emotions could cause illness, but also that they often determined the outcome of illness as well. They thought that people's attitudes shaped every aspect of their bodily experience and behavior, from health to sickness to recovery or death. Whether a person was generally healthy or sickly and how he or she reacted to illness were widely believed to be the result of those interactions.

All of the forces that lay white southerners believed caused disease were internal to the body. They believed that an individual's reaction to illness as well as the illness itself were caused by mind and body influencing each other. Miasmas, unhealthy locations, and the contagions of epidemics could all make people sick, but how people reacted to these exposures depended on internal forces. Likewise, the efforts of physicians in prescribing medicines and other treatments along with rest, changes in climate, travel, and similar alterations of routine could help, but most of the commonsense comments of whites suggest that they believed that the internal influences of mind over body and body over mind were central in shaping health and illness. Mind and body were a unit that together determined the individual's experience of illness or well-being.

White southerners' views of common sense had significant implications for their understandings of illness. Because mind and body worked together in their view, individuals could be expected to have some control over what happened to them. Having the right attitude when healthy helped a person stay healthy; incorrect ways of thinking could cause disease or prevent the person holding them from recovering. The level of personal responsibility inherent in these arguments seemingly contradicted the idea that whatever happened was God's will, but lay whites were not disturbed. Instead, they imposed a standard of cheerfulness in the face of illness on themselves and one another, even as they urged resignation. What they would not tolerate were expressions of negative attitudes such as grief or anger; their injunctions were for hope of recovery in this world and, if not, salvation in the next. Common sense in the face of illness demanded right thinking.[2]

What was common sense for whites, of course, was rarely common sense from the perspective of slaves. While most slaves shared the Christian beliefs of their owners, although with a different emphasis, they did not necessarily view the cause of illness as rooted in the internal interactions of mind and body. They believed instead that external forces, not internal ones, made them sick. They knew that they were often overworked, often hungry and cold and tired, often beaten or brutally treated in other ways, often forced to work when they were sick or pregnant, and they knew that these circumstances could and did make them sick. In addition, some slaves recognized the role of more specific external forces in making them sick, particularly the actions of conjure, voodoo, witchcraft, and other forms of magic deliberately invoked by one individual to cause harm to another. Yet this magic also depended on the connections between mind and body, for its practitioners recognized that its efficacy depended at least in part on the intended victim's acceptance of its very assumptions. Like whites, slaves rarely sought logical consistency in such matters and often held apparently contradictory beliefs without conflict. Even so, their definition of the commonsense origins of illness as external to the body defied that of the dominant culture and offered a mechanism for resisting its tendency to hold the individual's mind and body responsible for illness, rather than the circumstances in which he or she lived and worked.

Uncovering the commonsense perspectives of slaves and whites regarding the connections between mind, body, health, and sickness is challenging, given the unexamined—and in the case of slaves, often secretive—nature of such beliefs. Most of the time, southerners' beliefs can only be discerned from the almost inadvertent comments they made in the course of describing illness and its treatment. Not surprisingly, slaveholders were far more explicit in their explanations of such matters when discussing their slaves than they were in considering their own minds and bodies. They knew that slaves sometimes pretended to be sick and were determined to root out instances of shamming, but they were far more circumspect about considering the possibility that whites could deliberately manipulate the sick role. Yet their awareness of shamming forced them to acknowledge that similar behavior could also characterize the interactions of mind and body among whites. Slaves who accepted the premise that conjure could produce harm in others wondered if it would prove effective on whites or on slaves who did not share its assumptions. As a result of these uncertainties, comments about mind and body interactions in the historical record allow a more nuanced exploration than attention to unexamined common sense might otherwise permit.

In the slaveholding South as well as the rest of the nation, commonsense notions about the connections between mind and body influenced understandings of many aspects of life, not just health and sickness. Beliefs about those connections shaped ideas about race, sex, and class, about opportunity and destiny, about sexuality and marriage, about personality and identity. The focus here will be on understanding lay views of the ways common sense defined mind and body interactions in the cause, course, and treatment of disease.

## White Southerners View Mind, Body, and the Emotions

When lay white southerners commented directly about the connections between mind and body, it was often in the context of explaining why a particular individual was sick. They called on the received wisdom of Christianity mixed with common sense and concluded that difficult emotions were both cause and consequence of illness. For example, forty-four-year-old Joseph Milligan of Georgia wrote his wife Elizabeth, "My mind and my feelings have received shocks that have shaken my constitution to its center, and this with my sedentary occupation will break me down before many more years have come." He acknowledged that his "apprehensions" might be due to his "present indisposition" and that "returning health" might "prove them to be only the creation of the imagination," and added, "I have had so much distress to bear in days past both in mind & feeling, that I am primed to look at the dark side of things now."[3] Carolyn Clitherall of Alabama noted in her diary in 1853 that she had heard a sermon from Mr. Massey, whose "sallow complexion & thin visage, denote that his mind is not at ease, & his frame wearied with the constant drain upon his time & Person—."[4] Maria Bryan of Georgia often wrote her sister Julia Ann Bryan Cumming about her anxieties about their mother's health, noting on one occasion that "She is rather better, I think, and if she could only persuade herself of it she would be better still." On another, Bryan wrote that her mother was "benefitted by her journey, but she does not seem to think herself that her health is any better." On yet another, she wrote of her hopes that a new medicine would help her mother. "If it be a medicine which can 'minister to a mind diseased,' or, but its seeming effect upon the body, have a sanitary influence on the mind, I shall have hopes of her cure in time."[5] Virginia Campbell worried to her sister about their brother, fearing "that his feelings have some influence on his health." She asked whether he "apprehend[ed] a decline himself" and warned that he should not be allowed to "indulge the idea, it will be so certain to prove injurious." She added that "despondancy [*sic*] is such a foe to piety as well as to health that I would have it banished [from] the sickbed."[6] More explicitly than most, each of these writers acknowledged the links between a person's state of mind and bodily health and worried about the consequences of a disjuncture between them. Their comments reflect their commonsense ideas about the inseparability of mind and body and the individual's responsibility for right thinking in order to maintain or achieve health. Common sense demanded that people control their emotions.

White southerners who sought to explain illness more often made reference to the emotions caused by a specific event than to general expressions of the connections between mind and body. Because they were not developing theories but rather reflecting on individual circumstances when they wrote, such specificity is not surprising. Most of the time, the emotions said to cause illness were negative; among the most common were shock, grief, disappointment, and anxiety. White men and women believed that any of these emotions could cause the body to react inadvertently, suggesting that the emotions themselves were the cause of illness. Emotions did not always make people sick, but they certainly could do so, so prudent whites believed that keeping firm control over them was a prerequisite for good health, even in the face of adversity.

Emotions, however, could not always be controlled. Shock could not always be avoided, and thus illness was frequently attributed to it. When Mary Jeffreys Bethell of North Carolina learned of her sister's death after an illness lasting only a few hours, she noted in her diary that "it was such a shock to my feelings it [sic] my health suffered from it." Bethell reported that two weeks later she "was taken sick with a hemorage from the womb was confined to my bed two weeks and a month to the house."[7] Shock could also cause relapse from illness. Eliza Blanks's aunt "had a very severe spell of sickness and on her recovery she heard of the death of her son John from which she took a relapse and was very sick again."[8]

Shock was close kin to grief, which was also offered as the cause of illness. Virginia Campbell wrote her sister Margaret about their mother, who "has much to bear but what would I give if she were not so susceptible to deep sorrow. It surely will injure her health as well as peace."[9] Another woman who had been ill for some time was warned by friends that "suppressed grief is killing you" after she "made some exclamations" about her troubles in a feverish sleep.[10] Eliza DeRosset of North Carolina wrote her sister that when Euphemia Cutler died unexpectedly, surprising even her physician, the aunt who raised her was "almost heartbroken—has been in bed ever since and quite sick—entirely from grief the Doctor says sometimes with high fevers accompanied with delirium." DeRosset added that she "would not be surprised if it should prove a death blow to her."[11] Grief sometimes did kill those afflicted with it. Carolyn Clitherall wrote of her uncle's death in her memoir: "The nervous head-ache is an hereditary disease of our family—he was frequently attack'd with it, but since the death of my Aunt & the loneliness of his home, this disease had been more frequent, & terminated with Brain fever—."[12]

Grief was not far from disappointment, and that, too, could cause illness. Maria Bryan wrote her sister about a woman who "had been living in the hope of visiting her Mother in the Spring" but was surprised to discover that she was pregnant and so could not go. According to Bryan, "the disappointment was so great that it actually made her sick and she was obliged to go to bed." On another occasion, Bryan attributed her mother's illness to her brother's bad behavior, which was "enough to distress her."[13] Martha Dupree Treadwell of Alabama wrote her husband in 1859, "I have been sick for the few days untill today: though not bad sick, I expect it was caused by the non arrival of letters from you; but now that I have received them I feel well again."[14] Neither Bryan nor Treadwell acknowledged the manipulation inherent in their attributions of one person's ill health to the disappointing behavior of another.

Neither did Dolly Lunt Burge, who believed that her stepdaughter's constitution "contained the seeds of consumption" from the time that she left school. However, the young woman remained healthy until her fiancé left for war and ceased to write, which "forc[ed] into destructive action those seeds which had it not been for that love that passion, might have lain dormant for years."[15] Another woman also experiencing romantic unhappiness went to Charleston for her health, since "she has become of late very melancholy and her health has suffered."[16] Romantic difficulties of other sorts could also cause illness. After visiting Mrs. Telfair, whose young daughter had eloped at age fourteen and then been divorced, one gossip noted that "there is a report in town that her illness was occasioned by Bertas imprudence."[17]

Fear and anxiety were potent causes of illness and even death, according to many southern whites. Meta Morris Grimball, from low-country South Carolina, noted during the Civil War that one woman "died of consumption in Sumter brought on by anxiety at being in Charleston during the impending attack." On another occasion she wrote, "[T]his war has been the death of a great many old ladies."[18] Ann Turner of North Carolina wrote in her diary that August 1822 "has been with me a time of severe bodily suffering & mental agony doubts & fears at the approach of Death ware [sic] truly agonizing."[19] Maria Bryan mentioned a woman who "made herself very miserable and sick from uneasiness."[20] The unknown writer of an Alabama diary recognized the potential danger her emotions could cause. She noted, "I have been quite uneasy last night and this morning about a spider bite on my wrist, they told me so many stories of alarming results from the bite of poisonous insects that I almost imagined myself sick."[21] Emotions were powerful forces, but this woman was rare in her ability to acknowledge their influence over her own body; more often, whites recognized their impact in others, not themselves.

Insect bites were not the primary cause of fearful emotions dangerous to the health of southern whites; pregnancy and childbirth were.[22] Women recognized that these events could result in their deaths or the deaths of their babies. Even if both mother and child survived, serious injury could occur. Women had good reason to fear pregnancy and childbirth, yet they also recognized that fear and other negative emotions could cause them or their offspring harm. They advised one another and struggled themselves to keep their emotions in check so as to improve their chances of health. Because pregnancy and childbirth were so ubiquitous and so dangerous, they evoked some of the most adamant injunctions of common sense regarding attitude and behavior. For white women, whose control over their emotions was considered shaky under the best of circumstances, reproduction marked the occasion for extended anxieties about the ways in which body and mind could influence each other.

Although disease had a randomness about it that caused white southerners to warn against it in relatively general terms, they did not usually consider reproduction an illness. As a consequence, the importance of following the truths imparted by common sense was even greater than in cases of illness, for no one wanted pregnancy and childbirth to lead to harm for mother or child. Reproduction also elicited especially vehement injunctions about following the tenets of common sense because it was experienced solely by women, whose bodies and minds were widely assumed to be weaker than men's. White men were not alone in describing women's vulnerabilities; white women also considered themselves potentially in danger as a result of their own emotional states during pregnancy and childbirth. They worked hard to overcome their fears and to maintain a cheerful demeanor even as they fretted about their inability to control their emotions any more effectively than they could their swelling bodies.

Sarah Gayle of Alabama was among the most vehement of southern women who wrote about her fears during pregnancy and childbirth, confiding her anxieties about mind and body repeatedly to her diary. While pregnant for the fifth time, with three surviving children, she wrote, "[T]o dwell . . . on the suffering, the danger, the probably fatal consequences of the event before me is dreadful." During the same pregnancy, she vowed that she would "not let my situation weigh so heavily upon my mind" even though she was "dreadfully apprehensive" of the suffering to come. In fact, the child suffered convulsions and died a week after birth, while Gayle herself "grew more and more feeble" from "excessive anxiety." During her eighth pregnancy, when she was not yet thirty, she vowed to "struggle not only for cheerfulness, but for a more hopeful spirit—gloomy indeed will the time be in which the babe is beneath my bosom, unless some light spring up within me." Later in the pregnancy, she noted that she was suffering "turns of sickness," adding "it is not possible to retain any spring of spirits under these circumstances." That pregnancy probably ended in a miscarriage, for within a few months Gayle was pregnant again, complaining that her "mind [was] as still & inactive as this poor body." This pregnancy rendered her "an invalid now, all the time, scarcely able to lift my feet from the floor. My spirits are proportionately depressed, and I am all the time, as if to shed tears copiously,

would releive [*sic*] me more than any thing else." She added, "It is a dreadful
state to be in, but I cannot help myself." Gayle repeatedly struggled with gloomy
feelings during her pregnancies, noting on one occasion "the slightest matter
unnerves me, & my tears flow without control," and tried to console herself by
remarking, "[I]f I believed in presentiments, I should be completely wretched."
At such times, she regularly wrote of missing her dead mother, who "watched
every change in my countenance, whether caused by indisposition or low-spirits,
& nursed or reasoned & caressed me to myself again."[23] While other entries make
clear that Gayle felt the same unequivocal love for her own children, her words
reflect her ambivalence about her pregnancies and the emotional and physical
toll they took on her.

Gayle was not, of course, the only white southern woman to express her emotional and physical dismay during pregnancy, nor was she the only one to blur the
lines between the two sources of discomfort. Recently married and pregnant with
her first child, Penelope Skinner Warren of North Carolina wrote her absent husband that "every one takes great interest in me because I look so frail & delicate,
but if I had my choice I should rather have good health." Although she described
herself as sometimes feeling "very weak & badly," she noted, "I find that cheerful
spirits has an excellent affect on me." Only a week later, she told him "sometimes
when I feel excited in good spirits—it seems that I am doing wrong—& that evil
will follow but I endeavour to chase away such gloomy thoughts & not look for
evil until it comes." Still later she wrote, "[M]y spirits are generally very good
they could be much depressed if I chose to give way to dull feelings but I always
shake them off—for you told me not to suffer them to get the better of me that it
is injurious to my health & I have come to the same conclusion." She wrote her
cousin that she had "overcome all my idle fears & feelings . . . constant reasoning
with myself has brought me to my right senses."[24] Warren's positive thinking was
to little avail. The child was born less than four months later, but Warren died
within a month of the birth.

Women like Gayle and Warren implicitly recognized that their emotions influenced how they experienced their pregnancies, just as their pregnancies influenced
their emotions. Encouraged by friends and relatives to try to keep themselves
cheerful and to avoid dwelling on the trials to come, they believed that their minds
and bodies were inseparably connected, both shaped by the pregnancy that was
creating in them a physical and social transformation. Each woman tried to exert
deliberate control over her emotions, believing that doing so would help ensure
a problem-free pregnancy, a safe delivery, and a healthy mother and child. Each
knew that the pregnancy could end with her own death or that of the child, so
fear was not an unwonted emotion. The physical discomforts of pregnancy were
unpleasant, particularly for women who had to maintain their accustomed duties throughout, and culminated in the even more uncomfortable experience of
labor. Even if both mother and child survived, women knew that gynecological

accidents, including what physicians would call prolapsed uterus and vesico-vaginal fistula were not uncommon, resulting in chronic pain, unpleasant medical treatments, and even death. In the face of all these dangers, women tried hard to control their anxieties, believing that giving way to fear would be harmful.

Yet women could rarely control their emotions entirely; those who could not tried to turn their anxieties into beneficial lessons. Frances Bumpas, a North Carolina minister's wife, wrote in her journal, "I often think of the approaching critical period—its sufferings & its dangers. May I be prepared for the event whatever it may be." Pregnant again a year later, she wrote, "I have frequent thoughts of death. I do not think it ever seemed so near, as it has of late. My trying time is near."[25] Maria Bryan wrote of a conversation between two women that she overheard on a riverboat, in which one woman "said she hoped she would never have any more [children] for she suffered dreadfully. It was like death each time, and she said she sometimes felt right awful when she remembered the discontented and mumbling speeches she had made when her last child was born."[26]

Those women who could not find moral benefit in thoughts of death tried to find other ways to alleviate the worst of their fears. Some relied on their mothers. Mary Blount Shepard of North Carolina wrote her son-in-law that she could not visit in part because her daughter "Mary expects to be confined every day and I cannot think of leaving her at this time, she is very low-spirited and has taken up a notion that she will never get up again." Another of Shepard's daughters shared her sister's concerns, writing shortly after giving birth that "at such a time I am always depressed and all the kindness I can receive is not too much."[27] Meta Morris Grimball recalled "the feeling of nervous misery" she suffered after her twelve confinements, vowing that if she were "to begin life again," she would make different arrangements for her own comfort.[28] Each of these women struggled to control the emotions that she believed influenced the physical experience of pregnancy and childbirth even as she recognized that the physical changes her body underwent had an influence on her emotions. Minds and bodies were inextricably intertwined, and women tried to do what they could to ensure their health and that of their babies by maintaining the proper emotional and physical behavior.

Although lay white southerners did not offer elaborate distinctions between the ways in which men and women's minds and bodies interacted, they clearly thought that women's frequent experiences of pregnancy and childbirth demanded that they keep their emotions in close check. Because women were assumed to be more emotional than men, this required real effort on their part. Men's stronger bodies and minds were less vulnerable to begin with, while women's reproductive functions made them more subject to physical and emotional danger. As a result, white southerners were not surprised when women's bodies or minds gave way to illness. Here as everywhere else in southern society, assumptions about gender differences defined white women as weak and vulnerable, white men as strong and responsible. Lay assumptions were seemingly affirmed by the visible evidence of all too many women whose pregnancies and childbirths did leave them sick or injured.

Pregnancy and childbirth were not the only physical experiences that white southerners believed could influence a person's emotional state. Men, after all, got sick, too. Men's illnesses seemed more random because they were not tied to reproduction and their emotional control appeared stronger, so common sense dictated that they were typically healthier than women. While that was not necessarily true in reality, it was clearly the perception among lay southerners. Although they did not generally consider pregnancy or childbirth to be illnesses as such, they recognized that both made women more vulnerable to becoming ill and prevented them from doing their accustomed tasks at least some of the time. While common sense dictated that people think and act in ways that would preserve their health, few were able to live up to its demands; people did get sick. When they were sick, emotions could influence the outcome. Mind and body could not be separated. Illness was the direct result of the individual's inability to control his or her mind sufficiently, leaving the body itself vulnerable.

Just as emotions could cause illness in men and women and have an impact on its outcome, so, too, could illness transform emotions. People needed to control their emotions, but illness made doing so difficult, sometimes impossible. Both the sick and their families and friends recognized that illness could influence personality, sometimes making recovery even more difficult. Recently married Penelope Warren, who was sixteen years old and pregnant, wrote her husband shortly after he left for two months that "being absent from you has the same effect on me that sickness has[;] it perfectly subdues me—makes me as meek & gentle as possible."[29] More often, sick people reported that their illness made them depressed and fearful of death. Frances Bumpas noted in her diary, "Have not felt very well this week, which has made me somewhat sad." On another occasion she wrote, "I am not well & have been indulging in gloomy foreboding, but feeling this to be wrong, I have endeavoured to recover my wonted cheerfulness."[30] Such levels of self-awareness during illness were rare; more often, sick people refused or were unable to recognize the ways in which their physical experiences transformed them.

Friends and family were far more likely to recognize the ways in which illness influenced personality, sometimes even using a person's emotional state as a means of defining illness. Maria Bryan sympathized with a woman who "must have suffered a great deal." She doubted that anyone but God could "tell how much of gloom and irritability of temper, and apparent indolence might have originated in this [gynecological] disease long preying upon the vitality of health and cheerfulness and comfort."[31] Margaret Devereux of North Carolina wrote that her Aunt Harriet was still bedridden but was recovering from her illness: "[S]he has no fever tho' now and has got over her nervousness. . . . Her spirits are a great deal better, and she seems more calm now than she has done for some time."[32]

Young Sophia Peck of Alabama wrote her sister that "Aunt Clara has been very sick . . . she says she is entirely recovered now but I fear she is mistaken for her spirits appear to be very much depressed which is so unusual a thing with her that I cannot but attribute it to ill health."[33] John Berkley Grimball described George Morris's "horrible" suicide, noting that Morris "had suffered for two years under a severe liver affliction, which made him subject to the darkest depression." Grimball believed "beyond doubt his reason had given way, and he was not himself for many hours before he committed the deplorable act," adding, "our grief is mingled with amazement."[34] While Grimball may have been amazed that his friend's liver disease would cause him to commit suicide, his explanations fit neatly with those of other white southerners who believed that bodily illness influenced the emotions, sometimes far beyond the deliberate control of the suffering individual.

Among the most complex explanations for the connections between emotional and physical health were those of Ebenezer Pettigrew, a North Carolina planter. In 1832, he wrote his sister, "My health was never better than at this time. Distress & anxiety of mind it seems cannot Kill me." Although he had been exposed to the "awful disease" cholera, he did not fall sick, claiming, "my system & habits was equivalent to resist" it. He noted that "I have lost all fear of it" and that "at least 1/4 who die of it, die from fear." Here, Pettigrew implied that his mind and body were separate, since even though his emotional state was weakened he was able to control his fear and did not become sick with cholera. However, he told his sister that he had heard she was "rather desponding" and urged her "to let no such ideas dwell on your mind. . . . Our fears kill us, and if they do not they detress [sic] & make us miserable." This suggested that she might well succumb if she did not control her emotions, presumably because her mind and body were weaker and more closely intertwined than his. However, not trusting to the power of emotions to prevent illness entirely, he also offered her specific advice about avoiding cholera and "attack[ing] the premonotary symptoms."[35]

Pettigrew did recognize that mind and body influenced each other during illness, even when people made real efforts to control both. Several years after his exposure to cholera, when Pettigrew became sick enough to fear death, he apologized to a friend for not answering his letter, claiming, "[W]ith my bad health, my spirits declined and were exceedingly depressed." In spite of the "melancholy strain" of his letter, Pettigrew recovered. Some years later, he warned that no one should treat his daughter so "as to let her know that any thing was the matter with her" because "it is not well to talk of that disease to the person who has it, in as much as it is produced sometimes by sympathy."[36] He did not specify what disease his daughter had, but it may have been a form of chorea, from which another of his children and other family members suffered and died. Pettigrew's use of the word *sympathy* was ambiguous, underscoring the close connection he perceived between his daughter's mind and body. While he may have been warning of the dangers associated with treating her as an invalid, it is just as likely that he was referring to the influence her thoughts about the disease could have on her body. Pettigrew clearly believed that distress and anxiety might not kill, but that fear, despondency, and even suggestion could lead to diseases that would prove fatal. Implicit in his comments was the notion that his sister's and daughter's bodies were more likely to succumb to the power of their minds than was his own. His own momentary emotional weakness was the unfortunate result of his disease, while they were always physically and emotionally vulnerable because of their sex.

An unidentified woman diarist from Alabama was even more explicit about the ways in which illness could influence the emotions than Pettigrew, writing in 1835, "I thought poor Mrs S—— had the blues to day, and wondered that so good a person could be attacked by a malady confined to the repining, and the selfish, but indeed I was mistaken in my conjecture, she was ill, physically so, and I am vexed with myself for supposing such an absurdity."[37] Her assumption that depression was a disease caused either by physical or emotional disturbances reflects a common view of midcentury white southerners. So was the moral judgment inherent in her comments suggesting that those who succumbed to depression were emotionally weak and selfish unless their emotional state had physical origins. Likewise, Maria Bryan urged her sister to visit, suggesting that her sympathy might be beneficial for their father, who was depressed about debt. She worried that he "cannot stand long under his severe mental disquietudes, which, I plainly perceive, exercise a most unhappy influence upon all his bodily functions."[38] The chain of causation from debt to depression to disease was clear in her thinking.

By blurring the distinctions between mind and body as the source and site of illness, white southerners rejected any notion of a clear boundary between them. While they did not explicitly hold individuals deliberately responsible for becoming ill, they certainly recognized that attitude and belief played a part and thus held themselves and others to a high standard of emotional purity. They defined emotional purity differently for men and women, mostly because they considered women to be weaker and thus less capable of controlling mind and body than were men. Pregnancy and childbirth were particularly fraught with danger for women, who were necessarily held to a higher standard of moral rectitude than men. But both men and women were expected and expected themselves to adhere to the dictates of common sense. Only by having the right attitudes could people avoid illness; the wrong ones could make them sick and even die. At the same time, they recognized that being sick could itself cause negative emotions, which endangered the patient at least as much as the physical illness did. Here, too, women were more vulnerable because their minds were weaker and their emotions stronger than men's. Women and men might not be able to prevent themselves from becoming sick by behaving as they ought, but they were expected to try. Mind and body were seamless and circular; common sense taught that disease was an internal process that could be helped by medicine but that was ultimately in the domain of the individual and God.

When white southerners related such commonsense truisms about mind and body and their relationship to illness, they invariably assumed that the bodies in question were themselves white. To some extent, this was because the bodies under discussion were so, as most of the surviving evidence about common sense was related in the context of family, friends, and neighbors. At the same time, they struggled to find ways to apply what they considered common sense to their slaves' bodies and minds in order to prevent and cure their illnesses. Yet in the South, common sense was influenced by race; whites were not willing to extend to slaves what they believed to be true for themselves. As a result, they sometimes qualified commonsense observations about the interactions between mind and body in rather self-conscious ways. Generally unwilling to acknowledge the emotional experiences of slaves, whites assumed slaves' minds and bodies interacted in ways that would allow them to evade work by pretending to be ill, which they called shamming. If common sense as whites applied it to themselves required controlling negative emotions in order to avoid bodily illness, it meant exercising control by watching out for devious minds and bodies when applied to slaves.

Slaveholders' primary concern was always to keep their slaves at work, while still protecting their investment by keeping them alive and healthy. Plowden C. Weston instructed his overseer that "great care must be taken to prevent persons from lying up when there is nothing or little the matter with them." He insisted that "such must be turned out immediately" and even "those somewhat sick" be put to "lighter work, which encourages industry." He added that "nothing is so subversive of discipline, or so unjust, as to allow people to sham, for this causes the well-disposed to do the work of the lazy."[39] Planters who struggled to detect shamming also knew that while they might try to control slaves' bodies, at least from sunup to sundown, they had only limited influence over slaves' minds. As a result, their definitions of common sense and their views about what was reasonable to expect from an individual trying to stay healthy or recover from disease were rather different when applied to slaves.

Slaveholders also recognized that they had to acknowledge slaves' own views of health and illness, mind and body in order to intervene effectively. Most whites were aware that slaves did not share their understandings of what caused sickness and how to cure it, although for the most part they had only a garbled knowledge of what slaves actually did believe. Few whites were willing to recognize the health consequences of their own demands on slaves' bodies. Instead, they lamented what they considered the superstitions that impeded their efforts to cure slaves' ailments. Since slaveholders knew that they could not hope to control slaves' minds without acknowledging their perspective, slaveholders had no choice but to recognize that slaves' beliefs were different and to try to change them to conform to whites' own definition of common sense. Not surprisingly, they were rarely successful. Carolyn Clitherall acknowledged as much after she went to see her "faithful servant Jack," who had been sick and unable to work for six months. "A superstitious belief that some witchcraft had been practised upon him has been the cause of his disease, & the ignorance & credulity of his color sustain his belief."[40] While Jack (mal?)lingered, Clitherall considered her own beliefs common sense; his were superstition.

Clitherall was not the only slaveholder to lament the consequences of superstition among slaves. When cholera swirled around Tristrim Skinner's North Carolina home in 1849, he decided to remain at home for the summer, canceled the passes that allowed his slaves to visit the town, and took a variety of other precautions. He noted that word of the "sudden death" of two slaves on a neighboring plantation caused his slaves a "salutary fright" that he hoped would "be of great service" to them, a sign of his hope to impose his own version of common sense. A week later, he wrote his father of another neighbor who lost thirty-one slaves to cholera, fifteen of them men. According to Skinner, "several of his negroes died from alarm," although "several gentlemen," including the owner, told him the deaths were caused by "the use of pork killed during warm weather last winter & not well saved."[41] The owner and his neighbors refused to allow these slaves the same emotional latitude that they would have granted whites, nor were they willing to acknowledge the power of the slaves' emotions over their bodies. Whites might die of fright, according to many whites' informal comments, but slaves who seemed to do the same really died from bad meat. Slaveholders were reluctant to recognize slaves as having emotions powerful enough to cause illness and death, as was possible for whites, even though they believed that slaves' minds were weaker and so less under their deliberate control. Slaves who could not be made to control their emotions had to be denied the possibility of any but superstitious connections between mind and body.

Slaveholders who tried to understand the ways in which slaves' minds and bodies influenced each other had to find ways to distinguish real illness from shamming, or at least exaggeration. Sophia Watson wrote her husband that she had received many requests for medicine from the slaves on their Alabama plantation. She reported that "Hester about whom I was feeling so anxious when I last wrote you has gone out to work—Things are so much exaggerated when reported by negroes that I sometimes think I will believe nothing they tell me." She added, "If all had been true that they told me of Hester, it would scarcely have been possible for her to have been well now."[42] Maria Bryan also found a slave woman's condition "not so bad as was represented" after she suffered what "appears to be a nervous attack."[43]

Shamming remained a real concern, as South Carolinian John Peyre Thomas noted in his diary: "I whipped Lary myself today for feigning sickness, as I thought."[44] His last phrase suggests the degree of uncertainty that plagued all accusations of shamming, even those that slaveholders chose to punish. Margaret Devereux complained that she had had no cook for a week, because "Phillis either was or pretended to be not well enough to come to the kitchen."[45] The problem of shamming, or at least its potential, influenced slaveholders' understanding of the ways in which slaves' minds and bodies interacted with each other to cause disease. Shamming represented the deliberate invocation of illness by healthy slaves to avoid work or otherwise control their own lives, not the more subtle influence of mind over body that whites reserved for themselves. Whites believed that slaves wanted to appear sick, but they assumed that their own bodies and minds were incapable of such deliberate deception. They thought that there would have been no need for them to pretend to be sick, since they controlled their own lives.

White southerners clearly believed that their own minds and bodies were intertwined, even if those of slaves were not. Prudence thus demanded that white individuals work hard to control their emotions to avoid illness as much as possible and improve their chances of recovery when their initial efforts failed. Whites did not blame themselves for getting sick, but at least to some extent, they did hold themselves—or one another—accountable. They assumed that their slaves, whose emotions could not be controlled in the same way either by slaveholders or themselves, were instead liable to shamming. Thus slaves had to be held accountable in a very different manner from the way whites held themselves.

## Slaves' Views of Mind, Body, and the External Causes of Illness

Slaves, of course, did not hold themselves accountable for their illnesses.[46] Instead, they blamed other people, either the whites who controlled their labor and material environment or practitioners of witchcraft working at the behest of someone who wanted to harm them; the causes of illness were external to the body. As a result, where white people sought to control their own emotions, blacks tried to engage in preventive actions, by determining the intensity, pace, and timing of their work; shaping their own after-work lives; and guarding against the charms and countercharms of conjurers. Their version of the commonsense connections between mind and body interpreted them as quite separate, yet slaves engaged in a range of ritualized practices that they believed would protect them from harm.

Slaves' desire for health was not the sole or even the primary motivation for their efforts at autonomy. Autonomy was a goal in and of itself. Slaves who recognized overwork and poor living conditions as the source of illness believed that freedom might well bring better health, but this was hardly the most important reason they wanted to be free. Nevertheless, slaves knew that the very fact of being enslaved contributed to their experiences of illness and death. The problems that resulted could be emotional, physical, or both. An unnamed Tennessee woman recalled her brutal, violent mistress who was verbally and physically abusive, even preventing her mother from giving her dry moccasins to soothe her bloody, frostbitten feet. The woman added, "When I think back over what I came through I wonder that I am still living or why I didn't lose my mind. I was beat over the head and knocked around so much that my head and back stayed sore all the time." Even as a girl, she said, "I used to get sick a lot" and "was beaten so much that I don't see how I kept my right senses." However, she was grateful not to have lived on the adjoining farm, where she watched the owner "take his foot and kick poor women that were with child and cause them to have miscarriage right there in the field." When a baby was crying, she saw him "take his stick and knock its brains out and call for the foreman to come and haul off the nasty black rat."[47]

Such violent deaths were rare but vividly remembered by slaves and former slaves. A different unnamed woman interviewed by Fisk University remembered four people who were killed by whites, one "hit right in the forehead" who "fell down and never did come to," while another was whipped "one evening for the longest, and told . . . to get over the barb wire fence, and she said she couldn't, and he jerked her through by the hair, and she never did come to. She was a corpse in 10 minutes after they jerked her through." The third ran away with "a piece of long chain tied to his ankle"; when he was found "the flesh was swollen all over that chain . . . and it had to be sawed off." He died as a result.[48] Sophia Word remembered "two gals that killt themselfs." One "wuz found across the bed with a pen knife in her hand." The other's owner whipped her "most to death fer fergiting to put onions in the stew," after which she drowned herself.[49]

Clearly, the very fact of being a slave was dangerous to one's life, not to mention one's health, including mental health. Slaves who lived on the next plantation to one unnamed woman "did go crazy oned in a while; and they said it was 'cause they beat 'em so much." She claimed that when they "got like that," they were put in the asylum, but that the other slaves found them frightening. "They would go out in the woods and hide behind trees and things, and they would run from everything and everybody, jest scared, you know; they had been beat so much; why, they would run like a rabbit from a dog."[50] Her ambiguous language suggests that the slaves on both plantations were frightened by bad treatment; both were harmed.

Most slaves were not killed by whites, nor did they commit suicide or go crazy. Nevertheless, the very fact of being enslaved was harmful to their health. Because whites feared shamming, slaves were not allowed to define the subjective experience of their own bodies. Instead, whites acted as the gatekeepers of health and insisted on determining when slaves were too sick to work. Unwilling to admit slaves' own testimony about their bodily states, slaveholders dismissed the action of slaves' minds as much as they were able. They assumed instead that slaves' illnesses were located almost exclusively in their bodies, unmediated by their emotions. Similarly, they preferred to think that slaves' emotions could not make them sick. Slaveholders who intertwined their own minds and bodies uncoupled them when thinking about their slaves.

Slaves resentfully recognized their owners as gatekeepers of health and sickness. According to Amanda Jackson, who had been a slave in Georgia, "When you wuz too sick to go to de fiel' an' not sick enuff to be in bed you had to report to de white lady at de house—she could tell pretty much if you wuz sick an' she would work on you—if you did'nt git better den she would send fer de doctor."[51] According to George Womble, born around 1843 in Georgia, "Unless a slave was too sick to walk he was required to go to the field and work like the others."[52] Sometimes physicians performed the role of gatekeeper. Emmaline Heard, also from Georgia, remembered "if the doctor stated that the slave was well enough to work, they had to go to the fields."[53] Former slaves remembered that those who were legitimately sick did not have to work. Temple Pitts of Virginia recalled, "When we wuz sick we had de bes' doctor an' all de medicine dat he said we ought ter habe; an' we ain't wuck when we wuz sick nother."[54] Fleming Clark agreed, but added, "You had to be awful sick if dey didn't make you go out" to the fields to work.[55]

Slaves knew that their masters acted as gatekeepers because they were concerned about shamming. Most slaves denied that the practice occurred at all; those who admitted its existence thought it was rare. Both Jennie Kendricks and Amanda McDaniel of Georgia told Works Progress Administration (WPA) interviewers that they did not remember any shamming, while Isiah Green said that those who did pretend to be sick were quickly examined, revealing the truth.[56] Some slaves reportedly were successful at shamming, at least for a time. Louise Green, one of folklorist Elsie Clews Parsons's young informants early in the twentieth century, wrote a story about an "old man in slavery" who "told his master that he was cripple and couldn't work." He was allowed to "stay home to take care of his children," but he was found out and severely beaten when he was caught singing "I was fooling my master seventy-two years, And I am fooling him now."[57]

Charles Grandy, who had been a slave in Virginia, offered a more complex account of shamming that involved rewards as well as respite. "Anytime a slave got sick or had de misery, ole Marsa Tom would give him a dram of whiskey. Sometimes I'd go to Marsa Tom an' say, 'Marsa, I done got a terr'ble cole f'om someplace. Don't spec I gonna be able to work today.' Marsa laugh an' say, 'Come on, you black rascal. Nothin' wrong wid you. All you want is a drink of whiskey.' Den he give it to me." Grandy admitted that "sometime I go back to him de second or third time an' tell him de same thing. Sometime he remember he already give it to me an' sometime he don't. All depend on how much Marsa Tom done took hisself."[58]

For those able to get away with it, shamming could provide rewards even greater than having a drink or avoiding punishment or work, by offering the opportunity to manipulate those with power in more dramatic ways. In a volume of Gullah stories from the South Carolina coast, folklorist Ambrose Gonzales recounted the tale of a slave woman who carelessly tripped over a "cootuh," breaking the pitcher of water she had been carrying on her head so that the water "drap' 'puntop de gal two eye' en' run down 'e face en' gone een 'e mout.'" In spite of the broken pitcher, the woman's mistress did not punish her because the "missis t'ink de gal cry tuh dat, en' 'e missis sorry fuhr'um." Instead, the mistress gave the woman the broken pitcher, which she later broke into pieces to decorate her husband's grave.[59]

Shamming could be emotional as well as physical, directed at blacks as well as whites. In another story, Gonzales recounted the experience of a married woman who was given candy made from pine gum and molasses by a male friend. When her husband returned unexpectedly, her teeth were covered with the sticky stuff, but she was "smaa't 'nuf" to "biggin fuh moan. Uh moan, en' uh moan." When he asked her what was wrong, she "tell'um uh binnuh [was] walk roun' de fence en' uh walk 'puntop yalluh jacket nes' en' de t'ing 'ting me tuh dat. . . . Den uh biggin fuh cry." Her husband went to get medicine for her, which gave her time to get the sticky candy out from her teeth without him finding out about the other man, so that she "fool'um fuh true!"[60] In both stories, women pretended to be injured in order to avoid the wrath of someone more powerful than they were. The audience for them could enjoy the emotional rewards of outsmarting the mistress or a jealous husband without contemplating punishment from the more powerful master for actually shamming to avoid work.

Discussions of shamming are far more pervasive in the folklore of slavery than they are in the oral testimony of former slaves. This is perhaps because slaves who pretended to be sick in order to avoid work engaged in behavior the rest perceived as selfish and deceitful, even as they admired it. Shamming hurt the master by depriving him of labor, but it also hurt the other slaves who had to do additional work to pick up the slack and who were less likely to be believed when they were legitimately sick should the pretense be discovered. However, in the stories they told themselves about animals outwitting one another, shamming was a favorite technique. For example, many of the stories about Rabbit and other animals collected by Elsie Clews Parsons from blacks of the Sea Islands of South Carolina in 1919 show them pretending to be sick or injured in order to turn events to their favor. In one, Rabbit claimed to have a pain in his stomach in order to avoid Wolf finding out that he had eaten all of their butter. In another, Rabbit pretended to be sick in order to steal the fish that Fox had caught. In yet another, Rabbit pretended to be sick in order to convince Wolf to let him ride on his back to the dance, where he boasted about his riding horse.[61]

Even in folklore, shamming did not always have the relatively minor consequences of losing luxuries like butter or facing embarrassment at a dance. One of the stories recounted by Charles C. Jones Jr. has all of the animals working together to build a house and gather provisions for the winter. Rabbit promised to help, but when called upon to do so, he claimed that his wife was very sick and that he was needed at home to nurse her. Later, since "nutten mek um so merry es to lit offer tarruh [other] people," Rabbit slipped into the finished house and scared first Deer and then Lion into thinking he was "de Sperit" who had "tek persession er de house." Since the other animals were "faid fuh bus een de do," they all agreed to leave, and "dem yent fine out tel dis day dat eh been Buh Rabbit wuh fool um, an dat no Sperit bin day none tall."[62] Joel Chandler Harris offered the story of Miss Pa'tridge, who ate one of her own eggs, then "flew'd up, en fell down en flutter, en scramble 'roun' in de leaves" in order to scare Brer Rabbit from stealing the rest of her eggs. Partridge warned him that they were snake's eggs, "rank pizen!" and that he had best run away, allowing her to save the rest.[63] In these and similar stories, blacks warned one another that pretending to be sick, or even to nurse the sick, meant extra work and a dose of humiliation for everyone else, even if in real life it also offered the successful practitioner a measure of satisfaction at fooling the slaveholder. Slaves recognized shamming as part of their ongoing struggle against the demands of whites. Whites who served as gatekeepers denied slaves the right to define their own experiences, inviting the kind of vicarious trickery Rabbit and the other animals engaged in in these stories, if not the actual behavior.

Slaves who were less concerned with shamming than with the suffering of their bodies had their own views of health and sickness and their own ways of defining the connections between mind and body. Their view of common sense centered on the idea that good treatment and decent material conditions were conducive to health. According to Cicely Cawthon, who had been a slave in Georgia, "about the only things slaves needed to keep off diseases was good stout shoes on their feet, plenty to eat, good clothes, and when it started raining to quit work and come in."[64] Slaves who were not treated according to Cawthon's prescription could easily become sick. David Blount of North Carolina remembered working to clear new ground one cold day when a boy asked to warm himself by the burning brush and was denied permission by the overseer. "After awhile de boy had a chill. De oberseer don't care, but dat night de boy am a sick nigger." The master called a doctor, who diagnosed pneumonia, and later fired the overseer.[65] Slaves who were beaten easily recognized the ill effects. Rev. W. B. Allen, who had been a slave in Alabama, remembered that after a slave was beaten, masters and overseers would "rub salt and red pepper into his wounds, causing him to go into convulsions, developing a fever, resulting frequently in a state of coma lasting for several days."[66]

Slaves who were treated with a measure of decency recognized that masters had their own interests at heart in trying to keep slaves healthy. Genia Woodbury boasted about the careful treatment sick slaves were given on the South Carolina plantation where she lived, adding "dey ne'er didn't 'low de colored girls to work none tall 'fore dey wuz shape lak uh 'oman cause dey 'fraid dat might strain dey ne'ves."[67] One unnamed woman said, "[W]e didn't need so many medicines like they do now; we had more sense. We used to wear boots, and the women wore high top shoes, heavy yarn stockings, and all wool underwear, most all the year round."[68] Not all slaves were so well clothed or so healthy or had owners concerned about their nerves; far more often, overwork, inadequate diet, and poor living conditions made sickness a common experience.

Slaves sometimes wondered whether their own health was better or worse than that of whites, which was an important way of evaluating the consequences of slavery. Some thought that blacks were sicklier than whites. Ike Derricote remembered that during the Civil War there was such an "awful" outbreak of smallpox in Athens, Georgia, that they built a hospital "for all de folks dat was sick wid smallpox at one time." Since the pesthouse "warn't near large enough, . . . dey finally got to what dey used it jus' for de colored folks, 'cause it seemed dat smallpox went harder wid dem dan wid de white folks."[69] But Virginia Hayes Shepherd thought that in Norfolk, Virginia, where she and her family were sent to the wartime pesthouse, "more white folks died than Negroes. Negroes somehow seemed to get well."[70] Many blacks believed that the races were medically distinct. According to Auntie Rachel, "Mos' chillun boun' ter have whoopin' cough. Cullud chillun wouldn' have it, but dey all time ketch it from de white chillun!"[71] One of Ambrose Gonzales's informants told a story about his granddaughter, who "whimpered" that she had been scratched by a briar. The man laughed, asking, "[W]eh de debble you ebbuh know briah kin 'cratch nigguh' foot? You mus' be t'ink you is buckruh,[72] enty?"[73]

Former slaves interviewed by the WPA often claimed that slaves had been healthier than black people were in the present. Georgia Baker, who had been a slave in Georgia, said, "Slaves didn't git sick as often as Niggers does now days," which she attributed to the teas her mother made.[74] Neal Upson, also from Georgia, had a different explanation: "Folkses warn't sick much in dem days lak dey is now, but now us don't eat strong victuals no more."[75] Robert Shepherd was one of many who claimed, "Dere wasn't many folks sick dem days, 'specially 'mongst de slaves."[76] Sally Brown of Georgia agreed, noting, "We didn't need many doctors then fur we didn't have so much sickness in them days, and nachelly they didn't die so fast; folks lived a long time then."[77] Former slaves interviewed by Fisk University offered the same sorts of testimony. One man said, "Colored people didn't get sick and die like they do now. They had little things, but not serious diseases."[78]

Former slaves who insisted that they had been healthier than whites and sick far less often during slavery than later had been children during slavery. They were elderly when they made their claims. Their parents and grandparents, who worked hard to protect children from the rigors and deprivations of slavery, might well have offered a different assessment. By claiming not to have been medically harmed during slavery, elderly black interviewees were reflecting the rigors of a lifetime of hard work and often inadequate medical care as freed people. For the most part, they were reporting to white interviewers, who, they hoped, would help them obtain Social Security or other government benefits. Their testimony is more a reflection of the difficulties of using the slave narratives as sources for understanding the past than a reliable measure of the relative rates of illness among black people in slavery and freedom. It also reflects the difficulties slaves faced in having their illnesses recognized as such. One reason former slaves remembered being healthy so much of the time was because their bodily experiences were defined as such by whites, no matter how they felt subjectively. Since the definition of sickness was not having to work and children did not work as much as adults simply because they were children, former slaves may well have been correct in remembering that they experienced fewer illnesses as children than they did later in life. Children who survived into adulthood were less likely to have been sickly as children anyway. Even so, slaves were often sick, the result of overwork, poor living standards, inadequate nutrition, and insufficient medical care.[79] Their own definitions of common sense made clear that all too often, external factors beyond their control contributed to their poor health even when it was not acknowledged by whites. Those factors were less likely to be experienced and remembered by children than by their parents.

Since slaves could not control the external conditions of their lives to ensure standards that would keep them healthy or even define when they were not, they sought to improve their chances by manipulating their environment as best they could. Often, that meant following rituals and other behaviors that had been passed down from their ancestors to ensure good health and good luck as well to offer protection from harm. Folklorists have cataloged extensive lists of such practices, tracing some of them to their origins in African religions.[80] They appear in the oral histories from former slaves as well. Such practices focused on love and family, on work, on achieving success at any endeavor, and on health. They also were intended to avoid harm, including loss of love, health, or luck.

Staying healthy and protecting oneself required following a variety of rituals connecting mind and body. Among the most ubiquitous of such techniques was midwives' practice of placing something sharp under the bed of a woman in labor in order to cut the pains of childbirth. According to Sally Brown, "The granny would put a rusty piece of tin or a ax under the mattress and this would ease the pains. The granny put a ax under my mattress once. This wuz to cut off the after-pains and it sho did too, honey." Brown said women were allowed to sit up on the fifth day after giving birth, when "they tole us to walk around the house jest once and come in the house. This wuz to keep us frum takin' a 'lapse."[81] Shang Harris, however, believed that "dey didn't do nuttin' to cut de pains [of childbirth]—*you got to have dem*."[82] Childbirth was a particularly dangerous time for mother and child, demanding many rituals. Mason Crum, in his volume about people who spoke Gullah, noted that when a young woman died after childbirth, her baby was "passed over the coffin several times in order to make sure that it would survive and not be claimed in death by the spirit of its mother"; otherwise, the baby "could not be 'raised.'"[83]

Other rituals were intended to prevent sickness more generally. Alec Pope remembered that slaves "wore some sort of beads 'round deir necks to keep sickness away," while Green Willbanks, like Pope from Georgia, claimed "everybody wore buckeyes" for the same purpose.[84] Some behaviors were specific to a particular health problem. Mrs. Moore told a Fisk University interviewer that "you can't throw your hair out, if you did the birds got it and put it in their nest, and you would have headaches."[85] There were many other behaviors that offered protection as well as some actions that could be used by qualified people to cause harm. Mary Wright feared the poisonous bite of "a cross-eyed pusson er blue gummed niggers," either of which could cause death.[86] More than just bites could cause harm. Far more common were charms, ritual objects involving a wide variety of ordinary and exotic substances combined and dispersed in specific ways that could inflict harm on their unsuspecting recipients. If an illness were acquired in this way, ordinary medicine as practiced by whites could not cure; only a countercharm would do. Such charms and countercharms and the illnesses they caused and cured were the province of conjure (or root) doctors. Many slaves believed that conjure caused illness; common sense demanded protecting oneself from its dangerous effects. Former North Carolina slave Betty Cofer knew a man who "used to make charms, little bags filled with queer things. He called 'em jacks an' sold 'em to the colored folks an' some white folks too."[87] Since there were too many rituals to follow easily and the hidden dangers of charms lurked everywhere, slaves relied on conjure doctors and other experts to help them exert a measure of control over their lives.

Conjure and other varieties of witchcraft were a version of preventive medicine, designed to protect its practitioners against disease, accidents, injury, violence, and even bad luck. It was simultaneously proactive medicine, a way to make things happen for good or for ill. Both the ways conjure made people sick and the ways it could be used to prevent and cure illness were elaborately described in oral histories of former slaves and by collectors of folklore. Often, charms were used to make an enemy or a rival sick. Other times, witches did the damage by riding people as they slept; the testimony includes many ways of preventing or stopping this, such as keeping pins or sand by the door that the witch would have to count or sprinkling her skin with salt or pepper so that she could not return to it. The latter may have been an ironic reflection of the pepper some slaveholders sprinkled on the backs of slaves they whipped, in order to intensify the pain.

Those who did not adequately protect themselves could be harmed by the actions of witches. According to Sam Rawls, who had been a slave in South Carolina, "One old woman was a witch, and she rode me one night. I couldn't get up one night, and had a ketching of my breath and couldn't rise up. She held me down."[88]

Penny Williams from North Carolina was also ridden by a witch. "I wus in de bed, an' she thought dat I wus 'sleep. I feels her when she crawls up on my lef' leg an' stops de circulation. I knows how ter fox her do' so I gits up an' puts a knife under my pillow." Williams said that she continued to sleep with a knife "an' ain't had no mo' trouble wid witches ner circulation nother."[89] Some witches could simultaneously cause and diagnose disease in their victims. Former Georgia slave William McWhorter reported that "some folks say" that seeing a witch in the form of a black cat was "a sign your blood is out of order."[90] Charles Jones reported in a story that when you were sick, the devil "gone eensider you lucker a wurrum [like a worm], an eh gie you all sorter misry."[91] According to one of folklorist Newbell Niles Puckett's sources, witches were "supposed to afflict people with diseases and to transfer diseases from one person to another." Puckett thought that "any inexplicable or unexpected calamity . . . is often blamed on witchcraft," including pneumonia, "insanity, boils, ill luck in hunting or courting, death, [and] constipation." He attributed such beliefs to West African religions, which taught that the supernatural could "prevent and cure disease," "cause insanity or blindness," "cause sickness or death," "aid in childbirth," and "keep children healthy," among a long list of other things.[92] Some witches could even cause their victims to die. Anna Grant claimed that a conjurer "poisoned my ma and my two sisters," with something in a bottle she buried "under our fire chimney" so that "my ma nebber could eat anything that wuz cooked from that chimney." The sisters were poisoned "by putting snake dust in their clothes," which killed them. Not everyone died, according to Grant; "some conjured folks is confined to bed and is fixed just enough so dey will linger." Others were "fixed so dey'll walk on a stick" and still "others swelled up like dey got the dropsy."[93] Only a few were as sanguine as Georgia former slave Mary Colbert, who claimed "the dead can't harm you; its the living that make the trouble."[94] Most slaves believed that conjure could be both dangerous and beneficial; certainly it was a powerful source of sickness.

The extent of conjure's effectiveness was a matter of debate among slaves. As they tried to define common sense, they searched for its parameters in their efforts to explain the connections between mind and body, health and sickness. They wondered whether conjure worked on whites or even on blacks who did not believe in it. Some thought that it worked in tandem with Christianity, others that they were separate and contradictory. George White, who had been a slave in Virginia, offered a long list of ways to use roots to cure disease and make things happen. He believed that "dere's a root for ev'y disease . . . but you have got to talk wid God an' ask him to help out."[95] An unnamed informant for Fisk University claimed, "I don't believe in conjurers because I have asked God to show me such things—if they existed—and He came to me in person while I was in a trance and he said, There ain't no such thing as conjurers.'" The informant hedged his or her bets, however, adding, "I believe in root-doctors because, after all, we must

depend upon some form of root or weed to cure the sick."[96] David Goodman
Gullins of Georgia thought Christianity was central to understanding illness,
saying "it was a custom to hold prayer meetings in the quarters for the colored
sick."[97] For most slaves, though, conjure could easily coexist with Christianity;
the sensible thing to do was to accept help from both God and conjure and not
worry about the possibility of contradictions between them.

A more vexing question was the connection between conjure and the medical
practices of whites. According to Marrinda Jane Singleton, "the brewin' of certain
concoctions composed of herbs, roots and scraps of cloth was believed to wuk
charms or spells on the persons desired and yet not affected by other persons."
Such spells could not be removed by "medical science or skill"; instead, "only
similar methods to those used in castin' the spell could remove it." She added
that "Many of us slaves feared de charm of witchcraft more than de whippin' dat
de Marster gave. Dey would keep their tiny bags of charms closely hidden under
their clothes."[98] Her comments suggest that her Virginia master was at least suspicious of the practice of conjure.

The explanations and treatments provided by white doctors did not always
convince—or cure—those slaves who believed that conjure caused their ailments.
A few days after a white doctor bathed what Virginia Hayes Shepherd's father
believed to be a boil, "it burst and live things came out of the boil and crawled on
the floor. He thought he was conjured. He said an enemy of his put something
on the horse's back and he rode it and got it on his buttocks and broke him out."
Shepherd offered other ways that an enemy could "make you get sick, weak, and
the doctors couldn't do anything." Instead, you would have to send for the conjure
doctor, who had ways to "tell the victim the direction of the enemy."[99] White medicine was scarcely powerful enough to counteract conjure, even when prescribed
by physicians. White doctors sometimes recognized conjure's power, at least over
the minds of their patients. Charleston physician E. Geddings wrote of a slave
woman patient whom he diagnosed with a large tumor of the abdomen shortly
after she gave birth. He noted that the tumor, which grew so much "that she soon
became as large as before her confinement," and her inability to become pregnant
again "induced her to believe that she was *tricked* (bewitched)." Geddings's "attempts to influence the tumor by medical treatment, were unavailing," and she
continued to appear to be "in the last stages of pregnancy" until her death from
convulsions.[100] This woman's death would have been proof for many that conjure
was more powerful than the medicine white doctors could offer.

Conjure could raise complicated questions about slavery, race, and authority
for the slaves who believed in it. One of folklorist Orland Armstrong's informants
told of "an old gran'pap who led the revolt" against a cruel overseer. The man
"knew conjur" and so "made the rounds of the cabins, chanting incantations
against the overseer and passing on instructions for a meeting." There, "hoodoo
was said against the overseer that consigned him to the evil spirits for a speedy

death." A few days later, the overseer's horse fell, and the overseer died with the whip he had been brandishing "tangled about his broken neck." Armstrong also quoted Uncle Roger, who used conjure to help him run away. "When I run erway I had dat rabbit's foot an' I said de hoodoo over it. Conjured myself so de dogs couldn' smell me. Stayed out thar in de swamp three days, an' hy'ar 'em yelpin' an' hollerin' all roun.'" Roger claimed that he would not have been found had he been able to provide food and water for himself.[101] One unnamed former slave woman recalled that one night a man visited swinging a string with something on the end that stopped when it got to her father. "He said father was going to get whipped the next morning but he would keep him from getting the whipping. Sure enough the next morning they come got him, but they never touched him. They couldn', for that man had fixed it so they couldn't whip him." She added that although the man was a runaway slave, "he just went around keeping people from getting killed."[102]

Conjure was powerful, but it could not save everyone. An unnamed man said that there was "a Hoodoo nigger who could hoodoo niggers, but couldn't hoodoo masters. He couldn't make ole master stop whipping him, with the hoodooism, but they could make Negroes crawl to them."[103] Most conjure doctors probably followed his practice; it would have been far too dangerous to their reputations to promise protection from whites on a regular basis, to say nothing of the death of the overseer. Slaves' scarred backs bore mute testimony to conjure's limits as preventive medicine. Medicine as practiced by whites may have been unable to stop the harm conjure caused slaves, but even conjure could not reliably prevent white violence.

Some whites were aware of the power of conjure and used it to their advantage. Charles Jones retold the story of a man who was "berry tired long wuk" and so prayed aloud "dat Det would come an cahr way eh Mossa, an eh Mistis, an de Obersheer." Since the master heard about the prayer, he decided to put on a long white gown and go to the man's house, where the man "git skade, an tink duh Sperit." When asked, the master claimed to be death come for the man, who quickly escaped to the woods. The next day, he told everyone that "Det bin come fur um last night, but dat him bin dodge um." Even so, "arter dat nobody ebber yeddy [heard] um mek no mo prayer bout Det."[104] While this was almost certainly not a real event, it contained an important message about the power of conjure to serve whites' purposes as well as those of slaves.

A few whites even assumed the role of conjure doctors themselves. Ellen Trell, a former slave from North Carolina, reported that her mother "had a spell put on her and she lay in bed talking to herself and sweating draps of sweats as big as the end of my finger. She would groan and say, 'go away evil spirit, go away,' but the spell would not leave her until we went to a white witch doctor and got cured."[105] Patsy Mitchner knew a woman who had a similar experience. The woman "had a spell out on 'er an' it hurt her feet, but a ole white man witch doctor helped take de spell off, but I think it wus de Lord who took it off." Mitchner added that she was "a Christian an' I believes eberythin' is in his han's."[106] In a story published in the *Southern Literary Journal and Monthly Review* in 1837 and attributed to Professor H. J. Nott,[107] a white woman was "bewitched" by another white woman but was relieved when "a knowing man" who "doctored the whole neighborhood" told her what to do. Because of her "courage [and] presence of mind," she was able to follow his directions, leaving the "witch as hot as fire and entirely out of her senses." After the witch's death, it was "strange how many children got rid of fits, and old people of pains in the bones, rheumatisms and all sorts of ailments."[108] Conjure and witchcraft could both afflict and be cured by people of both races.

Powerful as it was, conjure, and the preventive and proactive medicine it inspired, could not regularly offer sufficient protection to slaves subject to the authority of white owners. Whites were simply too brutal, their control too strong, for conjure to provide effective immunity for slaves. It could neither prevent nor cure every ailment, but it allowed slaves to try to help themselves when white gatekeepers tried to define their bodily experiences and denied them respite from work. Although imperfect, conjure offered slaves a way to take action against the problematic options and limited control they had over their lives, not only because they were slaves, but also because of the very arbitrariness of life and death. For people who believed that the origin of illness was external to the body but were often unable to do very much about the conditions of their lives, conjure was a way to take an active role in their own health.

Conjure also offered slaves a way of thinking about interpersonal conflict within their own communities as well as within their bodies. Rather than addressing conflict directly, slaves could vent their anger by using charms to injure those whose behavior was troubling. Since slaves knew that living harmoniously was desirable, conjure provided them with a mechanism for addressing their grievances and protecting themselves at least to some extent from disappointment, sadness, and loneliness. As both explanatory system and means of solving difficulties, the common sense inherent in conjure effectively served the needs of slaves. It allowed individuals to take responsibility for shaping their own bodily and emotional experiences without blaming themselves for what they could not control.

However effective conjure was as preventive and proactive medicine, there were pains associated with slavery and with life that conjure could not cure. In particular, it was ineffective at easing the grief caused by separation from loved ones, whether due to sale or death. Former slaves recognized that neither conjure nor Christianity led directly to freedom from some sorrows. As a young boy, David Goodman Gullins watched as it required "three women to hold Charity on the bed while she was dying," which was "a very harrowing experience" that left him "so frightened" that he "slipped into unconsciousness." The doctor who was called "said that it was a thousand wonders that I ever came back"; a year later, the boy's hair turned white.[109] An unnamed woman reported, "Mama said she could tell when her chillen died. Everyone of them die, she said her nose would drop a drop of blood; and she said when the two boys died she went over to a neighbor's house and told her that they was dead 'cause her nose dropped a drop of blood."[110] Another said simply, "They sold my sister Ellen. My mother nearly died when they sold my sister."[111] For slaves as for whites, some sorrows of the mind could only be expressed in the body.

Laypeople of both races in the antebellum South struggled to make sense of illness and considered the extent to which individuals could control their own bodily experiences as well as their minds. Everyone was aware of the frailty of the flesh, yet members of each race had very different understandings of the origins of illness and how to prevent its ravages. White people urged one another to control their own emotions in order to keep their bodies healthy and to develop the right attitudes when they were not in order to recover. At the same time, they preferred not to believe that slaves' emotions were implicated in their illnesses. Instead, their primary concern was to prevent the shamming they were convinced was interfering with slaves' work. Slaves understood their illnesses to be the result of that work, along with violence and the often inadequate material conditions of their lives. Illness was also the result of conjure and witchcraft, which could be used by one person to inflict harm upon another. For members of both races, the mind influenced the body and the body influenced the mind, but in different ways. For whites, minds influenced the bodies in which they existed, while for blacks, other people's minds influenced what happened to their bodies. Whites saw the cause of disease as internal, blacks as external. Both tried to engage in what they considered commonsense behavior to try to protect themselves from illness, whites by controlling their own minds, blacks by protecting themselves against the influence of someone else's. By understanding themselves and their illnesses in these ways, southerners of both races influenced the ways physicians thought about and treated them. Prudent doctors knew that only by taking their patients' assumptions into account would they be able to treat them effectively.

# CHAPTER 7

# The Diseased Body

Antebellum physicians recognized that the connections between minds and bodies that were raced, sexed, and placed influenced how they could practice medicine in the South. Minds as well as bodies could make people sick; physicians with a professional interest in restoring them to health knew that their success depended on treating both. At the same time, they knew that slaveholders had a vested interest in understanding their slaves to be healthy unless suffering from the most obvious debility. The dichotomy caused physicians, along with their slaveholding employers, to consider the extent to which their slave patients were shamming. At the same time, physicians were well aware that on occasion any of their patients, not just slaves, could behave in ways that manipulated the sick role and challenged their authority. They considered white women particularly vulnerable to such behavior. Physicians concerned about shamming in slaves and resistance from whites looked to the interactions of mind and body to explain their patients' illness behavior. If southern physicians' efforts to define the body and understand the mind were motivated by their growing commitment to the science of medicine and thus to their own professional status, it also was formed by their desire to provide better care to their suffering patients.

People whose minds betrayed their bodies into illness or whose bodily illnesses led their already weak minds to unacceptable behavior caused their physicians no end of difficulty. The code of medical ethics adopted in 1847 by the fledgling National Medical Convention, which would become the American Medical Association, announced that "reasonable indulgence should be granted to the mental imbecility and caprices of the sick," even as physicians were told to "unite tenderness with *firmness*, and *condescension* with *authority*, as to inspire the minds of their patients with gratitude, respect and confidence."[1] Very few patients would have agreed with Maria Bryan of Georgia, who recognized that "the emotion and gratitude with which one regards a physician who has rendered them great and especial service, and relieved them from excruciating pain and hopeless sickness, is a strong and peculiar feeling." She thought that "our poor sex . . . often regard their physician and their clergyman as a sort of demigod because the one is the instrument of giving health to the body and the other to the soul."[2]

Determined to treat their patients' illnesses effectively, physicians knew that they had to take both sick minds and sick bodies into account. Often enough, that meant accommodating their patients' views of what was wrong and how best to treat it, even when physicians did not agree. For white women, it required assessing their reactions to being examined and to the treatment prescribed, as well as the reactions of their husbands. Physicians who considered women's minds weak and their bodies vulnerable nevertheless had to recognize that women had definite ideas about the diagnoses and treatments they would accept, an unwelcome but unavoidable intrusion into their practice. Similarly, physicians whose patients included slaves generally recognized that blacks had a different understanding of illness from their own, although they were seldom willing to accommodate it. They also recognized that slaves sometimes used illness as a means of avoiding both physical labor and punishment and so had to be on the alert for shamming.

In addition, physicians who believed that bodies and minds influenced each other had to consider their own influence in defining disease and shaping treatment for specific patients. Recognizing that disease was more than a strictly biological process, or at least not strictly rooted in the body itself, they knew that their own authority and prestige depended in part on their ability to manipulate patients' minds in ways that would help their bodies get well. Thus doctors could emphasize their own expertise as well as the expertise of science, making medicine an ever-increasing authority on how best to live. In the South, medical claims of authority over the interactions of mind and body allowed physicians yet another mechanism for keeping all categories of people in what they considered their proper place in society.

Doctors who believed that minds and bodies influenced each other knew that part of their responsibility as practitioners was to apply their knowledge of physiology and what today would be called psychology to curing their patients' ills. Because they could never be sure what originated in body and what in mind, because in their view the two could never be entirely separated, responsible physicians had to practice in ways that respected emotional influences on the body as well as the body's influence on patients' thoughts and behavior. Simon Abbott, a botanic physician in Charleston, South Carolina, claimed he had seen some "patients refuse medicine, merely because they did not know what it was; the mystery and technical name seemed an infringement on the very freedom of thought, and disgusted the sick with the prescription." Abbott knew that "small things will influence the condition of the sick," adding "the least shadow of concealment or deception, whispering, or doubtful looks, or the color of mystery, will distress the patient. If he loses confidence in his physician, it will aggravate his disease." Patients would be "reduced to the condition of the slave" if they had to "in profound ignorance receive with implicit faith whatever is offered."[3] Abbott recognized his obligation to appear certain about his expertise just as he wanted at least white patients to accede willingly to it based on their own more limited knowledge of medicine. He did not comment specifically on the feelings of slave patients.

Not all physicians agreed with Abbott's solution to the problem of the interplay between the minds and bodies of their patients. According to an anonymous allopathic critic of the *People's Medical Gazette,* a monthly botanic periodical published in Charleston, there was a real danger in its purpose of offering the public "such an amount of knowledge of medicine" that they could prescribe for themselves when necessary. He rejected the botanics' plan of informing the public that "issues of life and death are not in our hands, and that the actions of medicines are uncertain," because the public's "confidence in articles of the Materia Medica, as well as the skill of the physician would be impaired, if not utterly lost; and every one knows the value of *faith* and confidence in the treatment of disease."[4]

Patients' faith in their doctors and their prescriptions could play an important role in their recovery. Another allopathic physician, T. Bullard, believed that physicians' "hasty and sometimes premature announcement of their opinion that the case will terminate fatally and soon" was "unwise, inhuman, [and] barbarous, if not quasi murder." While he valued the "veracity, honesty, demanded of all, and none more than of the physicians," he did not believe that they should "wrest that hope from a fellow-being struggling upon the brink of the unknown hereafter." Even when the case was "certainly hopeless," patients "ordinarily, do not need to be told that their disease must end in death" because "the hour" could be "postponed by the lapse of months or years, and so postponed as much by hope as cod-liver oil and whisky." Bullard reminded physiologists of "the influence of the nervous system, guiding with royal hand all the functions of the organism; or how the emotions unduly excited, relax tissue and suspend secretion." He challenged anyone to say "that hope does not have a great influence in the recovery of the sick, or at least in the prolongation of life" and suggested that while physicians should not deceive their patients, it was "not always necessary to tell *all* we know or think."[5] Each of these physicians recognized the role that emotions played in illness and its cure; each was especially determined to harness the power of confidence in the physician and his prescriptions in the fight against disease.

But illness was a powerful adversary. It could cause a patient to refuse treatment or to reject medical advice. Physicians recognized that very refusal as itself a symptom of disease, part of what needed to be treated. Nowhere was this truer than for white women and slaves, whose mental and physical weaknesses left them vulnerable to misperceptions and the misbehaviors they caused. For physicians intent on perceiving the body in light of medical and scientific truths and then applying those truths to an increasingly empirically based treatment, the consequences of interactions between mind and body were necessarily part of their daily practice. At the same time, the observations of daily practice informed their theory as they sought to explain the unpredictability of bodies under their care by referring to the influences of nearly untreatable minds. Patients whose bodies did not respond to treatment, who did not get well when doctors thought they should, could be explained as continuing to suffer because of the power of their minds over their bodies. That power was sometimes difficult to see, but it could best be viewed in the behavior of white women suffering disorders of their reproductive organs. Here, where sympathy between brain and uterus was so powerful, doctors could plainly observe reasons why treatments they thought should cure sometimes did not. White women, whose weak minds and bodies left them vulnerable to an array of physical and emotional ills, were for the same reason likely to challenge the authority of physicians to examine and treat them.

## Medical Authority and White Women

Charles Meigs offered what one reviewer called "much good sense and truth" when he claimed "relations between the sexes are of so delicate a character, that the duties of a medical practitioner are necessarily more difficult when he comes to take charge of a patient laboring under any one of the great host of female complaints, than when he is called upon to treat the more general disorders." Meigs attributed the difficulty of treating women to "the embarrassment arising, from fastidiousness on the part either of the female herself, or of the practitioner, or both" and warned that this was responsible for "much of the ill success of treatment." Many diseases of women were so difficult to cure that women were either led to "some surprising cure" at the hands of a quack or "by gradual lapses of health and strength, down to the grave," even though "many of these cases are, in their beginning, of light or trifling importance." To avoid such an unwelcome outcome, Meigs advised physicians to prepare their minds and persons to raise themselves "above the grossness and sensuality of the corporeal nature, rendering the body the servant and the minister, not the tyrant of the soul and the heart."[6] Meigs believed that physicians needed to impose discipline upon their own male bodies as well as their patients' female ones.

Patients were far more likely to try to impose discipline upon their physicians. Their beliefs about what was wrong with them and insistence on setting the boundaries of acceptable diagnosis and treatment by male physicians frequently constrained what doctors could do in practice. Not surprisingly, at least from the perspective of those doctors, white women questioned their doctors' authority more often than did white men. Like the origins of disease itself, physicians also attributed this to the reciprocal influences of their minds and bodies, sometimes enhanced by the interference of others. For example, Alabama physician S. M. Meek wrote in the *Southern Medical and Surgical Journal* about his frustration with a white woman patient who suffered a hemorrhage from what he diagnosed as prolapsed uterus after she fell while standing on a chair. However, "some female friends more nice than wise, insisted that she should consult another physician, before she consented to the diagnosis." Because "the external appearance was perfectly natural," the second physician "decided most positively that . . . no prolapsus existed." He "therefore concluded . . . that her complaints were chiefly hysterical." Meek reported, "this being a much pleasanter suggestion to the patient and her husband," they accepted it, and she was treated with tonics and antispasmodics, typical remedies for hysteria. However, the woman's husband later called Meek back "in consequence of having himself made an investigation which proved to him" that she did indeed have a prolapsed uterus.[7]

Meek's vindication did not last long. He tried to convince "the discarded physician" that he had been wrong, without success. Meek had no better success treating his patient, who died after eight months because she was in a great "state of debility, and laboring under that dreadful train of nervous distresses, which generally attends the extremity of these cases when their proper treatment is too long delayed."[8] Meek believed this woman's hysterical symptoms to be the consequence of the prolapsed uterus that was her chief bodily affliction, but they also influenced the decision she and her husband made to listen to the advice of the physician who considered hysteria her primary complaint. Meek's use of the language of consent here is telling: The woman, her husband, and her friends, as well as by implication the second physician, assumed that patients could withhold their consent to diagnoses with which they disagreed, implying a right of choice Meek obviously found disconcerting.[9] Patients whose bodily diseases caused their minds to reject expert diagnoses lived in a state of circular logic that physicians could not easily break. Patients who resisted medical advice, or who chose to follow the wrong medical advice, were guilty of endangering their lives; in this case, Meek believed doing so cost this woman hers.

One of the most vexing ways white women resisted medical authority was by refusing to be examined. South Carolina physician E. C. Baker was called to treat an unmarried woman who had been suffering from what she thought was breast cancer, but what he diagnosed as vicarious menstruation. For two years, she had been given "every remedy that could be devised or 'heard of,' as curative of cancer . . . by all the '*old women*' of the neighborhood," but without success. "The girl now becoming seriously alarmed herself, consented finally, to have a physician called in, and the breast examined." Even then, the young woman would not permit Baker to examine her other breast. In spite of the woman's modesty, Baker illustrated the article with two drawings of her breast.[10]

More often, patients resisted vaginal examinations, whether manually, by speculum, or both. In doing so, they inadvertently echoed physicians' own doubts about the propriety of intimate examinations except under the direst circumstances. Here, the female mind and body of the patient collided with the male mind and body of the physician to create a social and medical conflict that reflected the still precarious authority of medicine. Physicians debated with one another as well as with their patients about the limits of their own behavior. Louis A. Dugas, professor of anatomy and physiology and later surgery at the Medical College of Georgia, tried to avoid placing "the patient under the disagreeable necessity of submitting to repeated manipulations highly revolting to delicacy, however much this may be tempered by reason."[11] Physicians were especially worried about the propriety of conducting vaginal examinations on unmarried white women, who were assumed to be virgins. According to an author in the *Southern Medical and Surgical Journal,* "no physical examination ought ever to be thought of in the unmarried female, without the physician is morally certain that severe disease exists in the vagina or womb."[12] One southern critic even took Charles Meigs to task for asking his patients "questions of the most delicate kind . . . which we in this part of the Union at least, are not in the habit even of asking married ladies, as it is information which can as readily and far less painfully to the feelings of the patients, be obtained from an attendant."[13] However, when Meigs described his own interactions with women patients, he was more circumspect. Suspecting that a laboring woman had a double vagina that would make it difficult for her to deliver, he at first "kept my own counsel" because he "suppos[ed] that such a revelation would not be agreeable to her." However, when he feared that her vagina was in danger of rupturing, he "explained to the monthly nurse, and to a relative of my patient" and "procured the requisite permission to expose the parts to an inspection."[14]

Like Meigs in this case, physicians knew that questions and examinations were often necessary. Alabama physician H. R. Easterling warned readers of the *Charleston Medical Journal and Review* that any doctor who suspected uterine disease but "avoids making the necessary examination, or at least does not remonstrate with the patient, and impress on her mind the importance of the examination, if objected to . . . deviates from the true principles which should be foremost in the mind of the medical man, and proves utterly recreant to the high trust confided in him." Easterling claimed to know of "instances on record when the innocent have been taunted and calumniated as respects her virtue, for a deceptive idea conveyed to the two [*sic*] eager mind by the untaught examiner, thereby giving a too hasty and incorrect diagnosis."[15] Virginia physician W. F. Barr similarly warned "that there is too much *fastidiousness* in the medical profession, resulting in the injury of patients." He believed that "the *false* modesty" that led some physicians to avoid use of the speculum caused "many a suffering female" to linger "out her days, on a bed of disease, which disease might have easily been cured." A wise physician, "influenced by a laudable spirit of philanthropy" and "a desire to *cure* his patients" as well as "a sense of *duty*" would use the speculum.[16]

John Stainback Wilson warned women that "no feelings of delicacy should prevent" them from submitting to being examined with a speculum; "so far from hesitating to do so, they should suggest it to their physician, should he fail to discharge his duty in this respect through negligence or any other cause." Wilson acknowledged that this was "a repulsive and disagreeable operation both to physician and patient," a "disagreeable duty" that he "would fain shun," but he nevertheless "condemn[ed] that false and extreme modesty that prevents women from submitting to an examination when health and even life itself are involved."[17]

Joseph Eve recognized those dangers and duties when he decided to examine a young woman suffering menstrual hysteria. He reported that he made "a careful digital and then a very cautious specular examination" with a particular instrument "well adapted for making examinations in cases of virgins."[18] In another instance, Eve rebuked critics of speculum use, arguing that he could not "perceive that it is any more indelicate to make a specular than a digital examination; it is the necessity of the case that renders either proper." He noted that "a truly sensible and delicate lady would submit to the one as readily as the other—indeed, were it not that a digital examination almost necessarily precedes the introduction of the speculum, the specular would involve less indelicacy than the other," especially if introduced "by the patient herself, or a female friend, and the physician only required to look through it."[19]

Doctors in daily practice could not rely on women to request examination by speculum or insert one for themselves; instead, they had to convince reluctant women that they must submit to direct examination by physicians even as they reassured themselves about the necessity of doing so. One of Joseph Eve's patients suffered "an offensive discharge from the vagina" after childbirth, caused by ulceration. He and a colleague tried to examine her with the speculum to determine the extent of the problem, but "before we could make a proper inspection, we were compelled to remove the speculum, for she became so excessively alarmed and agitated that we feared an hysteric convulsion would have been induced."[20]

James Green also had a patient for whom "the introduction of the speculum was so painful as to throw her into a spasmodic state." The "irritation" this produced led her to refuse "any more efficient medication" than general tonics until "the ulceration was nearly healed." Even so, Green noted, "it must be confessed there was little or no improvement in the general health, or in the local or sympathetic pains." Instead, "her symptoms . . . were severely exacerbated, without any evident cause, and she again became so discouraged as resolutely to decline any further treatment." Green viewed this as utter foolishness on her part, since "the intense vaginal sensibility was completely removed" due to "the curative pressure of the speculum." Instead, he attributed "the inefficacy of the treatment . . . to the obstinacy of the patient." The woman was better but not completely cured after a year of treatment, because of "the unmanageable character of the patient," her inability to tolerate most narcotics, and "a very feeble constitution."[21] Each of these women and the physicians who attempted to diagnose and treat her negotiated the limits of acceptable speculum use, with the patients generally reluctant to allow it until discomfort and fear of death caused them to submit.

Women's reluctance to allow their physicians to examine them with the speculum could have dire consequences. When a white woman "applied" to Georgia physician Z. E. Landrum "for treatment," he "suspected that a polypus[22] was doing the mischief," but he "could not consistently grant" the treatment she required, "because she was unwilling to submit to vaginal examination." Later he was called back and observed that she was in "extreme peril" because "her constitutional vigor had been blighted, and the resisting forces of life were rapidly succumbing." Although informed of another physician's diagnosis, Landrum "insisted on making the examination" for himself. Landrum discovered that she did indeed have polypus and recognized that she was "too evidently tending to death" from "that particular combination of prostration with excitement denominated irritative fever," the result of "the peculiar excitement engrafted on a constitution, enfeebled and depraved by the local contact and absorption of the foul and offensive effusions of a sloughing polypus." In other words, Landrum believed that the woman's early refusal to allow him to examine her directly had caused her disease to become worse, which was both cause and effect of illness of mind as well as body. He treated her for the tumor with an operation that he believed successful, although the woman died from what he considered an "incidental" cause.[23]

The speculum was not the only form of intervention rejected by white women and questioned by their physicians. L. A. Dugas noted that women suffering from prolapsed uterus were sometimes expected by their physicians to use the pessary[24] for extended periods of time, until "the patients, wearied with the remedy, as well as with the pertinacity with which its farther use was insisted upon, would announce themselves cured in order to get rid of the importunities of their adviser." He recognized that "the more unpleasant the prescription, the more apt will the patient be to practice deception," adding that "no prescription [was] more apt to be disregarded" than the pessary.[25] Paul Eve declared that the pessary was "highly injurious and properly forbidden" for a long list of reasons, including the fact that it was "exceedingly unpleasant to both physician and patient." He believed that "the very idea of a pessary is revolting to the female" and added, "they are to her a source of great moral as well as physical suffering."[26] Another medical writer "hope[d] to live to see the day, when the present fashion for pressaries [sic] and speculums will be toned down by judgment and discrimination, good taste and virtuous feeling."[27]

Physicians who could not agree about what constituted proper examination and care nevertheless criticized women for making decisions counter to their wishes. Here again, physicians attributed women's reluctance to follow their advice to the interplay of diseased bodies and minds, rather than the unpleasantness of the treatment, its cost, its impact on their ability to accomplish their duties, their lack of faith in its efficacy, or anything else. A reviewer noted Charles Meigs's belief that women suffering from prolapsed uterus would require "tedious and protracted" care, because "the fastidious delicacy of a female will always prevent her from disclosing to you her distress in its early stages."[28] A report of proceedings at the Medical Society of Augusta in 1837 warned physicians of "the very uniform disposition of females to make the best of their cases, and suffer them as far as possible, in the hope of avoiding a disagreeable course of treatment." For the same reason, physicians were told, women were "constantly incline[d] to avoid subsequent treatment whenever they enjoy such palliation of their distresses as to enable them to do so."[29]

Joseph Wright offered the most carefully developed analysis of the dangers of connections between a woman's mental state and her bodily affliction. He was particularly concerned about uterine disease, suggesting that women suffering from prolapse were even more influenced by these connections than those with other ailments. His comments are worth quoting at length, if only for the seamlessness with which he presented mind and body as influencing each other to cause disease and prevent cure. He warned his lay readers:

> Patients who labor under this disease have at first a great delicacy in letting it be known, and attempt to disguise it; but after a time they seem to have an inclination to take the advice of every quack and old women, however ignorant and contemptible, and are constantly consulting new physicians; but though fond of advice they seldom follow one course long enough to reap any benefit from it. Fickle and unsteady they fly from one thing to another till at length tired out with disappointment, and despairing of relief, they become a burden to themselves and surrounding friends. Would such persons, instead of hunting after medicines and flying from one physician to another, persist steadily in a proper plan, they might often render life easy and agreeable.

Wright noted that following his advice "requires more resolution than most women have, and they will swallow a drug because it is soon over and they expect immediate relief from it, but can by no means think of pursuing a plan that requires patience and perseverance." He added, "women most liable to this disorder are the luxurious and sedentary."[30] Prolapsed uterus was indeed a dangerous disease of mind and body.

Wright's comments are significant in part because of the manner in which he blurred the line between the disease and its impact on women's behavior. The woman's temperament, her habits of life, and the state of her uterus interacted to influence her disease and shape the ways in which she sought treatment for it. His implication was that the behavior was sign and symptom of the disease. According to Wright, women's obstinate refusal to comply with prescribed treatment was itself a symptom of the impact of disease on their minds, not simply a sign of bad behavior. His belief that women suffering from prolapsed uterus sought cures from a range of practitioners but were reluctant to commit themselves to the discipline necessary to effect a cure suggests the strength of the influence their bodies had over their minds. Wright's observations served as a warning to physicians to be vigilant as they sought to care for their female patients.

Physicians in actual practice were well aware of the truth of such warnings. Charleston physician Robert Bailey reported on a white woman patient whose nausea, vomiting, and other paroxysms during pregnancy he treated with "the infusion of cinchona" with apparent benefit. However, she "did not take it long enough to be of any permanent advantage, and during a cool change of the weather we had in June, she became worse and more debilitated"; in two months, she was dead.[31] Simon Sanders requested advice from Milton Antony, professor and editor of a medical journal, about a patient suffering prolapse and hemorrhage, because "to an operation, though it might promise the greatest success, she would not submit."[32] D. C. O'Keefe of Georgia also reported on "the error of not yielding immediate and implicit obedience to the physician's prescription." He attributed his patient's "long and needless suffering" to "her own reluctance to use the caustic" to cure her "urethral inflammation," for "fear of its severity."[33] Patients who showed no reluctance to challenge physicians' use of the speculum or the diagnosis offered also had no qualms about rejecting treatments they deemed unacceptable. While physicians considered such resistance part of the disease itself, their struggles against it were not always successful. At the same time, wary physicians also had to recognize that patients sometimes behaved coercively in other ways. Charles Hentz commented in his diary about Mrs. E., "a regular beggar—she promised her little boy that if he wd take physic, the Dr. wd. give him some cooked fish (i.e. dried herrings) when he came to town; & in the same way of bribe to little girl, that the Dr. wd. get her a pretty red dress—." Hentz promised himself that "I shall discourage such advances—."[34] Physicians in active practice could easily feel themselves besieged from all directions by recalcitrant and manipulative patients.

Not only were the physician's diagnosis, use of equipment, and prescriptions subject to evaluation and approval or disapproval by white women patients and their families, so, too, was his very person. A Charleston physician who reported the case of a woman suffering the effects of her husband's sexual brutality treated her for a time at her sister's request, until the woman's husband "desiring, as he said, to have an older physician than myself, employed one."[35] More often, white women themselves resisted the very bodily presence of male physicians. John H. Grant of South Carolina reported that while attending his first case of placenta previa,[36] he attempted "to pass the hand into the vagina," but the woman "commenced rotating her body with all the violence in her power, and imperiously demanded that I should desist, saying, 'Let me alone—let me die so, rather than do that.'" Grant added, "Of course, there was no alternative for me but to suspend operations. She would not again permit me to make another attempt."[37] Four days later, the woman delivered a dead child, but she survived. Grant thought the baby would have been born sooner had she allowed his interventions to continue.

Georgia botanic physician W. A. Beasley "reasoned with the patient, the husband and mother" to convince them to allow him to treat another woman whose placenta remained in her uterus after childbirth, in spite of "strong opposition from those who visited the patient, especially those opposed to our practice."[38] An allopathic physician suggested to his colleagues that it was necessary to test for the causes of parturient hemorrhage, warning "do not be satisfied with temporizing with digital examinations if they are not sufficient, but, explaining the necessity to your patient, pass the entire hand into the vagina . . . [and] the index finger well up into the cervical canal." He added that if there was no "immediate danger, you would not expose your patient to the annoyance and pain attendant upon this procedure; but far better would it be to err on that side, than by a culpable inactivity to remain ignorant of a point upon the knowledge of which so much will depend."[39] These physicians' attempts to reason with their patients implied a level of respect for their minds, or at least for the influence of those minds on their bodies, even though the physicians were certain they—and only they—could know what was best.

Joseph Milligan was quite explicit about these matters in the advice he offered his son, also a physician. The senior Milligan pronounced himself "sorry that your young patient is so very modest that she will not permit you to cup her on the loins and that her mother has so little self denial as to make the appearance of a blister a reason for not following your prescription." He suggested that his son speak to the mother "seriously and affectionately, and set before her the probable consequences of her refusal to follow your directions." Milligan lamented the presence of "a great many people of her character in the world, and especially in this country, and they embarras physicians very much in the discharge of their duties."[40] His solicitude for physicians embarrassed by their patients was not paralleled by a corresponding sentiment on behalf of his son's young woman patient, whose feelings, along with those of her mother, he viewed merely as obstacles to be overcome.

Not all physicians were even this solicitous regarding their patients' wishes or bothered to try to reason with them at all, even when the patients were white. When Georgia physician J. Dickson Smith encountered another woman with retained placenta, he "informed the patient that I must introduce my hand in order to remove" the placenta. When he tried to do so, he found "it impossible to introduce the hand, and so painful was the operation that the patient declared it *intolerable*." Smith decided that chloroform was in order, "and, despite the protestations of the patient and friends, I proceeded to administer it" and found the result "highly gratifying." He noted that without chloroform, "a *God send* in time of distress and emergency," he "should have had *very* great difficulty in relieving this patient" because "she would not have permitted the operation."[41] Smith, like many other physicians, found that women's emotional distress had to be subdued before he could treat their bodily afflictions.

## Physicians Negotiate Bodies and Minds

Physicians who struggled to convince their white women patients to submit to examinations and treatment believed that the women's diseased minds and bodies precluded their acquiescence in a circular pattern that frustrated physicians' efforts to cure them. At the same time, some doctors recognized the influence their own white and male minds and bodies could have in compelling cooperation. Convinced of their own superiority and authority, doctors were rarely reluctant to call on both when need be. Nowhere was this more apparent than in their efforts to treat white women suffering from hysteria, that perplexing amalgam of physical and emotional symptoms. Here, doctors brought to the bedside all of their knowledge about women's bodies, their minds, and the interactions between them, together with doctors' growing claims to authority over correct behavior. The result was an enhanced self-consciousness justifying their own interventions and diminished autonomy for their suffering patients.

Doctors called upon to treat hysteria in their women patients agreed that addressing the underlying uterine derangements was the necessary first step. Many would also agree that what British physician W. Camps called "moral treatment" was required. Moral treatment was the term nineteenth-century physicians used to describe care of the insane that eschewed physical forms of coercion in favor of more humane care. It generally involved trying to convince the patient to behave appropriately through a system of rewards and punishments, along with suitable amusements and distractions.[42] In the antebellum years, moral treatment was not generally prescribed for hysteria, which most physicians believed originated in the body, not the mind. Nevertheless, many physicians agreed that treatments of both mind and body were the most effective strategy for curing women suffering from it. Nor was moral treatment usually recommended during childbirth, although John Stainback Wilson called for the "moral management" of birthing women, which required removing "all sources of vexation and annoyance," respecting the woman's "whims and caprices," and making every effort "to animate her hopes, and inspire her with confidence."[43]

Hysteria presented a far greater challenge. Camps believed that hysteria, "which is almost, though not exclusively, confined to the female sex," could cause "a complete metamorphosis of the whole moral character." He warned that "nothing would be more injurious to a hysterical patient . . . than undue interference with personal liberty," restraint, or confinement. He described a woman suffering from the disease whose will "lost its controlling power," causing "great irritability of temper" and "very irregular and extraordinary phrases and actions of the body." Camps advocated the use of agents that would "improve the general health" and "act beneficially upon the mental state and condition of the patient."[44] Camps could urge other physicians to allow hysterical patients their liberty in part because he did not practice in a slave society, where slaves sometimes suffered from the disease but could not be granted any sort of freedom.

Joseph Wright, the southern author of a domestic medicine manual, placed less emphasis than Camps on the use of moral treatment in curing hysteria. While he noted that "nothing recovers a person sooner out of the hysteric fit than putting the feet and legs in warm water," he also thought that restoring menstruation or substituting "repeated bleedings" was necessary. Even so, he stated that "the cure depends chiefly upon the patient's own endeavors, and might often be accomplished were no medicines prescribed at all." He warned that "whenever physicians order medicine, patients will trust to it, and neglect their own exertions," adding that "patients who labor under this disease are generally very fond of taking medicines, and when they are not swallowing drugs they think their case neglected." Instead, Wright advocated "agreeable company, daily exercise, change of place, and a variety of amusements." Yet in spite of this advice, Wright supplied his readers with several prescriptions, including one for compounding "anti-hysteric pills," which were to be taken "twice a day: four at noon and at seven o'clock in the evening, drinking after them a wine glass of port wine."[45] Like that of other antebellum physicians struggling to cure hysterical patients, Wright's advice blurred the line between medical and moral treatments of a disease that underscored the connections between mind and body.

Physicians like Camps and Wright who advocated moral treatment of nervous diseases, or who considered the moral meaning of disease at all, almost never did so in the context of religion for either male or female patients. Committed to developing the science of medicine, they were reluctant to discuss matters that might otherwise fall under the heading of theology. Few reported encouraging patients to ensure salvation before their deaths, nor did any physician understand disease as God's punishment for improper behavior. To do so would have challenged their developing sense of scientific expertise as well as their convictions about the connections between mind and body. Joseph Milligan urged his son, also a physician, to offer dying patients "such comfort as you are able to bestow" at the same time that he encouraged them to trust God. "Have mercy on the souls of your patients, and let them not die in ignorance of the only means of Salvation."[46] But Milligan did not consider such attention part of the medical treatment his son provided. Only Alfred Folger, in his domestic medicine manual, assured "the reader that religion has a powerful effect upon the health of an individual." He noted that "the christian [sic] is enabled to bear with fortitude all the dispensations of Providence. . . . His mind being thus at ease, under all difficulties, he is not so subject to disease as the man who sinks in despondency under every misfortune."[47] Yet Folger took for granted the medical rather than the theological notion that a person's mind could influence the body's experience of illness, nervous or otherwise, and thus the need for intervention by physicians.

Physicians who considered moral treatment to be part of their responsibility struggled to provide it in a manner that those sick in mind and body would find acceptable. Establishing themselves as moral arbiters, they were convinced that conforming to the standards of society was best for their patients and part of the treatment expected by their patients' friends and families. Physicians also set high moral expectations for themselves. Charles Hentz noted in his diary a visit to a colleague, Dr. Telfair, commenting that he was "very sick from drinking—pity such a noble fellow & excellent physician should do so." Hentz characterized his wife's brother, a medical student in Charleston, as "a most generous, amiable young man; a universal favorite" who also drank enough to have "frequent attacks of delirium tremens." Hentz added that "he had an excellent mind—and might have been an ornament to society but for his unbridled & undisciplined appetites."[48] In an autobiography he wrote late in life, Hentz confessed his own early failings. In his first year as a doctor, he "had some trials that to one of my distrustful temperament—lacking self confidence all the time grievously—, were hard to bear." In one instance, he attended a woman "during a severe attack of fever—one that in after years I could have managed very easily." But because he was "inexperienced and timid," his patient "became unfortunately very badly salivated—,[49] the only patient that I ever had to suffer this misfortune." Hentz recalled that "it distressed me beyond measure—and it damaged my practice at the time very badly."[50] Hentz's comments were confined to private writings; physicians almost never confessed their mistakes or criticized one another publicly for their moral failings. They were only slightly less critical of one another for their failures in treating the sick, although they showed few limits when criticizing the philosophy and prescriptions of other medical sects.

On occasion, physicians of all sorts were willing to confess their personal reactions to the suffering bodies of their patients. Those reactions could reach such a level of moral and physical revulsion that they might well have had a difficult time disguising it in the sickroom. One anonymous physician admitted that prolapsed uterus was "so disgusting to the practitioner, that no inducement, but an insuperable sense of duty and an unavoidable sympathy with the sufferings and dangers of that sex which alone suffers it, can bring him to encounter the task." So "repugnant" was the doctor's task that he would "wish himself ignorant of every thing appertaining thereto, that he might honestly decline such service." However, this physician still believed he could "determine a clear and rational diagnosis and treatment."[51] Another, E. M. Pendleton, called to attend a seventeen-year-old slave woman in childbirth, acknowledged that "candour forces me to admit, that the examinations heretofore had been too casual" after he discovered that her pelvis had been deformed when she was a child.[52] Charles Hentz noted in his diary his frustration with Mrs. Skipper, who suffered from "a kind of hysterical convulsion, attendant upon an excruciating head ache." He was "puzzled about the case" because "she is a woman full of ailings." Hentz reported that "as a natural consequence . . . I was bothered & inclined to give up the profession in disgust," although he did prescribe medicine for her.[53]

Physicians whose own bodies and minds were repulsed by women's suffering or who were careless in their dealings with them were rarely able to acknowledge the consequences of their actions. They believed women's bodies and minds were weak, while they saw themselves as sympathetic yet disinterested men of science. Their patients, however, were not likely to miss the implications. When Joseph

Milligan wrote his sister, he could only lament his lot, saying, "[A] physician's life is a very uncomfortable one to say the least of it. The responsibility, anxiety, obstinacy of patients, & [the] ingratitude" of those whose lives he saved "render his path a thorny one—& a very crooked one too."[54] Midcentury medical practice was contested by patients in part because most physicians felt themselves entitled to comment on the connections between everyone's bodies and minds but their own, even as they remained largely oblivious of how their own physical and emotional reactions were perceived by their patients.

On some occasions, however, physicians did blame themselves for their patients' refusal to be treated. According to the editors of the *Southern Medical and Surgical Journal* in 1838, "[W]e have much blame to attach to most of American practitioners in relation to their management of those complaints of females which are peculiarly disagreeable, distressing and dangerous." While they could not say whether this blame was due to "wilful [sic] neglect of attention to those distresses, or from the great sin of torpid ignorance from obtuseness of intellect, or a wilful neglect of the study of them," they were sure that "the profession is far behind its progress in other particulars, in the understanding and the treatment of most of the uterine affections to which females are subject."[55] Another physician recognized that only "a very small proportion" of his colleagues had "that thorough knowledge of the female economy . . . to enable them to reason correctly for the prevention of disease." Furthermore, few of those "are sufficiently communicative, conscientious, and at leisure to enforce instructions on the too thoughtless and inconsiderate patients."[56] Those doctors seemingly had no difficulty ascribing the limits of their own knowledge to their patients' recalcitrance.

Physicians who studied gynecologic diseases were still all too likely to turn their attention to women's own responsibility for their illnesses as well as their failure to be cured of them. Many would have agreed with the view of a London physician reprinted in the *Southern Medical and Surgical Journal,* who commented on a patient in whom "the development of a malignant disease seem[ed], in great measure, to be influenced by the feelings or instinct of the patient."[57] In today's language, this might be considered blaming the victim. Few antebellum doctors were as pleased with their patients' emotional behavior or physical reactions to treatment as Joseph Eve was about one woman, whose "case exemplifies the happy effects of the most patient perseverance under the most adverse and discouraging circumstances. . . . Had this lady not possessed and exercised the most indomitable patience, she would have given up in utter hopelessness, long before a cure was accomplished." Eve had been called after several other physicians had treated the woman for more than two years; he diagnosed her with prolapsed uterus and cauterized her sixteen times, along with prescribing various medicines.[58]

Most physicians frustrated by their white female patients' determination to negotiate the parameters of acceptable treatment rather than submit to doctors' orders could only cluck their tongues and urge greater cooperation in the pages of their medical journals and textbooks—not the best locations for reaching their desired audience. Few women read such publications. Similarly, the code of medical ethics developed by the National Medical Convention in 1847 included a section on "obligations of patients to their physicians" that insisted "even the female sex should never allow feelings of shame or delicacy to prevent their disclosing the seat, symptoms and causes of complaints peculiar to them." Women were warned that "however commendable a modest reserve may be in the common occurrences of life, its strict observance in medicine is often attended with the most serious consequences, and a patient may sink under a painful and loathsome disease, which might have been readily prevented had timely intimation been given to the physician."[59] Again, few women, white or black, were likely to see this advice or the warning that accompanied it.

Authors of domestic medicine manuals aimed at the general public sometimes tried to respond to their colleagues' concerns by including passages addressing women's modesty with physicians. For example, Alfred Folger acknowledged that "there are many physicians, who are too mean and despicable to merit the confidence of a respectable lady" and advised his readers "not to lay your case before any physician, who has no regard for the feelings of a female, or respect for himself." In Folger's view, a good physician was "A GOOD MAN, posessing [sic] medical information," who would treat his patients "with becoming respect" and "never utter a word calculated to cause a blush on the cheek of modesty, or that would detract in the smallest degree from the dignity of a gentleman." Nevertheless, he worried that "many a fine amiable young lady, has been hurried from time to eternity, in consequence of her notions of delicacy having prevented her from applying to a physician for medical aid." He hoped that his work would "impress upon the minds of my fair young readers, the importance of throwing aside all false modesty, and consulting a good physician, whenever the health is much impaired, or in danger of being thus impaired."[60] John Stainback Wilson characterized the best doctor as one "who exhibits a practical common sense turn of mind in the ordinary affairs of life, who is attentive to his business, diligent in his studies, sober in his habits, and *who humbly prays for the Divine blessing on the means that he may use.*" In addition, women should seek physicians who "possess that refinement of manner, and that delicacy of feeling, which will secure the confidence and respect of his patients, and cause the most tender regard for the innate modesty of woman." The good physician "should not allow any mawkish sensibility to interfere with the necessary duties of his profession, but what is necessary, should be done as gently and as delicately as possible."[61]

Convinced that white women's attitudes about their bodies too often prevented them from receiving needed treatment, a few physicians suggested that the best solution would be for women themselves to become medical practitioners. However, the National Medical Convention's code of medical ethics explicitly warned patients against "self-constituted doctors and doctresses."[62] A vehement Thomsonian physician, John Roberts, objected "to the deleterious influence produced on the *mind* as well as the body, through preparations administered, and the paraphrenalia of professional attendance" on women in childbirth. He knew that "the delicate and modest female will shrink from the presence and touch of the male accoucheur, and, it has happened, that all the pangs of preparatory labor have subsided immediately on the appearance of the physician." Instead, he urged, "away with all this—give experienced females, their hands and nature is [*sic*] softer, they have no professional pride; let there be mirth and cheerfulness, and if necessary, sympathy; and, the result must be far more favorable in prospect than under this professional fear and gloom."[63]

While Roberts's thinking was shared by many doctors, few allopathic physicians were willing to accede to his solution. They were too concerned with their own professional credibility to be willing to share it with either Thomsonians or women. However, in 1854, the *Southern Medical and Surgical Journal* published an article by Alabama physician John Stainback Wilson in which he advocated for "Female Medical Education." While carefully circumscribing the limits of what he considered appropriate for women to do, he believed "their *sexual idiosyncracies* would afford material aid in the diagnosis, and perhaps, in the treatment, of certain sexual diseases." Wilson especially pointed to women's "*tact,* acumen and promptitude, combined with manual dexterity" as fitting them for obstetrics, which in any case did not require "the higher reasoning powers which are generally conceded to our own sex." A woman's own experience with "many of those sensations, physiological and pathological, normal and abnormal, which characterize the protean derangements of her sex, and render them so difficult of comprehension" would enhance her competence, as opposed to a male doctor, who "only has a theoretical knowledge of them." In addition, "the smallness of her hand, and the delicacy of her touch, fit her peculiarly for those manipulations so often required in parturition, many of which are extremely painful, and even impracticable, when performed by the clumsy hand of a male." Not only would allowing women to attend other women in childbirth relieve the male physician of "one of the most disagreeable and irksome branches of his profession," it would also provide employment for women in need. The most important reason of all, however, was because "*the safety and happiness, of a large portion, of the most refined and lovely women* (in the South particularly) DEMAND it."[64]

Wilson attributed that demand largely to modesty. He "deplore[d] the sad consequences of the morbid sensitiveness of females, in concealing those sexual secrets, which pertain to their nature, at the expense of health, and even life itself." This caused every southern physician to see "cases which have become incurable, on account of the reluctance of females to submit to the use of the speculum." Every physician "had cases which brought reproach upon himself and upon his profession, because he, in compliance with the natural aversion of females, failed to avail himself of the speculum and other means involving exposure, even when convinced of their almost indispensable necessity; and of the extreme uncertainty of being able to institute a successful plan of treatment without them." Diseases that now "linger along under an inefficient or palliative treatment" would be easily cured "were it not for the almost insuperable objections of the fair sufferers, to the inevitable exposure of their sexual secrets, to a male physician." Wilson advocated educating women "to treat all the '*purely sexual*' diseases"—and only those—as a way of avoiding the "ignorance and unskilfulness" of midwives and "'old grannies.'"[65] Wilson tried to forestall every objection, but his plan brought no response from his colleagues, although a few years later, William Hauser of the Oglethorpe Medical College urged that "physiology, ought to be taught in every school in the world, and to both girls and boys."[66]

In spite of the lack of enthusiasm for his suggestions, Wilson's reasons for advocating medical education for white women reflect a widespread consensus among doctors regarding the ways the attitudes of their female patients shaped their experiences of illness and their interactions with physicians. Doctors were enormously frustrated by white women's modesty and the influence it had on their experience of disease. Modesty did not cause illness, but like other emotions, it interfered with treatment, causing women to delay seeking professional help, to refuse intimate examination, and to reject the advice they were given once they submitted. White women who negotiated every aspect of their examination, diagnosis, and treatment with their physicians did so because both their bodies and minds suffered the influence of disease; physicians believed they had no choice but to treat both in tandem. Medicine could cure disease, but only if doctors could prescribe it and women complied. Too often, the diseases from which women suffered caused their minds to reject medical advice, a form of independent thinking doctors could only ascribe to pathology, the rejection and modesty only more symptoms to be treated. Yet doctors were notably reluctant to question the influence of their own minds and bodies. While doctors' still incomplete cultural authority meant that they were often frustrated by their female patients, the power granted to them as men inspired them to exhort their patients to submit. Often enough, they were successful. The struggle to define women's bodies and minds between male doctors and female patients did not begin on a level field. It only became more pronounced in favor of the former during the antebellum years.

## Medical Authority and Slaves' Minds and Bodies

Southern physicians attempting to understand white women's bodies and minds knew that they simultaneously had to consider the influence of race. Otherwise, their conclusions ran the risk of appearing to apply in like measure to black women. As before, reconciling sex and race was not easy. Physicians in daily practice knew that black women often enough displayed the same emotions, including modesty, with the same consequences that white women did. Yet they were reluctant to allow black women the same latitude in negotiating their own treatment that they did white women, in part because they had little choice but to allot slaveholders a voice as well. If slave women's minds influenced their bodies in parallel ways to whites,' then physicians knew that their practice would need to accommodate slaves' minds as well as their sick bodies. But slaveholders were not likely to tolerate in slaves the same sort of indulgence physicians provided for their wives and daughters, nor did physicians want to do so, forcing them to develop understandings of the connection between mind and body that took race into account as well as sex. Debating the extent to which slaves were subject to hysteria was one manifestation of their dilemma. More often, physicians in daily practice had to decide how much to take the sensibilities of their slave patients into account as they sought to treat their ailments.

According to A. P. Merrill, whose ideas about the "Distinctive Peculiarities of the Negro Race" helped shape southern medicine, "no class of people more urgently require, that the physician who attends them in their diseases, should rightly understand their mental characteristics; without which, indeed, it will be found impossible to secure their confidence, and inspire them with the hope of recovery, so essential to success."[67] He worried that slaves thought too often about "supernatural agencies" and had too much confidence in witchcraft, warning, "much of [their] diseases, proceeds from purely imaginary causes."[68] In spite of those anxieties, Merrill noted that slaves did not "experience much dread of the influence of contagion." Their religion made them "fatalists" who attributed life and death to God, uninfluenced by human agency. Even so, they were predisposed to disease by "apprehensions and forebodings of evil," which "depressed their vital energies." Merrill claimed "no people can be more completely under the influence of the mind in sickness, than the negro race."[69] Merrill's comments here suggest that while he believed there were few physiological explanations for different disease experiences for the races, any such differences could easily be attributed to psychological factors. A student at the Medical College of South Carolina reflected a similar perspective when he wrote of the "hygenical" advantages "of encouraging the naturally mirthful and fun-loving disposition of the Negro."[70] Both authors shared with most of the South's physicians a belief in the medical benefits of slavery for blacks.

Many physicians recognized that black women reacted to the experience of gynecologic care in ways quite similar to white women. For example, in an essay on "menstrual irregularities," Milton Antony, who believed that "perfect regularity *only* is compatible with perfect health," claimed that "most women will, on being asked if their monthly visitations are regular, answer affirmatively," even when they were not. Some did not understand the various "species of irregularity," while "a large majority in good society, and even amongst the blacks, are compelled by their native modesty and diffidence on this subject, to avoid every word they can." He warned that they might only say "the monosyllable *yes*, or *no*; and the latter is often avoided when it should not be, lest it should lead to the necessity of farther expression on the subject"; in fact, some could only shake their heads rather than use their voices to answer questions.[71] Antony clearly believed women of both races shared a reluctance to discuss menstruation, a sign of a shared female modesty. However, Alabama physician William Boling disagreed, justifying his detailed observations of births in which the child's shoulder presented first by saying, "my patients being negro women, many of whom are entirely indifferent as to the exposure of their persons, when suffering the pains of labor."[72] He did not, of course, bother to ask the women themselves how they felt about having their bodies exposed. John Stainback Wilson thought that all laboring women were "generally too much concerned about their 'pains,' and about getting out of their difficulties, to think much about exposure" of their bodies.[73]

Most physicians were more willing than Boling to take the feelings of slave patients into account, especially during childbirth, although they were rarely as solicitous of them as they were of white women. Paul Eve was invited by a colleague to examine a slave woman whose uterus had ruptured during childbirth, "but from her exhausted state and unwillingness to submit, he in kindness desisted."[74] Kindness was not the usual motive for physicians to accede to the wishes of slave patients. When William Post, a physician in South Carolina, was called to attend Nippy because she was hemorrhaging during childbirth, he found that the placenta was presenting first. None of his remedies was effective, so "as the negro was one of value, and a favorite servant, I deemed it best to request a consultation, as I was unwilling to assume all responsibility, especially as the case now assumed an ugly aspect." Before his colleague could arrive, however, the placenta was expelled and the hemorrhage ceased, so Post attempted to deliver the child with forceps. However, "the patient was so restless and unwilling, that after several ineffectual attempts, I desisted," especially because "there could be no doubt of the death of the foetus." Instead, he gave Nippy ergot, which helped her deliver the child, who was indeed dead.[75]

E. R. Feild, a Tennessee physician, also called for two physicians to consult when he discovered that his patient's fetus had "escaped" into her peritoneal cavity, presumably through a rupture in her uterus while in labor. Since one of the consulting physician's attempts to "introduce the hand through the rent, and return the foetus" was unsuccessful, they concluded there was only one option. The three physicians agreed "to state frankly to the patient and her mistress, her situation—the uncertainty of the event in case of an operation, and the certainty of death without one." Their actions indicate the limited extent to which they were willing to grant at least this slave woman control over her body similar to what other physicians routinely granted to white women. Feild reported that "the patient refused most obstinately, declaring that she 'would prefer death,' to use her own words, 'to being cut open.' We left her for a few minutes to prepare for the operation, having determined on it *nolens volens,* but insisted that her mistress and friends should persuade her to submit to the operation if possible." Soon after, they were told that she had agreed. Feild offered a young physician also present the opportunity to perform the operation "through courtesy." The young doctor agreed to do so only if the more experienced physicians would take responsibility, because he was not "satisfied in his own mind that the foetus had escaped from the womb" and "the patient strenuously refus[ed] to undergo another vaginal examination." They agreed, so the young physician operated and removed the child from "the position diagnosticated by us." In spite of the danger of "peritoneal inflammation," the woman survived; Feild was silent on the fate of the child, but it most likely died.[76]

Feild's account of this woman's case reflected the ambivalence with which physicians approached slave women patients. On the one hand, Feild and his colleagues wanted the woman's permission to examine and operate on her. They requested both her mistress and her friends to help convince her, implying that she had at least some right to make the decision for herself. On the other hand, they were clearly willing to proceed against her wishes, at least with the operation they believed was necessary to save her life. While they waited for her consent before proceeding, the extent to which she offered it voluntarily is open to question, even given the rather self-serving account Feild provided, since she apparently agreed to the operation but refused to be examined. It is hard to imagine exactly parallel events occurring with a white patient, not only because the husband and not the mistress would have been consulted, but also because the woman's wishes would have carried somewhat greater authority. Yet even a white woman facing death would likely have had her decision not to be treated overruled by a physician convinced that he knew what was best for her, because of the widespread belief that the influence of her emotions would prevent her from making the best choices about her body. Recall, for example, J. Dickson Smith, who considered chloroform a *"God send"* in a case of retained placenta because it allowed him to overrule his white patient's wishes.

Slave women were typically asked to give consent, no doubt because it was physically easier for the physician to administer treatment when slaves consented to it. As in the case of Feild's patient, the meaning of that consent was not the same as it was for white patients. In 1835, long before the advent of anesthesia, John Bellinger determined that a black woman had an ovarian tumor that had to be removed through her abdomen. He believed "the profession" was "becoming every year more favorable" about performing such operations because "a woman need not be gifted with unnatural capacity of endurance, in order to 'escape' its dangers." He reported that his patient "fully consented" to the operation, although partway through, "the patient, losing her self command, screamed and struggled violently—rendering it no easy task to control her movements and support the viscera." Bellinger "paus[ed] a few minutes, during which she became re-assured,"

then continued the operation, which she somehow survived. Another of Bellinger's patients, a black woman suffering from a uterine tumor that had caused
her health to fail "considerably," did not recover. The woman "had consented to
the operation, the dangers of which were distinctly explained to her, at the same
time that she was encouraged to hope that it would be successful." Although it is
impossible to know whether Bellinger would have used the same language had
his patients been white women, his enthusiasm for performing such operations
coupled with his claim that a white woman with similar tumors said she "desired
that their removal should be attempted," suggests some discrepancy.[77] Bellinger's
language suggests that he may have minimized the risks and the pain involved in
his explanations to the slave women. The white woman's use of the word *attempted*
implies a more tenuous agreement, perhaps because she was better informed.

The question of consent remained murky for midcentury physicians in their
dealings with all women, not just slaves. H. Steele, professor of obstetrics and diseases of women and children at Oglethorpe Medical College in Savannah, Georgia,
advocated curing prolapsed uterus by an operation to close "the lower third or half
of the vulva." However, he noted, "[I]t is rarely that females will submit to such
an operation, for, out of several cases which were fit subjects for it, I succeeded in
getting the consent of but one, upon whom I operated with success." Steele's case
was "a laboring negress, of the field, whose condition unfitted her for its tasks,
rendering her condition pitiable, and making her almost worthless to her owner."[78]
L. A. Dugas, professor of surgery at the Medical College of Georgia, noted that
such an operation was "repugnant to most women; but this is principally because
of an erroneous appreciation of its effects," adding that "it does not impede sexual
intercourse, nor even impregnation and parturition." He acknowledged performing it "with the happiest results" and expressed surprise "that it is not more common, especially upon our plantations" because it allowed "field hands, who were
utterly incapacitated for their duties" to be "restored to complete usefulness in
a short time."[79] Dugas's eagerness to operate on slave women in order to return
them to work suggests both a racially skewed approach to consent and perhaps
concerns about the risks of the operation. Since both black and white women
suffered from prolapsed uterus, Dugas's recommending the operation primarily
for slaves implies that he considered them lacking in value unless they were able
to work, making the operation worth the risk. On the other hand, he may have
considered the surgery not worth the risk to white women's more important lives.

Charles Hentz, a physician practicing in Florida, adopted a rather cavalier attitude toward obtaining consent from the women whose teeth he sought to pull.
In an 1852 diary entry he noted, "I pulled a tooth for a negro girl—Martha—after
much persuasion & botheration—; wishing to get Miss Green in the notion—she
having an aching 'ivory'—She concluded to bear the operation & bore it hero-
ically, whilst I extracted it with scientific skill—a large molar on the lower right
side."[80] Hentz did not say whether Martha's tooth ached as well as Miss Green's or

whether he used similar scientific skill with Martha. For all of these physicians, consent could easily shade into persuasion, persuasion into coercion, with the latter end of the continuum especially likely to be experienced by female slaves. Slaveholders determined to take advantage of physicians' claims that they could restore ailing slaves to usefulness were not likely to allow those slaves to refuse, no matter the pain and suffering involved or how doubtful the cure might be.

The extent to which black patients have been coerced into giving their consent or denied the opportunity to do so at all has become highly contentious in the decades since the Tuskegee study of untreated syphilis in black men was first exposed in the early 1970s.[81] However, the question of consent has a larger and even more complex history.[82] Much of the recent discussion has focused on the involuntary sterilization of thousands of men and women deemed unfit by the twentieth-century eugenics movement.[83] In the antebellum period, when the concept of consent was even more ambiguous than it was later, scholarly attention has focused on the black women J. Marion Sims experimented on in his native Alabama to find a surgical remedy for vesico-vaginal fistula.[84] Sims's repeated operations on a few slave women, some of whom he purchased while others were in effect donated to him because they were of no use to their own-ers, have become symbols of the exploitation of black women at the hands of the medical profession.[85]

While antebellum southern doctors preferred to obtain consent from each of their women patients, they did so as a means of addressing the emotional dimen-sion of her illness rather than because they believed that she had a real choice about what happened to her body. That they paid more attention to obtaining consent from white women was both a sign of their higher status in society and physicians' belief that white women were more vulnerable to the interplay of body and mind than were black women. Asking for consent was often a mechanism for preventing hysteria or worse in their already physically ill and emotionally vulnerable patients. Of course, physicians concerned about their professional reputations also knew that obtaining consent from white women was impor-tant for enhancing their image as kind and caring gentlemen; anyone who was considered brutal and unfeeling was not likely to gain the referrals necessary to sustain his practice.

Ironically, the question of consent was far more significant when the patient was dead. Physicians who wished to perform autopsies faced a degree of ambiva-lence from survivors, whose consent they normally had no choice but to request. Autopsies were helpful to physicians, who theoretically learned something from them that could help them know how to treat the next patient more effectively, but they were of no obvious benefit to the family. Both black and white fami-lies denied permission for autopsies. Joseph Eve reported matter-of-factly about Nancy, "a negro woman" who died after suffering convulsions during childbirth, that "permission could not be obtained to make a *post mortem* examination." He used almost the same language to describe what happened after a white woman died from the same cause: "[U]nfortunately, permission could not be obtained to make a post-mortem examination." Eve did not identify who refused his request in either case.[85] P. W. Harper of Georgia was not so reticent. When a slave woman under his care died during childbirth, he noted that "by the kind permission of her mistress, I made a *post mortem* examination." However, when a white infant was born with a "*hydrocephalus*" head with "the appearance of a pulpy mass," Harper and a colleague "with all of our persuasion . . . could not prevail on the parents to grant us the permission to puncture the head, to ascertain the quantity of water, and to make such other examinations as might be necessary."[87]

When given the chance, slaves also refused autopsies of their loved ones. According to Charles Witsell, a South Carolina physician, he would have liked to examine the body of a slave woman who died from an "enormous polypus of the uterus." In his report about the details of her case, he noted, "I regret extremely that I was unable to make a post mortem examination, (negroes in the country are much opposed to autopsies), and therefore cannot state the condition of the heart and veins."[88] However, neither persuasion nor permission was necessary to conduct an autopsy on the bodies of Henry and Jane, slaves "convicted of the crime of murder by poison" and executed in Charleston. Physician Myddleton Michel "requested that the internal organs of generation of the girl Jane should be closely inspected, supposing it possible that she was either menstruating or might be pregnant." Michel decided that she was not pregnant, but that "menstruation had only began a day or two." He used the opportunity "diligently" to search "this rare specimen" for the egg, "knowing that if discovered, this would be the only case of the kind recorded."[89] Michel's search for egg and scientific glory was unsuccessful, but he never questioned the access to the woman's body that her race and status afforded him.

Consent, whether for examinations, operations, or autopsies, was not the only mechanism by which canny physicians sought to turn their understanding of the influences of mind on body and body on mind to the medical advantage of their patients and themselves. Some also intentionally exploited their patients' beliefs, particularly when those patients were slaves. No one wrote more eloquently about this than Samuel Cartwright, whose descriptions of the extreme bodily differences between whites and blacks and the distinct diseases of slaves helped shape southern medicine. In an article published in the *New Orleans Medical and Surgical Journal* in 1854, Cartwright described the recommendations of a fellow physician for addressing an epidemic of typhoid dysentery among slaves in Alabama. Dr. Atchison's "plan consisted in making an impression upon the mind as well as the body, by breaking the chain of those superstitious influences which render epidemics so fatal among negroes, and at the same time to get [them] out of the infectious atmosphere causing any unusual sickness among them." Atchison accomplished this "by sending them back to an imitation of African barbarism in the neighboring fields, woods, and wilds, to lead a savage life."[90]

Cartwright reported adopting this plan during a cholera outbreak on a large sugar plantation. Once he brought the slaves into an open place in the swamp to live until the epidemic was over, he "drove the cholera out of the heads of all who had been conjured into the belief that they were to die with the disease." He did so by stripping, greasing with fat bacon, and then beating the "ashy-colored, dry skin conjurers, or prophets, who had alarmed their fellow-servants with the prophecies that the cholera was to kill them all, and who had gained, by various tricks and artifices, much influence over their superstitious minds." The beatings "broke the charm of the conjurers by converting them . . . into subjects for ridicule and laughter, instead of fear and veneration." Cartwright attributed the subsequent good health of the slaves to the good effects of "treat[ing] the negro like a negro."[91]

Cartwright believed that the original "frightful mortality" of dysentery among the slaves was "more in the mind than in the body." They had been treated with conventional medicines that should have been effective in curing the disease, but the treatment was not effective because "there was nothing in the treatment addressed to the mind." He thought that after a few deaths among the slaves, "superstition and panic . . . raise their hideous heads and become executioners, outstripping by far the disease itself." The slaves died "from that mental affection which might be termed a *cholera of the mind,*" the result of "a splinter of superstition run into [their minds] from the appearance of cholera . . . with as much certainty as tetanus from a splinter in the foot." Slaves could die from this "tetanus of the mind" with only "the veriest pretense of a disease, and sometimes without any apparent bodily infirmity at all." Instead, their "excessive mortality" was the result of "this singular mental affection," which could not be cured by conventional medical treatment. Because "they very commonly have some undefined or indefinite notion that they are conjured, bewitched, or from some cause of other, inevitably doomed to die," even the best medical treatment would be counteracted. "They see in the remedies, given to cure them, the agents of the sure and certain destruction that awaits them." Cartwright warned that "when panic struck . . . they will often hold the most nauseous medicine in their throat, for hours together, without swallowing it, waiting for an opportunity to spit it out."[92]

Cartwright's insistence that large numbers of slaves succumbed to the suggestions of conjurers, rather than dying as a consequence of disease upon their bodies along with their refusal to swallow the prescribed medicine, reflected his belief in the power of their minds over their bodies. Cartwright's plan to break the power of the conjurers also, of course, removed them from the sources of contagion, a factor he scarcely considered. Instead, he focused on slaves' weak control over their bodies and minds. Unlike white men, who could be counted on to think and behave more rationally, slaves easily fell victim to the suggestions of others, as a result literally dying of fright. Only the white, male physician, with his superior mind and body in control of medical knowledge, could attempt to persuade them, even through coercive means, to think differently about their illnesses and thus remain alive. Cartwright's assumptions about bodies and minds defined not only how he understood illness and its cure, but also how he thought medicine should be practiced.

For physicians concerned about mind and body interactions in their slave and white patients, the difficulty was not just coercing reluctant patients to cooperate with medical authority, but also determining when the patient was merely pretending to be sick. This was most common in the case of slave patients, who were all too frequently accused of shamming, even when their illness was hard to deny. But on occasion, whites could be accused of shamming as well. In 1860, the *Medical Journal of North Carolina* printed an article about a white woman in Ohio who was a "pauper, . . . much trouble to the authorities, and a great expense to the people." Her physicians were at first baffled by the "*black lumps*" she claimed to pass from her vagina. One doctor was called "to remove one of the woman's 'black balls,' but while doing so she had a terrible convulsive fit," so he refused to continue. Another gave her opiates, "which the poor woman assured him acted like a charm in calming the constitutional irritation attending such a harassing 'irregularity' as she was subject to, and completely controlling the distressing convulsions." Two more physicians, determined to find out what was wrong, attended while she delivered one of the balls, "during which procedure the woman assimilated acute pain, and very nearly went into one of her 'convulsions.'" Convinced that "she was of the 'genus homo' known to the naturalists as 'humbugs,'" the doctors nevertheless gave her opium but examined the ball and found it was made of dough and contained sewing thread. "His suspicions . . . now confirmed," one doctor concluded "there was no physiological function by which thread was secreted; *ergo,* the woman has been simulating a queer disease, in order to obtain opium." Her ruse had been successful for ten years, but "she now found that her narcotic supplies were to be cut off." She then claimed to suffer "falling of the womb," which was also discovered to be a ruse when the physician pulled "a *bullock's rectum*" and another ball of dough from her vagina. The woman confessed, and the report concluded "no more trouble was had with her afterwards: she was furnished with a little opium, in diminished doses, and in course of time her bad habit was broken up."[93] Unusually detailed for an account of shamming, perhaps because the patient was white and not from the South, this woman's case demonstrates both the ease with which women could pretend to be sick—she convinced the doctors for ten years before her ruse was revealed—and the advantages of doing so. She not only was able to get opium, she was given medical attention and the invalid status that allowed her to receive public charity

Devious patients could engage in other activities designed to fool the unwary physician. Tomlinson Fort noted that "it would appear, that nothing could be plainer than the fact, that a patient threw up blood by vomiting." But truth could be complex, he warned, because "cases have occurred in which fraudulent attempts to prove the presence of this disease, by crafty, wicked, or insane persons." Sometimes people "secretly swallowed" blood "from other sources . . . that it might be thrown up in the presence of witnesses."[94]

Slave women were unlikely to insert balls of dough or other objects into their vaginas or swallow blood in order to be counted among the sick. Since illness was ubiquitous, such dramatic gestures were rarely necessary. Nevertheless, wary slaveholders and the physicians they hired constantly suspected shamming, because sickness could bring respite from work, better food, and other advantages that were otherwise unavailable. As a result, slaves whose complaints of illness were assumed to be shamming were denied treatment, often with surprising consequences. For example, South Carolina physician Joseph Quattlebum successfully treated a slave woman for "a complication of diseases" related to prolapsed uterus, so that she was able to return to work as a plantation nurse and eventually to the fields. Several months later, believing herself pregnant, the woman "was seized with pain in the abdomen, which she complained of . . . as excruciating." She suffered for two days, "but as she had previously deceived her master he did not call in a physician, thinking that she was doing the same again." Instead, she was given domestic remedies but died the next day, from what Quattlebum's autopsy revealed to be an ovarian pregnancy. [95] Such incidents caused prudent physicians and slaveholders to be wary. Charles Hentz wrote about a difficult nighttime ride through a thunderstorm to see one patient, then being awakened at two o'clock in the morning to see another, "a negro woman of bro. Russ, who sent word she was about to die—a 'deceptions' negress—cries 'wolf' where there is no wolf—; Hamilton [the overseer] & I went to her cabin—I gave her dose of morphine & returned to my couch—12 miles—."[96]

On occasion, however, slaves could claim to be well when physicians considered them sick, a circumstance that complicated physicians' practice. Hentz wrote in his medical journal about three visits to the "Mulatto girl Ann," whose long list of symptoms first included "fever . . . tongue furred—papillae prominent—red around edges." The next day he found her "panting & tremulous—pulse very quick, tongue &c as before," while on the third he thought her "very sick—pulse very quick, & with a tremulous thrill." Nevertheless, Hentz recorded that on the first visit, Ann "says she feels very well," while on the second and third, she "says she feels 'smart.'"[97] He offered no explanation of her apparent reluctance to consider herself sick or to be treated by him.

Most of the time, physicians considered behavior they found objectionable in their slave patients to be the result of organic disease of mind and body, occasionally even such bizarre diseases as drapetomania (running away) and dysoesthesia

Ethiopis (rascality) discussed in chapter 1. However, shamming could in itself be considered a disease by harried physicians trying to strike a balance between the needs of their slave patients complaining of bodily ills and those of slaveholders determined to keep their labor force at work. According to M. D. McLoud, whose medical thesis at the Medical College of South Carolina focused on the "medical treatment of Negroes," the "observant Physician" would not dispute "that their complaints demand at the hands of the physician a more careful investigation than those of whites."[98]

McLoud believed "the nature of the daily avocations of the negro is frequently so disagreeable that sickness is feigned in order to escape the unpleasant tasks assigned to him." Even though the slaves' symptoms might be "anomalous," the slaveholder would give "medicines for days in succession, but no good result will follow." This was because "the negro prefers to take the medicine until the time when more agreeable work is to be done on the plantation; he then recovers rapidly and soon is at work again." The physician had the responsibility of "detect[ing] the imposture," which was "a most difficult task; one which requires all his discrimination and acuteness." The physician "must therefore be on his guard, he must note carefully all the evidences of disease" and make appropriate inquiries into various bodily functions. In addition, doctors should "notice the garrulity or silence of the patient, whether he complain much or little; the position he lies in and the degree of derangement of the nervous system evinced by his rising and walking." Only then could the physician decide if the patient "be actually sick."[99]

According to McLoud, the physician "must be careful to let no word drop which would cause the negro to think that he is suspected of imposition; but on the contrary he must sympathize with him in his afflictions, and draw from him every symptom which he would wish to notice." This would encourage the patient to place "the most implicit confidence in his skill and ability" and thus "relate with wonderful garrulity and exaggeration a host of contradictory symptoms and complaints." If this allowed the physician to "pronounce with confidence his opinion," he risked losing "the good will of his patient, but at the same time gain the most profound admiration of his talents from both Master and Negro." McLoud noted that "the garrulity of a sick negro is a good evidence of imposture; the loud groans and exclamations, ejaculations, tossing and turning rapidly in his bed are all circumstances which should excite suspicion." Doctors knew that "in cases of acute pain; the patient will lie as still as possible and talk as little as possible," so "the contrary demeanour will therefore be looked upon as a prima facia [sic] evidence of the absence of acute pain." McLeod knew that there were good reasons for slaves to pretend to be sick. They were especially likely to feign colic on plantations where it was treated with whiskey—less so when Epsom salts were offered. He recommended treating colic with "some nauseous compound" to "prevent imposition on that score."[100]

McLoud was especially wary of slaves who feigned "concusion of the brain," which he thought they did "through anger and malevolence." This was alarming to masters, "as they only feign this when they are beaten for their negligence." McLoud recounted the experience of a slave whose master struck him on the head with the butt of a whip for sleeping at his post of carriage driver, causing him to fall "back speechless." Alarmed, the master called the physician, who found "the negro was still stupid but exhibited some signs of intelligence" and that he had eaten and had good pulse and pupils and no swelling of the head. "The conclusion of the Physician was, that there was nothing the matter except a stubbornness of disposition which should be corrected immediately by the whip." This cured the slave "almost immediately; to the great relief of the Master, who was much alarmed at the idea of having killed his negro."[101]

McLoud warned that it was "not infrequent for negroes to dessemble [*sic*] an attack of epilepsy," which he thought they could "feign with so much exactness that it is almost impossible to distinguish the feigned from a real attack." He offered the example of a woman whose attack in the fields was treated by the master with undiluted ammonia, the "pungency" of which "caused an immediate resolution of the fit and she started up in alarm. Her mouth suffered severely, there has been no recurrence of the fit since." The physician of another woman whose epilepsy was considered suspicious told her master "to have her back stripped and with a cowskin or hickory switch to scourge her on the spine," which marked the end of her disease.[102]

Recognizing that "such impostures . . . are well known to every practicing [*sic*] Physician," McLoud nevertheless acknowledged that it was "repugnant to humanity to leave an apparent sufferer without attempting for their relief," which left doctors "often imposed upon." Physicians "look upon apparent suffering as real," but after prescribing, the "almost immediate recovery of the patient from what seemed an alarming condition, first leads to a suspicion of the truth." Physicians learned from such experiences, in part because "every planter is well aware of this universal disposition to deception, and if his physician does not appear to be aware of the same, his confidence in his judgment immediately abates." Both professional ambition and professional prudence required sensitivity to the dangers of impositions. McLoud also argued that "the very great difference in the mode of Living between the blacks & whites would naturally lead us to suppose that there ought to be some difference in the treatment of their diseases," including their ability to tolerate bleeding, cathartics, and stimulants.[103]

McLoud's attempt to explicate physicians' difficulties with slaves who sometimes feigned illness reflects a rather perplexed sense of their responsibility for understanding the connections between slaves' minds and bodies. On the one hand, he knew that the physician needed to be skeptical of slaves' complaints and could even resort to trickery if necessary to detect them in shamming. The slaveholder who employed him expected no less. At the same time, McLoud knew that sometimes slaves really were sick. McLoud's dilemma was shared by all southern physicians; it was at the heart of southern medicine.

Slaves who feigned illness in order to obtain respite from work and enjoy benefits not ordinarily available to them exposed the contradictions at the core of southern physicians' efforts to understand the connections between body and mind—for everyone, not just slaves. If slaves pretended to be sick, was this not a rejection of their proper role and thus a sign of mental weakness, itself a form of illness? Were slaves who pretended to be sick in fact suffering from hysteria, a legitimate disease in physicians' eyes, or something like it? Were they mentally ill? Was it ever possible to distinguish with absolute certainty between mental and physical illnesses? What about white women and their difficult reproductive organs and even more difficult emotions? What were the consequences of making the wrong decision about these matters, especially when it came to slave patients? For physicians bent on enhancing their credibility as well as building their practice, the latter question was particularly resonant. Understanding the connections between mind and body was central to their effectiveness as physicians, a reality only the foolish or most inexperienced among them ignored. For southern physicians committed to defining the body in ways that both conformed to the assumptions and met the needs of their society, attention to white women's modesty and slaves' shamming was necessary not only for professional success, but also for understanding the essence of the bodies and minds under their care. The essence of the ideal southern practitioner was not just one who could cure disease, but one who could probe the secrets of mind and body well enough to tell the difference between legitimate and false illnesses and then negotiate his patients' responses effectively enough to cure them. As arbiters of all forms of bodily legitimacy, physicians claimed for themselves the power to define health as well as illness, mind as well as body, for everyone in the South.

Recognizing the power that came with the responsibility of defining relations between mind and body, physicians increasingly appropriated for themselves the right to define morality and proper social relations. No longer were they content to leave to ministers the right to judge acceptable human behavior and to God such abstract notions as conscience, free will, and destiny. By articulating the connections between mind and body, physicians expanded the power of medicine from the beating heart to the feeling heart, from the mechanical brain to the thinking brain. In doing so, they expanded their reach into every corner of individual existence and claimed for themselves the right to act as influential arbiters of the social order as well. They would only develop these powers more fully as time passed.

# The Body Politic

In the March 1853 *Charleston Medical Journal and Review,* T. S. Hopkins, a physician from Waynesville, Georgia, published an article called "A Remarkable Case of Feigned Disease," in which he offered "the history of the case" of Nat, a slave man. Nat, who was forty-five years old, was sent for treatment of "pain in the side and *fits.*" Dr. Hopkins "diagnosticated [*sic*] functional derangement of the liver," for which he prescribed several treatments. A few days later, he "was summoned in haste to see Nat in a *fit,*" which was different from what Hopkins expected, as "there was no spasm or muscular rigidity whatever . . . no throbbing of carotid or temporal arteries, no heat of head, change of pulse, respiration or appearance of eyes, from a state of health." After several types of treatment, Nat was soon "himself again," but two days later "he had another *fit.*" As before, Hopkins put Nat's feet "into a tub of warm water," but without effect, so he began pouring boiling water into the tub. "In a few seconds he showed signs of life by attempting to remove his feet," but Hopkins seized Nat "by the knees" and "forced his feet again into the water, where I held them, until my patient becoming stronger than myself, I left him." Hopkins also treated Nat with blue pill, cups, and blisters, all of which Nat said left him "feeling 'like another man.'"[1]

At the same time, Hopkins agreed to hire Nat from his master for a couple of months, which apparently pleased him. However, the master "requested me to give him up" after a month, and Hopkins agreed. He "watched the countenance of Nat when the news was announced, and if it had been the reading of his death warrant he could not have looked more wo-begone." Nat predicted that before he was home a month, he would "be worse off than ever." In fact, Hopkins reported, in "*less* than a month he was brought to my house in a cart, from which he seemed unable, without assistance, to reach the sick-house. He wore the most pitiable, haggard, and friendless aspect I ever beheld," and was "the very 'picture of despair.'" For the first time, Nat told Hopkins that he "lived very unhappily" because "his master treated him badly." Nat said that "he was kept from his wife and children, whom he loved very dearly, and unless his master would sell him to the gentleman who owned them, he could never recover." Indeed, as soon as he had returned home, "the same old *fits* and pain in the side returned in a more aggravated form than ever," and the fits continued almost daily for the three weeks Nat remained with Hopkins for treatment as well.[2]

Hopkins described Nat during those weeks as "at times taciturn and melancholy" and weeping "like a child," with "tears *flowing freely*" when "addressed in sympathizing tones." At other times, he was "as restless and fidgetty [*sic*] as an old maid after witnessing a marriage ceremony." Since Hopkins was unable to "relieve him of what I considered his *hysterical symptoms*," he "ordered him to return to his master." At that point, Nat claimed that "he was *witched*" and asked to be sent to Dr. Jones, "one of these characters who sometimes attain a degree of *eminence* in the 'backwoods,' in consequence of the magic power they possess in casting out devils from man as well as beast." Nat's owner denied his request, and he was sent home. Soon after, Hopkins learned that Nat was not only "*vomiting pins*" but that more pins could be felt in the same regions of his body that had been so painful before; the pins were removed by "cut[ting] down upon" his flesh.[3]

When Nat believed that he had been sold to his wife's owner, "every unpleasant symptom disappeared." He "continued in the enjoyment of *perfect* health" for two-and-a-half years, when he had to have another pin removed. Hopkins noted that "the cause of this relapse was the discovery that he was *hired* and not sold." Hopkins also learned that two years before he began treating Nat, he had suffered "a severe Cephalalgia,[4] which deprived him of sleep, and *threatened,* at one time, permanent insanity." At that time, "a piece of twine several inches in length and tied into numerous knots" was pulled from his "meatus auditorius"[5] with forceps. Hopkins noted that Nat "persists in denying most positively any agency whatever on his part in the introduction of the thread and pins into his person, and contends that the several acts were committed whilst he slept." Hopkins was not convinced, noting that "the manner in which the pins were introduced" intended to protect his stomach, and the absence of heads on those under his skin would be "sufficient to remove" any doubt.[6]

Hopkins introduced Nat's story to the medical journal's readers in terms of hysteria. While he recognized that "to assert that *man* enjoys an entire immunity from hysteria, would be opposing high authority," he also knew that "such cases are sufficiently uncommon, to be classed among the exceptions to the rule which makes it a disease peculiar to woman." However, after presenting Nat's story, Hopkins abandoned the idea of hysteria and instead began his interpretation by wondering "were the *pins* present when he first came under my treatment, and if so, were they the cause of those symptoms?" Hopkins's complex explanation suggested that the "pin irritation was suppressed" by the sore mouth and gums caused by Nat's treatment with blue pill. He claimed he was "satisfied in my own mind that there was no *pin disease* at this time," but rather that Nat's "liver affection" was "the result of a severe attack of climate fever." Since Hopkins cured that with the several prescriptions and Nat was "compelled to return again to his master," he "resorted to artifice for the accomplishment of his cherished object," to be sold. Hopkins surmised that in order to "aggravate the symptoms, and by way of *frightening* his master into a compliance with his desire, he *swallowed* a *few*" pins to make the master think "the sooner he got rid of him the better." Hopkins concluded his account by remarking that "it is difficult to say whether this man is most deserving of our condemnation or approbation. If it be the simple desire to change masters, certainly he merits the former; if it be devotion to his family, from [whom] he has been separated, he is worthy of the latter. In such a case, the end would justify the means."[7]

Hopkins's presentation of Nat's experience offers rich insight into the political significance of different definitions of the body for slaves, slaveholders, and physicians in the antebellum South. Nat recognized that claiming to be suffering from pain and fits offered him respite from work, and indeed he was able to arrange months away from the fields while under medical treatment. Even more significant was his deliberate—and undoubtedly painful—invocation of illness in order to escape his master's bad treatment and instead live with his wife and children, at least temporarily. (Hopkins does not indicate what finally happened to Nat after his "game of 'push pin'" was discovered.[8]) Nat depended on the sympathies of a regular physician at first, but when that proved insufficient to accomplish his goal, he claimed he needed the aid of a conjure doctor to rid his body of the consequences of witchcraft. He tried to enlist Hopkins's aid in this effort, which failed in part because Hopkins, a regular physician, did not accept the premises of conjure. Nat's effort to turn to an alternate system of medicine when the first did not accomplish his purposes was a familiar strategy for slaves. In all of this, Nat's owner was the gatekeeper, deciding when Nat could be treated by Hopkins and when he had to return to work; the owner also made the decision not to allow Nat to be treated by the conjure doctor. Nat's efforts to use his body in ways both literal (by harming himself with pins and knotted string) and figurative (by invoking illness in the form of pain and fits) in order to live with his family rather than allow it to be used by his owner to labor in the fields suggest his awareness of the power of the body in defining slavery.

Hopkins also recognized the power of the body in defining slavery, in his case the medicalized body. Hopkins did not suspect that Nat was shamming at first, nor did he consider that even his first illness was deliberately invoked to suit his purposes. Rather, Hopkins believed that his successful cure of Nat's original liver disease and climate fever enabled him to turn to pins and fits as a way of influencing his life. He sustained this belief even after he learned of Nat's earlier deception with the knotted string in his ear. Hopkins did not see Nat's illnesses as evidence of shamming until overwhelming evidence left him little choice, but even then he understood Nat's original problem in strictly medical terms.

Slaves were inclined to illness; his responsibility as a physician was to try to diagnose and cure that illness and only incidentally to investigate it. His concluding
comments about Nat deserving either condemnation or approbation reflect his
sense of responsibility for the physical and emotional well-being of at least this
individual slave. His sympathy for Nat's desire to live with his wife and children
marked him as perhaps more generous than most, but nowhere in his account
did he question the validity of race differences or the legitimacy of slavery.

Nat's story was not only about race from Hopkins's perspective; it was also
about sex and gender. Nat's black, male body and Hopkins's white, male one
were opposites in the South's racial system but were aligned in its gendered one,
although Hopkins believed Nat's body to be much closer to a woman's than was
his own. Hopkins began the article with a brief discussion of the possibility that
a man could suffer from hysteria and tried hard to relieve Nat of his "*hysterical
symptoms.*" He clearly viewed Nat's tears and desire for sympathy as atypical and
inappropriate behavior for an adult man, even a black one. Even his metaphor
about "figetty" old maids speaks to his assumptions about sex and sex differences. Since he did not initially consider the possibility of shamming, an activity
exclusively practiced by slaves in the view of antebellum physicians, Hopkins
had few options other than to define Nat's illness as hysterical—that is, to put
it into the category of female diseases. To do so fit neatly with the widespread
belief that both slaves' and white women's bodies were inferior to those of white
men and thus more likely to succumb to diseases of all sorts. Slaves' and white
women's bodies were vulnerable to the influence of their minds; both were weak
and impressionable. As a result, both fared best when kept under the authority
of white men, whose bodily characteristics suited them for power. The politics of
sex as well as race were rooted in the medicalized body in the antebellum South.

Among the most interesting aspects of Hopkins's account of Nat's illness was
the nearly invisible tension between Hopkins the physician and Nat's owner, Mr.
R. M. The two men held some views in common, the most important of which
was that the slaveholder had the ultimate right to determine what happened to
his slaves. Hopkins ordered Nat to return to his owner when he was unable to
cure him, although he knew that Nat was reluctant to go. R. M. told Nat that he
had been sold to his wife's owner, a deception with which Hopkins colluded.
However, their perspectives differed in important ways. Hopkins believed in
Nat's illness and wanted to cure him, while R. M. simply wanted his body to be
available to labor in the fields. The two white men also differed about how long
and where Nat should be under treatment, a signal for medicine's potential to
humanize slavery in what would turn out to be its final years. Hopkins did not
wish to abandon slavery, but he was capable of sympathizing with Nat's physical
suffering as well as with his desire to live with his family, while his owner was not.
Not dramatic enough to be elevated to the status of a disagreement over slavery,
the differences between the ways the slaveholder and physician viewed Nat's body

suggest the potential power of medicine to challenge as well as to reify the South's institutions. It was, of course, a potential seldom realized in daily practice.

Hopkins's presentation of Nat's story demonstrates the ways in which the politics of the South were rooted in the raced and sexed bodies of its inhabitants. Slavery and subordination could not have existed without bodily difference; politics reflected the body. The raced and gendered meanings of individual bodies were a reflection of the politics of southern society, just as society reflected the politics of the body. Medicine as theorized and practiced by physicians and as understood by laypeople offered a way to define raced and gendered characteristics of the body. Those characteristics preserved slavery and subordination and were consequently central for the culture and identity of the region. Southern politics depended on elaborate theories of bodily difference to sustain its institutions.

In all of this, medicine served to define bodies and minds and their characteristics with the growing authority of science; science and medicine reinforced each other. Not only did this enhance the cultural authority of doctors, it also enhanced the legitimacy of the South's political institutions. The irony, of course, is that these arguments were circular and self-serving yet made without a great deal of self-reflection by physicians. An even greater irony is that physicians made them by recognizing the humanity of slaves and acknowledging the suffering of their bodies. For slaveholders threatened by increasing challenges in the antebellum years, physicians offered a new way to justify slavery and the race and gender subordination upon which it depended. Nat, along with his wife and children, may have enjoyed occasional respite when sick due to the growing intervention of physicians, but the medical theories and practices advanced in the antebellum years only reinforced the legitimacy of the subordination of slaves and white women.

# NOTES

## Introduction

1. William C. Bellamy, "History of a Case of Insanity with Hemorrhage from Some Unknown Source Escaping from the Urethra," *Oglethorpe Medical and Surgical Journal* 3 (July 1860): 77. On case reports and other medical narratives and their power to shape perception and reality, see Thomas W. Laqueur, "Bodies, Details, and the Humanitarian Narrative," in Lynn Hunt, ed., *The New Cultural History* (Berkeley: University of California Press, 1989), 176–204; Steven M. Stowe, "Seeing Themselves at Work: Physicians and the Case Narrative in the Mid-Nineteenth-Century American South," *American Historical Review* 101 (February 1996): 41–79; W. F. Bynum, Stephen Lock, and Roy Porter, eds., *Medical Journals and Medical Knowledge: Historical Essays* (New York: Routledge, 1992).

2. Bellamy, "History of a Case of Insanity," 77–79.

3. Ibid., 78–79.

4. For discussion of black men and women as healers, see for example Leslie A. Falk, "Black Abolitionist Doctors and Healers," *Bulletin of the History of Medicine* 54 (Summer 1980): 258–72; Martia Graham Goodson, "Medical-Botanical Contributions of African Slave Women to American Medicine," in Darlene Clark Hine, ed., *Black Women in American History: From Colonial Times through the Nineteenth Century*, 4 vols. (Brooklyn, N.Y.: Carlson, 1990), 2:473–84; Gertrude J. Fraser, *African American Midwifery in the South: Dialogues of Birth, Race, and Memory* (Cambridge, Mass.: Harvard University Press, 1998); Wilbur H. Watson, ed., *Black Folk Medicine: The Therapeutic Significance of Faith and Trust* (New Brunswick, N.J.: Transaction Books, 1984); Loudell F. Snow, *Walkin' Over Medicine: Traditional Health Practices in African-American Life* (Boulder, Colo.: Westview, 1993).

5. The literature on southern medicine is vast and growing; see James O. Breeden, "States-Rights Medicine in the Old South," *Bulletin of the New York Academy of Medicine* 52 (March–April 1976): 348–72; John Duffy, "Medical Practice in the Ante Bellum South," *Journal of Southern History* 25 (1959): 53–72; Kenneth F. Kiple and Virginia Himmelsteib King, *Another Dimension to the Black Diaspora: Diet, Disease, and Racism* (New York: Cambridge University Press, 1981); Martha Carolyn Mitchell, "Health and the Medical Profession in the Lower South, 1845–1860," *Journal of Southern History* 10 (1944): 424–46; Ted A. Rathbun, "Health and Disease at a South Carolina Plantation: 1840–1870," *American Journal of Physical Anthropology* 74 (1987): 239–53; Ronald L. Numbers and Todd L. Savitt, eds., *Science and Medicine in the Old South* (Baton Rouge: Louisiana State University Press, 1989); Joseph I. Waring, *A History of Medicine in South Carolina, 1620–1825* (Columbia: South Carolina Medical Association, 1964); Joseph Ioor Waring, *A History of Medicine in South Carolina, 1825–1900* (Columbia, S.C., 1967); Richard H. Shryock, "Medical Practice in the Old South," *South Atlantic Quarterly* 29 (April 1930):

160–78; Todd L. Savitt and James Harvey Young, eds., *Disease and Distinctiveness in the American South* (Knoxville: University of Tennessee Press, 1988); Jeffrey R. Young, "Ideology and Death on a Savannah River Rice Plantation, 1833–1867: Paternalism amidst 'a Good Supply of Disease and Pain,'" *Journal of Southern History* 59 (November 1993): 673–706; Steven M. Stowe, *Doctoring the South: Southern Physicians and Everyday Medicine in the Mid-Nineteenth Century* (Chapel Hill: University of North Carolina Press, 2004); Sharla M. Fett, *Working Cures: Healing, Health, and Power on Southern Slave Plantations* (Chapel Hill: University of North Carolina Press, 2002); Kay Moss, *Southern Folk Medicine* (Columbia: University of South Carolina Press, 1999); Steven Stowe, "Obstetrics and the Work of Doctoring in the Mid-Nineteenth Century South," *Bulletin of the History of Medicine* 64 (1990): 540–66; John Harley Warner, "The Idea of Southern Medical Distinctiveness," in Judith W. Leavitt and Ronald L. Numbers, eds., *Sickness and Health*, 2nd. ed. (Madison: University of Wisconsin Press, 1985), 53–70; Richard Steckel, "A Peculiar Population: The Nutrition, Health, and Mortality of American Slaves from Childhood to Maturity," *Journal of Economic History* 46 (1986): 721–41; Sally McMillen, "Antebellum Southern Fathers and the Health Care of Children," *Journal of Southern History* 60 (August 1994): 513–32; Martin Kaufmann, "Medicine and Slavery: An Essay Review," *Georgia Historical Quarterly* 63 (1976): 380–90; James O. Breeden, *Joseph Jones, M.D.: Scientist of the Old South* (Lexington: University Press of Kentucky, 1975).

6. The literature on science, medicine, and women's bodies is vast; see for example Andrew Scull and Diane Favrean, "'A Chance to Cut Is a Chance to Cure': Sexual Surgery for Psychosis in Three Nineteenth Century Societies," in Steven Spitzer and Andrew T. Scull, eds., *Research in Law, Deviance, and Social Control*, vol. 8 (Greenwich, Conn.: JAI Press, 1986), 3–39; Janet Moore Lindman and Michele Lise Tarter, eds., *A Centre of Wonders: The Body in Early America* (Ithaca, N.Y.: Cornell University Press, 2001); Barbara Bair and Susan E. Cayleff, eds., *Wings of Gauze: Women of Color and the Experience of Health and Illness* (Detroit: Wayne State University Press, 1991); Lynda Birke, *Feminism and the Biological Body* (New Brunswick, N.J.: Rutgers University Press, 2000); Regina Morantz, "Making Women Modern: Middle Class Women and Health Reform in Nineteenth Century America," *Journal of Social History* 10 (June 1977): 490–507; Nancy Sahli, "Sexuality in Nineteenth and Twentieth Century America: The Sources and Their Problems," *Radical History Review* 20 (Spring/Summer 1979): 89–96; Elizabeth Fee and Nancy Krieger, eds., *Women's Health, Politics, and Power: Essays on Sex/Gender, Medicine, and Public Health* (Amityville, N.Y.: Baywood, 1994); Mary Jacobus, Evelyn Fox Keller, and Sally Shutleworth, eds., *Body/Politics Women and the Discourses of Science* (New York: Routledge, 1990); Susan Bordo, *Unbearable Weight: Feminism, Western Culture, and the Body* (Berkeley: University of California Press, 1993); Dorothy Roberts, *Killing the Black Body: Race, Reproduction, and the Meaning of Liberty* (New York: Vintage, 1997); Catherine Gallagher and Thomas Laqueur, eds., *The Making of the Modern Body: Sexuality and Society in the Nineteenth Century* (Berkeley: University of California Press, 1987); Rima D. Apple, ed., *Women, Health, and Medicine in America: A Historical Handbook* (New Brunswick, N.J.: Rutgers University Press, 1990); Maureen Milligan and Ellen S. More, eds., *The Empathic Practitioner: Empathy, Gender, and Medicine* (New Brunswick, N.J.: Rutgers University Press, 1994).

7. The biological basis of class would become central to medical discussion later in the nineteenth century and into the twentieth, when the eugenics movement began to define poverty as one of the characteristics of those it deemed unfit to reproduce.

8. On medical sects, see especially James C. Whorton, *Nature Cures: The History of Alternative Medicine in America* (New York: Oxford University Press, 2002); John S. Haller Jr., *The People's Doctors: Samuel Thomson and the American Botanical Movement, 1790–1860* (Carbondale: Southern Illinois University Press, 2000); Norman Gevitz, ed., *Other Healers: Unorthodox Medicine in America* (Baltimore: Johns Hopkins University Press, 1988); John Haller, *Medical Protestants: The Eclectics in American Medicine, 1825–1939* (Carbondale: Southern Illinois University Press, 1994).

9. On medical education, see Regina Morantz-Sanchez, *Sympathy and Science: Women Physicians in American Medicine* (New York: Oxford University Press, 1985); John Duffy, "Sectional Conflict and Medical Education in Louisiana," *Journal of Southern History* 23 (1957): 286–306; William Rothstein, *American Medical Schools and the Practice of Medicine: A History* (New York: Oxford University Press, 1987); Daniel Kilbrick, "Southern Medical Students in Philadelphia, 1800–1861: Science and Sociability in the 'Republic of Medicine,'" *Journal of Southern History* 65 (November 1999): 697–732.

10. "Code of Medical Ethics," *Southern Medical and Surgical Journal* 3 (September 1847): 537–48; "Code of Medical Ethics," *Southern Journal of Medicine and Pharmacy* 2 (September 1847): 573–85; "Medical Ethics," *Medical Journal of North Carolina* 2 (February 1859): 389–99; see also Morris Fishbein, *The History of the American Medical Association, 1847–1947* (Philadelphia: Saunders, 1947).

11. H. R. Easterling, "The Effects of Uterine Diseases on the Constitution—Their Diagnosis and Treatment—With Remarks on the Importance of Instituting a Physical Exploration as a Means of Diagnosis," *Charleston Medical Journal and Review* 10 (July 1855): 475; see also S. N. Harris, "Observations on Some of the Opinions Generally Received among Medical Men," *Charleston Medical Journal and Review* 7 (November 1852): 750–51.

12. The editor, quoting Dr. James Henry Bennet, in "Inflammation and Ulceration of the Neck of the Uterus in the Virgin Female," *Southern Medical and Surgical Journal* 3 (November 1847): 669.

13. Gunning S. Bedford, *Clinical Lectures on the Diseases of Women and Children,* 2nd. ed. (New York: Samuel S. and William Wood, 1855), 64 and passim; see also "[Introduction to] 'Chloroform Applied to Midwifery, as well as Surgery, in Augusta, Ga.," *Southern Medical and Surgical Journal* 4 (April 1848): 251; Octavius A. White, "A New Hysterotome," *Southern Medical and Surgical Journal* 15 (September 1859): 641.

14. Richard H. Shryock, "Empiricism versus Rationalism in American Medicine, 1650–1950," *Proceedings of the American Antiquarian Society* 79 (1969): 99–150; John Harley Warner, *The Therapeutic Perspective: Medical Practice, Knowledge, and Identity in America, 1820–1885* (Cambridge, Mass.: Harvard University Press, 1986); John Harley Warner, "The Fall and Rise of Professional Mastery: Epistemology, Authority, and the Emergence of Laboratory Medicine in Nineteenth Century America," in Andrew Cunningham and Perry Williams, eds., *The Laboratory Revolution in Medicine* (New York: Cambridge University Press, 1992), 110–41.

15. Roy Porter, *Flesh in the Age of Reason: The Modern Foundations of Body and Soul* (New York: Norton, 2003).

16. See for example Michael T. Taussig, "Reification and the Consciousness of the Patient," *Social Science and Medicine* 14B (1980): 3–13; Charles Rosenberg and Janet Golden, eds., *Framing Disease: Studies in Cultural History* (New Brunswick, N.J.: Rutgers University Press, 1992); Michel Foucault, *The Birth of the Clinic: An Archaeology of Medical Perception,* trans. A. M. Sheridan Smith (New York: Vintage, 1973); Kathryn Montgomery Hunter,

*Doctors' Stories: The Narrative Structure of Medical Knowledge* (Princeton, N.J.: Princeton University Press, 1991); Arthur L. Caplan, James J. McCartney, and Dominic A. Sisti, eds., *Health, Disease, and Illness: Concepts in Medicine,* part 2 (Washington, DC: Georgetown University Press, 2004); Elaine Scarry, *The Body in Pain: The Making and Unmaking of the World* (New York: Oxford University Press, 1985); Rafael Campo, *The Healing Art: A Doctor's Black Bag of Poetry* (New York: Norton, 2003); Arthur W. Frank, *The Wounded Storyteller: Body, Illness, and Ethics* (Chicago: University of Chicago Press, 1995); Susan Sontag, *Illness as Metaphor and AIDS and Its Metaphors* (New York: Anchor Books, 1989); Nancy M. P. King and Ann Folwell Stanford, "Patient Stories, Doctor Stories, and True Stories: A Cautionary Reading," *Literature and Medicine* 11 (Fall 1992): 185–99.

Individual diseases also have cultural histories; see for example Anne Fadiman, *The Spirit Catches You and You Fall Down: A Hmong Child, Her American Doctors, and the Collision of Two Cultures* (New York: Farrar, Straus, and Giroux, 1997); Howard I. Kushner, *A Cursing Brain?: The Histories of Tourette Syndrome* (Cambridge, Mass.: Harvard University Press, 1999); Paula A. Treichler, *How to Have Theory in an Epidemic: Cultural Chronicles of AIDS* (Durham, N.C.: Duke University Press, 1999).

## Chapter 1. Constructing Race

1. The literature on early theories of anthropology and other ways of understanding race and race differences is extensive; see, for example, William Stanton, *The Leopard's Spots: Scientific Attitudes toward Race in America, 1815–1859* (Chicago: University of Chicago Press, 1960); Londa Schiebinger, *Nature's Body: Gender in the Making of Modern Science* (Boston: Beacon Press, 1993); John S. Haller Jr., *Outcasts from Evolution: Scientific Attitudes of Racial Inferiority, 1859–1900* (Urbana: University of Illinois Press, 1971); Cynthia Eagle Russett, *Sexual Science: The Victorian Construction of Womanhood* (Cambridge, Mass.: Harvard University Press, 1989), ch. 1; Stephen Jay Gould, *The Mismeasure of Man,* rev. ed. (New York: Norton, 1996); Nancy Leys Stepan and Sander L. Gilman, "Appropriating the Idioms of Science: The Rejection of Scientific Racism," in *The Bounds of Race: Perspectives on Hegemony and Resistance* (Ithaca, N.Y.: Cornell University Press, 1991), 72–103; Jonathan Marks, *Human Biodiversity: Genes, Race, and History* (New York: Aldine de Gruyter, 1995); Waltraud Ernst and Bernard Harris, eds., *Race, Science, and Medicine, 1700–1960* (New York: Routledge, 1999); T. W. Todd, "Anthropology and Negro Slavery," *Medical Life* 36 (1929): 157–67; Thomas Holt, "Marking: Race, Race-Making, and the Writing of History," *American Historical Review* 100 (February 1995): 1–20; Seymour Drescher, "The Ending of the Slave Trade and the Evolution of European Scientific Racism," in Joseph Inikori and Stanley Engerman, eds., *The Atlantic Slave Trade: Effects on Economies, Societies, and Peoples* (Durham, N.C.: Duke University Press, 1992), 361–96; Thomas F. Gossett, *Race: The History of an Idea in America,* new ed. (New York: Oxford University Press, 1997); Scott L. Malcomson, *One Drop of Blood: The American Misadventure of Race* (New York: Farrar, Straus, and Giroux, 2000).

2. The language used by participants in this debate can be confusing. Most of the time, they used the word *Americans* interchangeably with *Indians* to refer to the native population of the continent; those with white skin living here who were the descendants of Europeans were generally called "Europeans." The term *African* could be used to describe both people living on that continent and their descendants in the United States; they were never included in the category "American."

3. For a turn-of-the-tenth-century Arab version of light-skinned peoples as underdone in the womb and dark-skinned as overdone, with the ideal as "neither half-baked dough nor burned crust, but between the two," see Malcomson, *One Drop of Blood,* 139.

4. Even in the mid-nineteenth century, medical observers identified a range of body types, based in part on the balance of the four humors (blood, phlegm, yellow bile, and black bile) they contained. For a clear statement of this theory, see Londa Schiebinger, *The Mind Has No Sex?: Women in the Origins of Modern Science* (Cambridge, Mass.: Harvard University Press, 1989), 161–62.

5. John Harley Warner, *The Therapeutic Perspective: Medical Practice, Knowledge, and Identity in America, 1820–1885* (Princeton, N.J.: Princeton University Press, 1997, 1986); Paul Starr, *The Social Transformation of American Medicine* (New York: Basic Books, 1982); Owsei Temkin, "The Scientific Approach to Disease: Specific Entity and Individual Sickness," in *The Double Face of Janus and Other Essays in the History of Medicine* (Baltimore: Johns Hopkins University Press, 1977), 441–55; Phyllis Allen, "Etiological Theory in America Prior to the Civil War," *Journal of the History of Medicine and Allied Sciences* 2 (1947): 489–520.

6. Richard Shryock, "Empiricism vs. Rationalism in American Medicine, 1650–1950," *Proceedings of the American Antiquarian Society* 79 (1969): 99–150.

7. Gould, *The Mismeasure of Man,* 75; see also Stanton, *The Leopard's Spots,* 25–27, 101.

8. Lester D. Stephens, "Scientific Societies in the Old South: The Elliott Society and the New Orleans Academy of Sciences," in Ronald L. Numbers and Todd L. Savitt, eds., *Science and Medicine in the Old South* (Baton Rouge: Louisiana State University Press, 1989), 57–58; Joseph I. Waring, "Charleston Medicine 1800–1860," *Journal of the History of Medicine and Allied Sciences* 31 (July 1976): 330.

9. Stanton, *The Leopard's Spots,* 24–44, esp. 32; Haller, *Outcasts from Evolution,* ch. 1. For women's skulls, see Elizabeth Fee, "Nineteenth-Century Craniology: The Study of the Female Skull," *Bulletin of the History of Medicine* 53 (1979): 415–33; Nancy Leys Stepan, "Race and Gender: The Role of Anatomy in Science," in Sandra Harding, ed., *The "Racial" Economy of Science* (Bloomington: University of Indiana Press, 1993), 359–76. For phrenology, see Peter McCandless, "Mesmerism and Phrenology in Antebellum Charleston: 'Enough of the Marvelous,'" *Journal of Southern History* 58 (May 1992): 199–230; Michael Shortland, "Courting the Cerebellum: Early Organological and Phrenological Views of Sexuality," *British Journal for History of Science* 20 (1987): 173–99.

10. Thomsonian medicine was one of various medical sects popular in the mid-nineteenth century. Following the teachings of Samuel Thomson, it offered "vegetable," or plant-based, remedies in opposition to the "mineral" poisons of so-called regular physicians; see John S. Haller Jr., *The People's Doctors: Samuel Thomson and the American Botanical Movement, 1790–1860* (Carbondale: Southern Illinois University Press, 2000).

11. Andrew Combe, "Anatomy and Physiology: Remarks on Tiedeman's Comparison of the Negro Brain, with Those of the European," *Southern Botanic Journal* 2 (August 18, 1838): 193, 195.

12. For the clergy, see Moses Ashley Curtis, "The Unity of the Races," *Southern Quarterly Review* 7 (April 1845): 372–448. Much of this debate occurred in a series of essays in the *Southern Medical Journal,* 1850–51; see also Reginald Horsman, *Josiah Nott of Mobile: Southerner, Physician, and Racial Theorist* (Baton Rouge: Louisiana State University Press, 1987); Lester D. Stephens, *Science, Race, and Religion in the American South: John Bachman and the Charleston Circle of Naturalists, 1815–1895* (Chapel Hill: University of North

Carolina Press, 2000), ch. 9–10. For the views of the South's premier woman intellectual, see L[ouisa] S[usannah] M[cCord], "Diversity of the Races: Its Bearing upon Negro Slavery," *Southern Quarterly Review* 19 (April 1851): 392–419.

13. The term *mulatto* was in wide use at midcentury to describe a person with one (pure) white and one (pure) black parent; see chapter 4.

14. For Nott, see Stanton, *The Leopard's Spots;* Horsman, *Josiah Nott of Mobile.*

15. Nott sometimes called these types species, arguing that each race qualified as a separate species; see J. C. Nott, "Unity of the Human Race: A Letter Addressed to the Editor, on the Unity of the Human Race," *Southern Quarterly Review* 9 (January 1846): 1–57.

16. Josiah Clark Nott and George Robins Gliddon, *Types of Mankind; or, Ethnological Researches, Based upon the Ancient Monuments, Paintings, Sculptures, and Crania of Races, and upon Their Natural, Geographical, Philological, and Biblical History* (Philadelphia: Lippincott, Grambo, 1854), 49–61 and passim. Nott developed some of his ideas more fully in "Influence of Anatomy on the March of Civilization," *New Orleans Medical and Surgical Journal* 15 (1858): 64–77.

17. Nott and Gliddon, *Types of Mankind,* 49, 53.

18. Ibid., 63, 67, 77, and passim.

19. Like many midcentury ethnologists, Nott was unsure how to classify Egyptians and was somewhat contradictory in his assessments, vacillating between categorizing them as African and Caucasian.

20. See chapter 4 for his views on "hybridity."

21. Nott and Gliddon, *Types of Mankind,* 180, 182, 185, 260, 411–12; on the similarities of Africans to the orangutan and chimpanzee, see also 457.

22. J. C. Nott, "An Examination into the Health and Longevity of the Southern Sea Ports of the United States, with Reference to the Subject of Life Insurance, [Part 2]," *Southern Journal of Medicine and Pharmacy* 2 (March 1847): 136–38; part 1 in *Southern Journal of Medicine and Pharmacy* 2 (January 1847); see also Josiah C. Nott, "Statistics of Southern Slave Population," *DeBow's Review* 6 (November 1847): 275–89.

23. J. C. Nott, "Liability of Negroes to the Epidemic Diseases of the South," *Southern Medical and Surgical Journal* 14 (April 1858): 254.

24. James O. Breeden, "States-Rights Medicine," *Bulletin of the New York Academy of Medicine* 52 (March–April 1976): 355–56.

25. Samuel A. Cartwright, "The Diseases and Physical Peculiarities of the Negro Race," *Charleston Medical Journal and Review* 6 (September 1851): 643–52; this was originally published in the *New Orleans Medical and Surgical Journal* in 1851. On Cartwright, see especially James D. Guillory, "The Pro-Slavery Arguments of Dr. Samuel A. Cartwright," *Louisiana History* 9 (1968): 209–27; Thomas Szasz, "The Sane Slave: An Historical Note on the Use of Medical Diagnoses as Justificatory Rhetoric," *Journal of American Psychotherapy* 25 (1971): 228–39.

26. [Samuel A. Cartwright,] "Cartwright on the Diseases and Physical Peculiarities of the Negro Race," *Oglethorpe Medical and Surgical Journal* 3 (January 1861): 271–72 and passim. In spite of similar titles, this is a different article from Cartwright's article in the *Charleston Medical Journal and Review.*

27. Ibid., 272–74.

28. In fact, slave infants died at higher rates than did white infants from a variety of causes, which puzzled many physicians. The matter also has garnered attention from

historians; see Sally G. McMillen, "'No Uncommon Disease': Neonatal Tetanus, Slave Infants, and the Southern Medical Profession," *Journal of the History of Medicine and Allied Sciences* 46 (July 1991): 291–314; Richard H. Steckel, "A Dreadful Childhood: The Excess Mortality of American Slaves," *Social Science History* 10 (Winter 1986): 427–65.

29. Cartwright, "Cartwright on the Diseases and Physical Peculiarities of the Negro Race," 275–76.

30. Ibid., 275–79.

31. "Cartwright on the Diseases, etc., of the Negro Race," *Charleston Medical Journal and Review* 6 (November 1851): 829–33.

32. "Cartwright on the Diseases and Physical Peculiarities of the Negro Race, Concluded," *Charleston Medical Journal and Review* 7 (January 1852): 89–98.

33. James T. Smith, "Review of Dr. Cartwright's Report on the Diseases and Physical Peculiarities of the Negro Race," *New Orleans Medical and Surgical Journal* 8 (September 1851): 731.

34. [D. J. Cain and F. Peyre Porcher, eds.], "The Review of Cartwright on the Diseases, etc., of the Negro Race," *Charleston Medical Journal and Review* 6 (November 1851): 895; "Cartwright on the Diseases and Physical Peculiarities of the Negro Race, Concluded," 89–90.

35. The question of the racial specificity of disease went beyond the antebellum South's discussion of black and white; see, for example, on specifically Jewish illnesses, Howard I. Kushner, *A Cursing Brain?: The Histories of Tourette Syndrome* (Cambridge, Mass.: Harvard University Press, 1999), 50.

36. In the mid-nineteenth century, fevers were considered specific diseases rather than symptoms of disease as they are today. Each fever was considered a separate disease, although it could sometimes shift to another in the course of the illness; see Phyllis Allen Richmond, "Glossary of Historical Fever Terminology," in Gert H. Brieger, ed., *Theory and Practice in American Medicine: Historical Studies from the Journal of Medicine and Allied Sciences* (New York: Science History Publications, 1976), 105–6; see also chapter 3.

37. D., "Review of *Indigenous Races of the Earth*," *Southern Medical and Surgical Journal* 14 (January 1858): 18–26; quote 22.

38. E. D. Fenner, "Acclimation; and the Liability of Negroes to the Endemic Fevers of the South," *Southern Medical and Surgical Journal* 14 (July 1858): 458.

39. Steven M. Stowe, *Doctoring the South: Southern Physicians and Everyday Medicine in the Mid-Nineteenth Century* (Chapel Hill: University of North Carolina Press, 2004), 217.

40. Fenner, "Acclimation," 452–53, 458.

41. Margaret Humphreys, *Malaria: Poverty, Race, and Public Health in the United States* (Baltimore: Johns Hopkins University Press, 1989); Todd L. Savitt, *Medicine and Slavery: The Diseases and Health Care of Blacks in Antebellum Virginia* (Urbana: University of Illinois Press, 1978).

42. Thompson McGown, *A Practical Treatise on the Most Common Diseases of the South: Exhibiting Their Peculiar Nature, and the Corresponding Adaptation of Treatment* (Philadelphia: Grigg, Elliot, 1849), 27, 28, 294, also 310, 315.

43. Tomlinson Fort, *A Dissertation on the Practice of Medicine: Containing an Account of the Causes, Symptoms, and Treatment, of Diseases* (Milledgeville, Ga.: Federal Union Office, 1849), 141, 9.

44. John Stainback Wilson, "Peculiarities and Diseases of Negroes: Food, Clothing,

and General Rules of Health," *DeBow's Review* 28 (May 1860): 597. This series of articles was reprinted from *American Cotton Planter and Soil of the South.*

45. John Stainback Wilson, "Peculiarities and Diseases of Negroes," *DeBow's Review* 29 (July 1860): 115.

46. *Miasma* refers to the vapors that arose from decaying animal or vegetable matter, often in marshy or other low-lying areas. It was widely believed to cause disease, especially malaria and other fevers; see Charles Rosenberg, *The Cholera Years: The United States in 1832, 1849, and 1866* (Chicago: University of Chicago Press, 1962).

47. [D. F. Nardin], "The Cholera—No. II" *Southern Botanic Journal* 1 (April 7, 1837): 97. Nardin was the editor of this journal, published from 1837 to 1839, before its move to Augusta, Georgia. Although Nardin was the "chief" proponent of Thomsonian medicine in Charleston, he enrolled in the Medical College of Charleston in 1837–38; see Waring, "Charleston Medicine 1800–1860," 332.

48. Cachexia was defined by one nineteenth-century medical writer as "a depraved habit with great paleness" and by another as "a bad habit or condition of the system . . . in which the *red corpuscles* are more or less *below* the natural standard . . ."; Fort, *A Dissertation on the Practice of Medicine,* 727; McGown, *A Practical Treatise on the Most Common Diseases of the South,* 424, see also 595–98

49. Editor's introduction to W. M. Carpenter, "Observations on the Cachexia Africana, or the Habit and Effects of Dirt-Eating in the Negro Race," *Southern Medical and Surgical Journal* 1 (March 1845): 126.

50. On hookworm, see Alan I. Marcus, "The South's Native Foreigners: Hookworm as a Factor in Southern Distinctiveness," in Todd L. Savitt and James Harvey Young, eds., *Disease and Distinctiveness in the American South* (Knoxville: University of Tennessee Press, 1988), 79–99.

51. Carpenter, "Observations on the Cachexia Africana," 126–37.

52. Ibid.

53. Ibid.; of course, whites could and did suffer from the same nutritional deficiencies and other maladies that caused dirt eating. For more on slaves' diet and its consequences, see Sam Bowers Hilliard, *Hogmeat and Hoecake: Food Supply in the Old South, 1840–1860* (Carbondale: Southern Illinois University Press, 1972); Kenneth F. Kiple and Virginia Himmelsteib King, *Another Dimension to the Black Diaspora: Diet, Disease, and Racism* (New York: Cambridge University Press, 1981); Savitt, *Medicine and Slavery,* 86–103.

54. Editor's introduction to Carpenter, "Observations on the Cachexia Africana," 137.

55. S. L. Grier, "The Negro and His Diseases," *New Orleans Medical and Surgical Journal* 9 (January 1853): 757–58.

56. Daniel Drake, "Diseases of the Negro Population," *Southern Medical and Surgical Journal* 1 (June 1845): 341. On Drake, see Conevery Bolton Valencius, *The Health of the Country: How American Settlers Understood Themselves and Their Land* (New York: Basic Books, 2002); Frank Barrett, "Daniel Drake's Medical Geography," *Social Science and Medicine* 42 (1996): 791–800; see also Grier, "The Negro and His Diseases," 757–58.

57. Andrew R. Kilpatrick, "Scraps from My Case Book," *Southern Medical and Surgical Journal* 1 (June 1845): 308.

58. Fort, *A Dissertation on the Practice of Medicine,* 596.

59. John Stainback Wilson, *Woman's Home Book of Health: A Work for Mothers and for Families* (Philadelphia: J. B. Lippincott, 1860), 243, 283.

60. Jno. Evans to George Jones, June 15, 1854, George Noble Jones Papers, Duke University.

61. Cartwright, "Cartwright on the Diseases and Physical Peculiarities of the Negro Race," 290–92. Cartwright's writings were widely reprinted; he also regularly repeated himself. Most of his work originally appeared in the *New Orleans Medical and Surgical Journal.* Mental alienation and other maladies that today would be called mental illnesses are discussed in Peter McCandless, *Moonlight, Magnolias, and Madness: Insanity in South Carolina from the Colonial Period to the Progressive Era* (Chapel Hill: University of North Carolina Press, 1996).

62. Cartwright, "Cartwright on the Diseases and Physical Peculiarities of the Negro Race," 290–92.

63. Smith, "Review of Dr. Cartwright's Report on the Diseases and Physical Peculiarities of the Negro Race," 733.

64. Cartwright, "Cartwright on the Diseases and Physical Peculiarities of the Negro Race," 292–95.

65. Ibid., 295–96.

66. Ibid., 271, 293–94, 285–86, 299; see also M. D. McLoud, "Hints on the Medical Treatment of Negroes," medical thesis, Medical College of South Carolina, March 1850, 1, Waring Medical Library, Medical University of South Carolina, Charleston.

67. Scrofula is now recognized as tuberculosis of the lymph glands, yaws as a tropical disease; historians generally view phthisis as another name for consumption; dyspepsia was the term used for what today would be considered any one of a range of digestive ailments.

68. Cartwright, "Cartwright on the Diseases and Physical Peculiarities of the Negro Race," 280–90.

69. A. P. Merrill, "An Essay on Some of the Distinctive Peculiarities of the Negro Race [No. I]," *Southern Medical and Surgical Journal* 12 (January 1856): 21–25.

70. Note Merrill's use of heat, or rather its absence, as a means of characterizing body type. In suggesting that blacks' bodies were cold, he made an implicit analogy with those of (white) women; ibid.; see also Schiebinger, *The Mind Has No Sex?*, 211–13.

71. Merrill, "An Essay on Some of the Distinctive Peculiarities of the Negro Race [No. I]," 27–36.

72. Wilson, "Peculiarities and Diseases of Negroes: Food, Clothing, and General Rules of Health," 597–99; Wilson, "Peculiarities and Diseases of Negroes," 113.

73. A. P. Merrill, "An Essay on Some of the Distinctive Peculiarities of the Negro Race, No. II," *Southern Medical and Surgical Journal* 12 (February 1856): 80–81.

74. Ibid., 82–90.

75. Ibid.

76. A. P. Merrill, "An Essay on Some of the Distinctive Peculiarities of the Negro Race, No. III," *Southern Medical and Surgical Journal* 12 (March 1856): 147–50.

77. H. L. B[yrd], "African Race—Re-Opening of the Slave Trade," *Oglethorpe Medical and Surgical Journal* 1 (August 1858): 191–93.

78. H. L. B[yrd], "African Slave Trade," *Oglethorpe Medical and Surgical Journal* 1 (February 1859): 392–93.

79. Merrill, "An Essay on Some of the Distinctive Peculiarities of the Negro Race, No. II," 83.

80. Merrill, "An Essay on Some of the Distinctive Peculiarities of the Negro Race, [No. I]," 24–25.

81. Ibid., 25–26, 34–36.

82. Cartwright, "Cartwright on the Diseases and Physical Peculiarities of the Negro Race," 297–98.

83. Samuel A. Cartwright, "How to Save the Republic, and the Position of the South in the Union," *DeBow's Review* 11 (August 1851): 186, 194; see also [Samuel A. Cartwright], "Dr. Cartwright on the Caucasians and the Africans," *DeBow's Review* 25 (July 1858): 45–56. Cartwright was among the most vehement defenders of slavery among the medical profession; Stowe argues that he was less interested in exploring race differences than in supporting the institution; see Stowe, *Doctoring the South,* 215–18.

84. The author was similarly critical of Cartwright's theories regarding defective atmospherization, calling on various medical authorities and his own experience to support his position; "Cartwright on the Diseases, etc., of the Negro Race," 834–42.

85. Ibid.

86. Cain and Porcher, "Review of Cartwright on the Diseases, etc., of the Negro Race," 894.

87. This point is made frequently by Stephens, in *Science, Race, and Religion in the American South,* in which he writes about a Charleston circle of naturalists; see also Horsman, *Josiah Nott of Mobile.*

88. On slaves' view that whites treated them like animals, see Mia Bay, *The White Image in the Black Mind: African-American Ideas about White People, 1830–1925* (New York: Oxford University Press, 2000).

89. Samuel Gaillard Stoney and Gertrude Mathews Shelby, *Black Genesis: A Chronicle* (New York: Macmillan, 1930), 4–5, 13, 46–47. Like many folkloric sources, this one reflects the collectors' choices of how to record language and speech patterns, in this case Gullah (see xxiv). Some chose to use dialect, others to use more standard English words and grammar. Neither decision could accurately reflect actual speech, which remains one of the difficulties of using folklore as a source for history.

90. Archibald Rutledge, *God's Children* (Indianapolis: Bobbs-Merrill, 1947), 106.

91. Gus Rogers, in George P. Rawick, gen. ed., *The American Slave: A Composite Autobiography,* 19 vols., vol. 6, *Alabama* (Westport, Conn.: Greenwood, 1978-), 335–36. The story is also discussed in Lawrence W. Levine, *Black Culture and Black Consciousness: Afro-American Folk Thought from Slavery to Freedom* (New York: Oxford University Press, 1977), 84.

92. Stoney and Shelby, *Black Genesis,* 165–71.

93. Newman Ivey White, gen. ed., *The Frank C. Brown Collection of North Carolina Folklore,* 7 vols. (Durham, N.C.: Duke University Press, 1961); vol. 6 of the collection, Wayland D. Hand, ed., *Popular Beliefs and Superstitions from North Carolina,* 97.

94. Elsie Clews Parsons, *Folk-Lore of the Sea Islands, South Carolina* (Chicago: Afro-Am Press, 1969; reprint of Cambridge, Mass.: American Folk-Lore Society, 1923), 104–5; brackets in original.

95. Newbell Niles Puckett, *Folk Beliefs of the Southern Negro* (Chapel Hill: University of North Carolina Press, 1926), 569–70.

96. Annie B. Boyd, in Rawick, *The American Slave: A Composite Autobiography,* 19 vols., suppl. ser. 1, suppl. ser. 2 (Westport, Conn.: Greenwood, 1978-), vol. 16, *Kentucky,* 59, also 64, 106; see also Henry C. Davis, "Negro Folk-Lore in South Carolina," *Journal*

*of American Folk-Lore* 27 (July–September 1914): 248. The same belief was also reported among whites and in other parts of the South; see Hand, *Popular Beliefs and Superstitions from North Carolina*, 97.

97. Carrie Pollard, *The American Slave*, vol. 6, *Alabama*, 318.

98. *The American Slave*, vol. 16, *Kentucky*, 64; Puckett, *Folk Beliefs of the Southern Negro*, 460–61; Elwyn A. Barron, "Shadowy Memories of Negro Lore," *The Folklorist* 1 (1892): 50.

99. Barron, "Shadowy Memories of Negro Lore," 52–53.

100. Davis, "Negro Folk-Lore in South Carolina," 244.

101. Joel Chandler Harris, *Uncle Remus: His Songs and His Sayings*, new and rev. ed. (New York: Grosset and Dunlap, 1921), 166–68.

102. Levi Pollard, in Charles L. Perdue Jr., Thomas E. Barden, and Robert K. Phillips, eds., *Weevils in the Wheat: Interviews with Virginia Ex-Slaves* (Charlottesville: University of Virginia Press, 1976), 233.

## Chapter 2. Constructing Sex

1. The literature on such matters is vast; see, for example, Naomi Zack, "The American Sexualization of Race," in Naomi Zack, ed., *Race/Sex: Their Sameness, Difference, and Interplay* (New York: Routledge, 1997), 145–55; Lynda Birke, *Feminism and the Biological Body* (New Brunswick, N.J.: Rutgers University Press, 1999); Judith Lorber, *Gender and the Social Construction of Illness* (Thousand Oaks, Calif.: Sage, 1997); Londa Schiebinger, *Nature's Body: Gender in the Making of Modern Science* (Boston: Beacon, 1993); Sander Gilman, *Difference and Pathology: Stereotypes of Sexuality, Race, and Madness* (Ithaca, N.Y.: Cornell University Press, 1985).

2. This point is elaborated most completely in Thomas Laqueur, *Making Sex: Body and Gender from the Greeks to Freud* (Cambridge, Mass.: Harvard University Press, 1990).

3. Gunning S. Bedford, *Clinical Lectures on the Diseases of Women and Children*, 2nd ed. (New York: Samuel S. and William Wood, 1855), 6, 100.

4. H. R. Easterling, "The Effects of Uterine Diseases on the Constitution—Their Diagnosis and Treatment—With Remarks on the Importance of Instituting a Physical Exploration as a Means of Diagnosis," *Charleston Medical Journal and Review* 10 (July 1855): 467.

5. Larkin G. Jones, "On the Peculiarities of the Female: The Physiological Changes Produced by Conception and the Treatment of Some of the Most Important Diseases Consecutive to Parturition," MD thesis, Medical College of South Carolina, 1829, Waring Medical Library, Medical University of South Carolina, Charleston.

6. Joseph F. Wright, *A Practical Treatise on the Management and Diseases of Infants and Children, with Some of the Diseases Peculiar to Females, and Their Treatment* (Macon, Ga.: Joseph Clisby, 1859), 135–36.

7. Bedford, *Clinical Lectures on the Diseases of Women and Children*, 98.

8. Jones, "On the Peculiarities of the Female."

9. Wright, *A Practical Treatise on the Management and Diseases of Infants and Children*, 132.

10. Samuel K. Jennings, *A Compendium of Medical Science, or Fifty Years' Experience in the Art of Healing* (Tuscaloosa, Ala.: Marmaduke J. Slade, 1847), 197.

11. Tomlinson Fort, *A Dissertation on the Practice of Medicine: Containing an Account of the Causes, Symptoms, and Treatment of Diseases, and Adapted to the Use of Physicians and Families* (Milledgeville, Ga.: Federal Union Office, 1849), 548, 552, 610, 613–16.

12. J. A. E., "Review of *Females and Their Diseases: A Series of Letters to His Class,* by Charles D. Meigs," *Southern Medical and Surgical Journal* 4 (May 1848): 289.

13. L. L. Hill, "'Treatise on Women' Submitted to the Examination of the Faculty of the South Carolina Medical College for the Degree of M. Dr.," 1837, Waring Medical Library.

14. He meant white women, of course; Samuel Cartwright, "How to Save the Republic, and the Position of the South in the Union," *DeBow's Review* 1 (August 1851): 4.

15. Hill, "Treatise on Women."

16. "Review of *Elements of Health, and Principles of Female Hygiene,* by E. J. Tilt," *Charleston Medical Journal and Review* 8 (September 1853): 658.

17. See, for example, Judith Walzer Leavitt, *Brought to Bed: Childbearing in America 1750 to 1950* (New York: Oxford University Press, 1986), ch. 3, esp. 71.

18. Bedford, *Clinical Lectures on the Diseases of Women and Children,* 99.

19. Catharine Beecher, *Letters to the People on Health and Happiness* (New York: Harper and Row, 1855); see also Kathryn Kish Sklar, *Catharine Beecher: A Study in American Domesticity* (New York: Norton, 1973).

20. "To the Ladies," *The Southern Botanic Journal Devoted to the Dissemination and Support of the Thomsonian System of Medical Practice* 2 (January 19, 1839): 367.

21. "Of Physicians," *Southern Botanico-Medical Journal* 1 (March 1, 1841): 110.

22. Wright, *A Practical Treatise on the Management and Diseases of Infants and Children,* 131.

23. J. McF. Gaston, "Treatment of Menorrhagia with Ergot," *Charleston Medical Journal and Review* 12 (July 1857): 459.

24. "Review of *Elements of Health,*" 661.

25. J. A. Eve "Medical Intelligence: Letter from Professor J. A. Eve," *Southern Medical and Surgical Journal* 4 (April 1848): 253.

26. W. K. Griffin, "Midwifery," *Southern Botanico-Medical Journal* 1 (March 15, 1841): 123–24.

27. Bedford, *Clinical Lectures on the Diseases of Women and Children,* 99.

28. Jennings, *A Compendium of Medical Science,* 134–35.

29. John Stainback Wilson, *Woman's Home Book of Health* (Philadelphia: J. B. Lippincott, 1860), 312–13.

30. H[enry] L[ee], "Editorial Department," *Southern Botanico-Medical Journal* 1 (April 15, 1841): 194.

31. Simon B. Abbott, *The Southern Botanic Physician* (Charleston: for the author, 1844), 44, 46.

32. M. Antony, "An Essay . . . on the Cause of Abortion," *Southern Medical and Surgical Journal* 3 (March 1839): 333; [Milton Antony], "Monthly Periscope: Prolapsus Uteri," *Southern Medical and Surgical Journal* 3 (April 1839): 436–37; [Milton Antony], "Monthly Periscope: Medical Electricity," *Southern Medical and Surgical Journal* 3 (September 1839): 765–67; Wilson, *Woman's Home Book of Health,* 173, 273–74.

33. Antony, "An Essay . . . on the Cause of Abortion," 339.

34. H. L. B[yrd], "Hoop-Skirts, Women, Exercise, &c.," *Oglethorpe Medical and Surgical Journal* 1 (August 1858): 194–95; see also Wilson, *Woman's Home Book of Health,* 178–79.

35. Wilson, *Woman's Home Book of Health,* 264.

36. D. T. Tayloe, "A Case of Strangulated Umbilical Hernia," *Medical Journal of North Carolina* 3 (October 1860): 527.

37. A. P. Merrill, "An Essay on Some of the Distinctive Peculiarities of the Negro Race [No. I]," *Southern Medical and Surgical Journal* 12 (January 1856): 30–1.

38. H. W. Moore, "A Thesis on Plantation Hygiene," Medical College of the State of South Carolina, February 1856, Waring Medical Library.

39. Robert Battey, "Vesico-Vaginal Fistula," *Southern Medical and Surgical Journal* 15 (December 1859): 823–24. Battey was the inventor of a surgical repair for this problem, known as Battey's operation, that brought him both renown and notoriety; see Deborah Kuhn McGregor, *From Midwives to Medicine: The Birth of American Gynecology* (New Brunswick, N.J.: Rutgers University Press, 1998).

40. "Review of *Elements of Health*," 659; see also J. A. E., "Review of *Females and Their Diseases*," 191.

41. Byrd, "Hoop Skirts, Women, Exercise, &c.," 195–97.

42. Wilson, *Woman's Home Book of Health*, 86–87, 161.

43. J. M. Dill, "Observations Principally on the Acute Form of Cholera Infantum, Read before the Medical Society of South Carolina," *Carolina Journal of Medicine, Science, and Agriculture* 1 (January 1825): 37–38.

44. *The American Lady's Medical Pocket-Book, and Nursery Adviser* (Philadelphia: James Kay, Jun. and Brother; Pittsburgh: John I. Kay, 1833), 59, 67.

45. R. A. Kinlock, "Remarks on 'Snuff Chewing,' and a Mode in Which It May Affect the Pulmonary Organs," *Charleston Journal of Medicine* 5 (July 1850): 451.

46. "Intemperance," *Southern Botanico-Medical Journal* 1 (15 June 1841): 283.

47. Wilson, *Woman's Home Book of Health*, 100–101.

48. W. H. Coffin, *The Art of Medicine Simplified, or a Treatise on the Nature and Cure of Diseases* (Wellsburg, Va.: W. Barnes, 1853), 146.

49. James Ewell, *The Medical Companion, or Family Physician*, 9th ed., rev. and enl. (Philadelphia: Carey, Lea, and Blanchard, 1836), 372–73; see also Wright, *A Practical Treatise on the Management and Diseases of Infants and Children*, 131.

50. J. A. Eve, "Letter to the Editor, on the Use of Chloroform in Obstetric Practice," *Southern Medical and Surgical Journal* 4 (April 1848): 253.

51. A. G. Goodlett, *The Family Physician, or Every Man's Companion . . . Adapted to the Southern and Western Climates* (Nashville, Tenn.: Smith and Nesbit, 1838), 18–19.

52. Wright, *A Practical Treatise on the Management and Diseases of Infants and Children*, 132.

53. [L. A. Dugas], "Editorial and Miscellany: Remarks upon the Use of Pessaries in the Treatment of Prolapsus Uteri," *Southern Medical and Surgical Journal* 9 (September 1854): 569.

54. The clearest statement of the postwar view is in Edward H. Clarke, *Sex in Education; or, a Fair Chance for Girls* (Boston: James R. Osgood, 1874).

55. Wright, *A Practical Treatise on the Management and Diseases of Infants and Children*, 34–35.

56. T. L. Ogier, "Hereditary Disposition," *Southern Medical and Surgical Journal* 4 (August 1848): 488.

57. "Review of *Elements of Health*," 668.

58. William Hauser, "Pre-Natal Influences," *Oglethorpe Medical and Surgical Journal* 2 (November 1859): 217.

59. John Stainback Wilson, "Female Medical Education," *Southern Medical and Surgical Journal* 10 (January 1854): 5–6.

60. *The American Lady's Medical Pocket-Book,* 28.

61. Wed. [March] 1855, Mary Hort Diary, *American Women's Diaries: Southern Women* (New Canaan, Conn.: Readex Film Products, 1988); original at South Caroliniana Library, University of South Carolina.

62. Christine Jacobson Carter, ed., *The Diary of Dolly Lunt Burge, 1848–1879* (Athens: University of Georgia Press, 1997), 43.

63. May 27, 1850, Martha E. Crawford Diary, *American Women's Diaries: Southern Women;* original at Perkins Library, Duke University.

64. Carolyn Elizabeth (Eliza) Burgwin Clitherall, family reminiscences, vol. 3, *American Women's Diaries: Southern Women;* original at Southern Historical Collection, University of North Carolina.

65. "Black Cohosh," *Southern Botanico-Medical Journal* 1 (February1, 1841): 64.

66. Wilson, *Woman's Home Book of Health,* 55.

67. Samuel Cartwright, "Address of Samuel A. Cartwright, M.D., of Natchez, Mississippi; Delivered before the Medical Convention, in the City of Jackson, January 13, 1846," *New Orleans Medical and Surgical Journal* 2 (May 1846): 732.

68. Simon H. Sanders, "Monthly Periscope," *Southern Medical and Surgical Journal* 3 (April 1839): 431.

69. "Of Physicians," *Southern Botanico-Medical Journal* 1 (March 1, 1841): 110–11.

70. H. Steele, "The Pessary and Other Mechanical Means in Prolapsus Uteri," *Oglethorpe Medical and Surgical Journal* 1 (October 1858): 208.

71. [L. A. Dugas], "Editorial and Miscellany: Remarks upon the Use of Pessaries in the Treatment of Prolapsus Uteri," *Southern Medical and Surgical Journal* 10 (September 1854): 568–69.

72. Joseph A. Eve, "A Report on Diseases of the Cervix Uteri," *Southern Medical and Surgical Journal* 13 (November 1857): 518.

73. E. M. Pendleton, "On the Comparative Fecundity of the Caucasian and African Races," *Southern Journal of Medicine and Pharmacy* 6 (May 1851): 354.

74. G. K. Holloway, "Remarkable Case of Fibro-Schirro Cartilaginous Enlargement of the Ovaria," *Southern Medical and Surgical Journal* 2 (July 1838): 714–15.

75. The child was "delivered by the perforator, crotchet and blunt hook"; "Review of *An Elementary Treatise on Midwifery, or Principles of Tokology and Embryology,*" *Southern Medical and Surgical Journal* 3 (October 1838): 57.

76. "Editorial and Miscellaneous: Review of *The People's Medical Gazette,*" *Charleston Medical Journal and Review* 9 (January 1854): 126–27.

77. Jones, "On the Peculiarities of the Female."

78. "Review of *Elements of Health,*" 660.

79. "Review of *The People's Medical Gazette,*" 125.

80. Hill, "Treatise on Woman."

81. Wilson, *Woman's Home Book of Health,* 52, 281.

82. See, for example, Winthrop D. Jordan, *White over Black: American Attitudes toward the Negro, 1550–1812* (Chapel Hill: University of North Carolina Press, 1968); Philip D. Curtin, *The Image of Africa: British Ideas and Action, 1780–1850* (Madison: University of Wisconsin Press, 1964).

83. See, for example, Kathleen Brown, *Good Wives, Nasty Wenches, and Anxious Patriarchs: Gender, Race, and Power in Colonial Virginia* (Chapel Hill: University of North Carolina Press, 1996).

84. Merrill, "An Essay on Some of the Distinctive Peculiarities of the Negro Race [No. I]," 23.

85. J. B. Hughes, "Syphilis of New-Born Children," *Medical Journal of North Carolina* 3 (May 1861): 253–68.

86. Robert Gooch, *A Practical Compendium of Midwifery* (Philadelphia: E. L. Carey and A. Hart, 1832), 44.

87. Wright, *A Practical Treatise on the Management and Diseases of Infants and Children,* 161.

88. Sam[ue]l L. Strait, "Remarks on Neuralgia," *Southern Journal of Medicine and Pharmacy* 1 (September 1846): 487.

89. Pendleton, "On the Comparative Fecundity of the Caucasian and African Races," 351–56.

90. See Darlene Clark Hine, "Rape and the Inner Lives of Black Women in the Middle West: Preliminary Thoughts on the Culture of Dissemblance," *Signs: Journal of Women in Culture and Society* 14 (Summer 1989): 912–20.

## Chapter 3. Placed Bodies

1. James O. Breeden, "States Rights Medicine in the Old South," *Bulletin of the New York Academy of Medicine* 52 (March–April 1976): 348–72.

2. See the introduction for southern medicine; see also Nicolaas A. Rupke, *Medical Geography in Historical Perspective, Medical History,* suppl. 20 (London: Wellcome Trust Center for the History of Medicine at UCL, 2000); Conevery Bolton Valencius, *The Health of the Country: How American Settlers Understood Themselves and Their Land* (New York: Basic Books, 2002); A. Cash Koeniger, "Climate and Southern Distinctiveness," *Journal of Southern History* 54 (1988): 21–44; Philip Curtin, *Death by Migration: Europe's Encounter with the Tropical World in the Nineteenth Century* (New York: Cambridge University Press, 1989); Joyce E. Chaplin, *Subject Matter: Technology, the Body, and Science on the Anglo-American Frontier, 1500–1676* (Cambridge, Mass.: Harvard University Press, 2001); Charlene M. Boyer Lewis, *Ladies and Gentlemen on Display: Planter Society at the Virginia Springs, 1790–1860* (Charlottesville: University Press of Virginia, 2001).

3. J. Dawson, "The Substance of Some Remarks Made before the Columbus Scientific Association, on Ethnology," *Oglethorpe Medical and Surgical Journal* 2 (November 1859): 265.

4. James M. Green, "Cases of Inflammation and Ulceration of the Cervix Uteri," *Charleston Medical Journal and Review* 8 (January 1853): 41.

5. John Stainback Wilson, *Woman's Home Book of Health: A Work for Mothers and for Families* (Philadelphia: J. B. Lippincott, 1860), 152–53.

6. Samuel K. Jennings, *A Compendium of Medical Science; or, Fifty Years' Experience in the Art of Healing* (Tuscaloosa, Ala.: Marmaduke J. Slade, 1847), 220–22.

7. Thomas Denman, *An Introduction to the Practice of Midwifery,* from the 6th London ed., 3rd American ed. (New York: Carville, 1829), 373.

8. Margaret Humphreys, *Malaria: Poverty, Race, and Public Health in the United States* (Baltimore: Johns Hopkins University Press, 2001), 46.

9. Fevers were among the most commonly diagnosed illnesses in the South from colonial times until well into the nineteenth century. Doctors identified many different kinds of fevers, including yellow, remittent, periodic, congestive, autumnal, malignant, bilious,

typhus, putrid tertian, spotted, dengue, and so on. Today, many of these would likely be diagnosed as malaria, with yellow fever, typhoid, and typhus also recognized as distinct diseases; see Phyllis Allen Richmond, "Glossary of Historical Fever Terminology," in Gert H. Brieger, ed., *Theory and Practice of American Medicine: Historical Studies from the Journal of Medicine and Allied Sciences* (New York: Science History Publications, 1976), 105–6; Gordon Harrison, *Mosquitoes, Malaria and Man: A History of the Hostilities since 1880* (New York: E. P. Dutton, 1978).

10. For ways physicians and laypeople interpreted the varying susceptibility of different kinds of bodies to yellow fever, see Jo Ann Carrigan, "Privilege, Prejudice, and the Strangers' Disease in Nineteenth-Century New Orleans," *Journal of Southern History* 36 (November 1970): 568–78; see also Margaret Humphreys, *Yellow Fever in the South* (New Brunswick, N.J.: Rutgers University Press, 1991).

11. Historians disagree about the prevalence of deadly malaria in seventeenth-century Virginia, although it was present in South Carolina in the 1680s; Humphreys, *Malaria*, 22–26; see also Lawrence Fay Brewster, *Summer Migrations and Resorts of South Carolina Low-Country Planters* (Durham, N.C.: Duke University Press, 1947), 3–5; H. Roy Merrens and George D. Terry, "Dying in Paradise: Malaria, Mortality, and the Perceptual Environment in Colonial South Carolina," *Journal of Southern History* 50 (November 1984): 533–50.

12. Humphreys, *Malaria*, 14–20, quote 17; see also Erwin Ackerknecht, *Malaria in the Upper Mississippi Valley, 1760–1900* (New York: Arno Press, 1977, orig. pub. 1945); Brewster, *Summer Migrations and Resorts of South Carolina Low-Country Planters;* Philip Curtin, "Epidemiology and the Slave Trade," *Political Science Quarterly* 83 (1968): 191–216; Jill Dubisch, "Low Country Fevers: Cultural Adaptations to Malaria in Antebellum South Carolina," *Social Science and Medicine* 21 (1985): 641–49; Julia Floyd Smith, *Slavery and Rice Culture in Low Country Georgia, 1750–1860* (Knoxville: University of Tennessee Press, 1985).

13. Edward Delony, "Original Communications: A Letter to the Editors," *Southern Medical and Surgical Journal* 1 (October 1836): 257–59; see also Thomas Fuller Hazzard, "St. Simons' Island," *Southern Botanic Journal* 2 (May 26, 1838): 101.

14. S. M. Meek, "An Essay on Female Diseases, and the Use of the Pessary in Uterine Displacements," *Southern Medical and Surgical Journal* 2 (August 1837): 26.

15. "[Review of] *Indigenous Races of the Earth* . . . by J. C. Nott and Geo. R. Gliddon," *Southern Medical and Surgical Journal* 14 (January 1858): 20.

16. E. D. Fenner, "Acclimation; and the Liability of Negroes to the Endemic Fevers of the South," *Southern Medical and Surgical Journal* 14 (July 1858): 454–60.

17. Dawson, "The Substance of Some Remarks Made before the Columbus Scientific Association, on Ethnology," 260–61.

18. A. P. Merrill, "An Essay on Some of the Distinctive Peculiarities of the Negro Race [No. I]," *Southern Medical and Surgical Journal* 12 (January 1856): 25.

19. Dawson, "The Substance of Some Remarks Made before the Columbus Scientific Association, on Ethnology," 260.

20. A. P. Merrill, "An Essay on Some of the Distinctive Peculiarities of the Negro Race, No. II," *Southern Medical and Surgical Journal* 12 (February 1856): 81–82.

21. A. P. Merrill, "An Essay on Some of the Distinctive Peculiarities of the Negro Race, No. III," *Southern Medical and Surgical Journal* 12 (March 1856): 147.

22. Daniel Drake, "Diseases of the Negro Population," *Southern Medical and Surgical Review* 1 (June 1845): 342–43.

23. Quoted in Victor H. Bassett, "Plantation Medicine," *Journal of the Medical Association of Georgia* 29 (March 1940): 115.

24. Merrill, "An Essay on Some of the Distinctive Peculiarities of the Negro Race [No. I]," 30.

25. Quoted in "[Review of] *Indigenous Races of the Earth*," 20.

26. J. C. Nott, "Liability of Negroes to the Epidemic Diseases of the South," *Southern Medical and Surgical Journal* 14 (April 1858): 253–54.

27. Life insurance companies' efforts to use statistics to calculate liability were in their infancy. They were more likely to base their decisions on a particular location's reputation for healthiness than anything else; see James H. Cassedy, *American Medicine and Statistical Thinking, 1800–1860* (Cambridge, Mass.: Harvard University Press, 1984).

28. Nott, "Liability of Negroes to the Epidemic Diseases of the South," 253–54.

29. Fenner, "Acclimation," 453–58.

30. Drake, "Diseases of the Negro Population," 342; see also Frank Barrett, "Daniel Drake's Medical Geography," *Social Science and Medicine* 42 (1996): 791–800.

31. Merrill, "An Essay on Some of the Distinctive Peculiarities of the Negro Race, No. II," 86–87.

32. Ibid., 87–88.

33. Merrill, "An Essay on Some of the Distinctive Peculiarities of the Negro Race, No. III," 147–48.

34. Ibid., 148–50, 155.

35. Ibid., 155.

36. Nott, "Liability of Negroes to the Epidemic Diseases of the South," 253.

37. Merrill, "An Essay on Some of the Distinctive Peculiarities of the Negro Race [No. 1]," 25.

38. Ibid., 27–30.

39. Ibid., 30–31.

40. Ibid., 31–34.

41. Ibid., 28, 33.

42. John Stainback Wilson, "Peculiarities and Diseases of Negroes: Food, Clothing, and General Rules of Health," *DeBow's Review* 28 (May 1860): 597–99, originally published in *American Cotton Planter and Soil of the South*.

43. John Stainback Wilson, "Peculiarities and Diseases of Negroes," *DeBow's Review* 29 (July 1860): 112–13, originally published in *American Cotton Planter and Soil of the South*.

44. Bassett, "Plantation Medicine," 115.

45. Joseph A. S. Milligan to Octavia Camfield, October 3, 1848, Milligan Family Papers, *Southern Women and Their Families in the Nineteenth Century: Papers and Diaries*, ser. A, *Holdings of the Southern Historical Collection, University of North Carolina, Chapel Hill*, pt. 5, *Alabama, South Carolina, Georgia, and Florida Collections*, consulting ed. Anne Firor Scott (Bethesda, Md.: University Publications of America, 1991).

46. Samuel A. Cartwright, "The Diseases and Physical Peculiarities of the Negro Race," *Charleston Medical Journal and Review* 6 (September 1851): 645; see also Daniel Stahl, "The Sectional Teachings of Medicine," *Southern Medical and Surgical Journal* 5 (September 1849): 545–50. For views of historians, see John Duffy, "Sectional Conflict and Medical Education in Louisiana," *Journal of Southern History* 23 (1957): 289–306; John Harley Warner, "A Southern Medical Reform: The Meaning of the Antebellum Argument for Southern Medical Education," *Bulletin of the History of Medicine* 57 (Fall 1983): 364–81.

47. Merrill, "An Essay on Some of the Distinctive Peculiarities of the Negro Race, No. II," 90.

48. James W. Taylor, "An Address, Delivered on the First Anniversary of the Charleston Medical Society of Emulation, Held Friday, 2d December 1825," *Carolina Journal of Medicine, Science, and Agriculture* 1 (1826): 84–85.

49. [Thomas Y. Simons and William Michel], "Case of Amputation of a Portion of the Inferior Maxillary Bone, Performed by Benjamin B. Simons, M.D.," *Carolina Journal of Medicine, Science, and Agriculture* 1 (July 1825): 283.

50. Edward Deloney, "A Letter to the Editors," *Southern Medical and Surgical Journal* 1 (October 1836): 257–59.

51. [Samuel A. Cartwright,] "Address of Samuel A. Cartwright, M.D., of Natchez, Mississippi; Delivered before the Medical Convention, in the City of Jackson, January 13, 1846," *New Orleans Medical and Surgical Journal* 2 (May 1846): 730.

52. Cartwright, "The Diseases and Physical Peculiarities of the Negro Race," 645–46.

53. Ibid.; see also Samuel A. Cartwright, "Remarks on Dysentery among Negroes," *New Orleans Medical and Surgical Journal* 11 (September 1854): 162.

54. "Reviews: Cartwright on the Diseases, etc., of the Negro Race," *Charleston Medical Journal and Review* 6 (November 1851): 836.

55. "Reviews: Cartwright on the Diseases and Physical Peculiarities of the Negro Race, Concluded," *Charleston Medical Journal and Review* 7 (January 1852): 92–93.

56. Ibid., 92–95.

57. J. C. Nott, "Medical Schools," *New Orleans Medical and Surgical Journal* 14 (1857): 353–54. I am indebted to Cynthia Melendy for obtaining a copy of this for me.

58. Ibid., 356.

59. Ibid., 356–57.

60. Reginald Horsman, *Josiah Nott of Mobile: Southerner, Physician, and Racial Theorist* (Baton Rouge: Louisiana State University Press, 1987), ch. 10.

61. A Baltimore M.D., "To the Editor of the Medical Journal of North Carolina," *Medical Journal of North Carolina* 3 (August 1860): 460–61.

62. Ibid.

63. Ibid., 461–62.

64. "Negro Hospital," *Charleston Medical Journal and Review* 15 (November 1860): 850–51.

65. William Peirce to Ellen [Nell] Peirce, November 5, 1852, January 28, 1853, Ellen E. Peirce Papers, Duke University.

66. Joseph Eve, "Notes to a Report on Diseases of the Cervix Uteri," *Southern Medical and Surgical Journal* 14 (February 1858): 97.

67. He of course meant only white women, although he did not say so; Wilson, *Woman's Home Book of Health,* 153.

68. Meek referred to the loss of tone in the muscles and ligaments that hold female reproductive organs in place, which was the proximate cause of prolapsed uterus.

69. Meek, "An Essay on Female Diseases," 26–27.

70. Denman, *An Introduction to the Practice of Midwifery,* 218, 375–76, 640–41.

71. T. L. Ogier, "Removal of a Fibrous Tumor from the Uterus, Including a Portion of the Cervix Uteri," *Charleston Medical Journal and Review* 7 (February 1852): 155.

72. B. W. Harder, "Case of Extra Uterine-Pregnancy, Complicated with General Anasarca and Ossification of the Uterus," *Oglethorpe Medical and Surgical Journal* 1 (August 1858): 142–43.

73. "Reviews: *The History of Prostitution . . .,*" *Charleston Medical Journal and Review* 14 (January 1859): 77–78.

74. H. L. B[yrd], "Northern White Slavery and Southern Black," *Oglethorpe Medical and Surgical Journal* 2 (March 1860): 426–28.

75. 3rd Sabbath, June 1847, Diary of Lucila Agnes McCorkle, William Parsons McCorkle Papers, *Southern Women and Their Families in the Nineteenth Century: Papers and Diaries,* ser. A, *Holdings of the Southern Historical Collection, University of North Carolina, Chapel Hill,* pt. 5, *Alabama, South Carolina, Georgia, and Florida,* ed. Anne Firor Scott (Bethesda, Md.: University Publications of America, 1991).

76. December 12, 1853, Mary Jeffreys Bethell Diary, *Records of Ante-Bellum Southern Plantations from the Revolution through the Civil War,* ser. J, *Selections from the Southern Historical Collection, Manuscripts Department, Library of the University of North Carolina at Chapel Hill,* pt. 13, *Piedmont North Carolina,* gen. ed. Kenneth M. Stampp (Frederick, Md.: University Publications of America, 1992).

77. E. L. Skinner to Tristrim Skinner, January 11, 1847, Skinner Family Papers, *Records of Ante-Bellum Plantations,* ser. J, pt. 12, *Tidewater and Coastal Plains North Carolina.*

78. April 12, 1858, June 3, 1858, Priscilla Beall McKaig Journal, McKaig Family Papers, *American Women's Diaries: Southern Women* (New Canaan, Conn.: Readex Film Products, n.d.), original at Allegany County Historical Society.

79. E[liza DeRosset] to Mary DeRosset Curtis, October 2, 1838, Moses Ashley Curtis Family Papers, University of North Carolina.

80. Eleanor Douglass to Mary Hall, August, ca. 1821, Eleanor Hall Douglass Papers, Duke University.

81. Ellen C. Ewing to Aunt, March 30, 1859, Thomas Ewing Papers, Duke University; see also August 18, 1845, Frances Bumpas Journal, Bumpas Family Papers, University of North Carolina.

82. October 24, 1855, Carolyn Elizabeth (Eliza) Burgwin Clitherall Diaries, *American Women's Diaries,* original at Southern Historical Collection, University of North Carolina.

83. Sarah McCulloh Lemmon, ed., *The Pettigrew Papers,* vol. 2, *1819–1843* (Raleigh: North Carolina Department of Cultural Resources, Division of Archives and History, 1988), 607.

84. Young A. Smith to Washington Smith, March 25, 1849, Washington M. Smith Letters, Duke University.

85. G. M. Wilkins to [John] Berkley Grimball, 1843, Grimball Family Papers, *Records of Ante-Bellum Southern Plantations,* ser. J, pt. 3, *South Carolina.*

86. G. M. Wilkins to [John] Berkley Grimball, 1843, Grimball Family Papers.

87. March 17, 1844, John Berkley Grimball Diary, *Records of Ante-Bellum Plantations,* ser. J, pt. 3.

88. Sophia Watson to Henry Watson, August 4, 1848; see also September 8, 1848, Henry Watson Jr. Papers, *Records of Ante-Bellum Plantations,* ser. F, *Selections from the Manuscript Department, Duke University,* pt. 1, *The Deep South.*

89. Personal Reminiscences, Carolyn Clitherall, *American Women's Diaries,* vol. 5.

90. Tristrim Skinner to Eliza H. Skinner, August 15, 1850, Skinner Family Papers, *Records of Ante-Bellum Southern Plantations,* ser. J, pt. 12, *Tidewater and Coastal Plains North Carolina.*

91. Lewis, *Ladies and Gentlemen on Display.*

92. Joseph A. S. Milligan to Octavia Camfield, April 18, 1848, Milligan Family Papers.

93. Joseph Milligan to Elizabeth Camfield Milligan, August 20, 1844, Milligan Family Papers.

94. April 8, 1834, John Berkley Grimball Diary, *Records of Ante-Bellum Southern Plantations,* ser. J, pt. 3.

95. Sophia Peck to Eliza Peck, March 28, 1838, Henry Watson Jr. Papers, *Records of Ante-Bellum Plantations.* Peck would later marry Henry Watson and worry about his return from the North in the fall.

96. D. Johnson to Hall, February 25, 1825, Eleanor Hall Douglass Papers, Duke University.

97. January 28, 1864, Mary Jeffreys Bethel Diary, *Records of Ante-Bellum Plantations,* ser. J, pt. 13.

98. Margaret Devereux to Ellen Mordecai, September 28, 1847, Margaret Mordecai Devereux Papers, *Records of Ante-Bellum Plantations,* ser. J, pt. 12.

99. Arabella Bolton to Caroline Lawrence, July 24, 1846, Bedinger-Dandredge Family Papers, Duke University.

100. Penelope S. Warren to Thomas Warren, September 2, 1840, Skinner Family Papers.

101. Mary Jane Milligan to Joseph A. S. Milligan, February 29, 1848, Milligan Family Papers.

102. Henry M. Burns to Joseph Milligan, April 15, 1836, Milligan Family Papers, *Southern Women and their Families,* ser. A, pt. 5.

103. Emily A. Rutherfoord to John Rutherfoord, September 9, 1834, John Rutherfoord Family Papers, Duke University.

104. Martha Dupree Treadwell to E. W. Treadwell, September 15, 1861, E. W. Treadwell Papers, Duke University.

105. Carol Bleser, ed., *Tokens of Affection: The Letters of a Planter's Daughter in the Old South* (Athens University of Georgia Press, 1996), 176.

106. November 25, 1837, May 1, 1851; see also December 25, 1837, John Berkley Grimball Diary.

107. Kate [Meares] to mother, August 8, 1854, DeRosset Family Papers, University of North Carolina.

108. Mother to Katie [Meares?], 1858, Meares-DeRosset Family Papers, University of North Carolina.

109. E[liza DeRosset] to Mary DeRosset Curtis, May 24, 1837, Moses Ashley Curtis Family Papers, University of North Carolina.

110. Tristrim Skinner to Joseph Skinner, September 23, 1850, Skinner Family Papers, *Records of Ante-Bellum Plantations.*

111. Martha Dupree Treadwell to E. W. Treadwell, September 15, 1861, E. W. Treadwell Papers, Duke University.

112. April 21, 1858, John Berkley Grimball Diary, *Records of Ante-Bellum Plantations;* see also April 19, 1844, September 15, 1844, August 23, 1850, March 6, 1854, April 5, 1854, December 5–20, 1854, September 21, 1856; Lemmon, *The Pettigrew Papers,* 158–59, 190, 196, 210–11, 333–39.

113. September 6, 1856, Frances Jane (Bestor) Robertson Diaries, *Southern Women's Diaries,* original at Alabama Department of Archives and History.

114. August 10, 1833, Sarah Haynesworth Gayle Diary, *American Women's Diaries,* original at University of Alabama Library.

115. Lemmon, *The Pettigrew Papers,* 301.

116. E[liza DeRosset] to Mary and Ashley Curtis, January 1, 1850, Moses Ashley Curtis Family Papers, University of North Carolina.

117. Lemmon, *The Pettigrew Papers,* 91.

118. January 30, 1861, Margaret Ann "Meta" Morris Grimball Diary, *Records of Ante-Bellum Plantations,* ser. J, pt. 3.

119. August 22, 1834, John Berkley Grimball Diary.

120. Dropsey, or dropsy, refers to edema, which could range from swelling in the extremities to what we might today consider congestive heart failure.

121. August 7, 1840, October 15, 1859, John Berkley Grimball Diary, *Records of Ante-Bellum Plantations.*

122. For example, Sophia Watson to Henry Watson, June 19, 1848, Henry Watson Jr. Papers, *Records of Ante-Bellum Plantations.*

123. Lights were lungs.

124. Reuben Rosborough, *The American Slave: A Composite Autobiography,* gen. ed. George P. Rawick (Westport, Conn.: Greenwood, 1974), vol. 3, 4:46–7.

125. Newbell Niles Puckett, *Folk Beliefs of the Southern Negro* (Chapel Hill: University of North Carolina Press, 1926), 263.

126. Elsie Clews Parsons, *Folk-Lore of the Sea Islands, South Carolina* (Chicago: Afro-Am Press, 1969; reprint of Cambridge, Mass.: American Folk-Lore Society, 1923), 132.

## Chapter 4. Ambiguous Bodies

1. M. Antony, "An Essay on the Subject of Maternal Influence on the Foetus in Utero," *Southern Medical and Surgical Journal* 3 (November 1838): 67.

2. On medical jurisprudence, see James C. Mohr, *Doctors and the Law: Medical Jurisprudence in Nineteenth-Century America* (Baltimore: Johns Hopkins University Press, 1993). On determining death, see Jan Bondesman, *Buried Alive: The Terrifying History of Our Most Primal Fear* (New York: Norton, 2001); Michael E. Bell, *Food for the Dead: On the Trail of New England's Vampires* (New York: Carroll and Graf, 2001). On policing the boundaries between the races, see Ariela J. Gross, "Litigating Whiteness: Trials of Racial Determination in the Nineteenth-Century South," *Yale Law Journal* 108 (October 1998): 109–88; Ian F. Haney Lopez, *White by Law: The Legal Construction of Race* (New York: New York University Press, 1996).

3. Shamming will be discussed more fully in chapter 5.

4. Ariela J. Gross, *Double Character: Slavery and Mastery in the Antebellum Southern Courtroom* (Princeton, N.J.: Princeton University Press, 2000), esp. ch. 5.

5. I am grateful to Steven Stowe for raising these issues for me and for his helpful comments on an early version of part of this chapter.

6. See, for example, Michael P. Johnson and James L. Roark, *Black Masters: A Free Family of Color in the Old South* (New York: Norton, 1984); Adele Logan Alexander, *Ambiguous Lives: Free Women of Color in Rural Georgia, 1789–1879* (Fayetteville: University of Arkansas Press, 1991).

7. J. C. Nott, "An Examination into the Health and Longevity of the Southern Sea Ports of the United States, with Reference to the Subject of Life Insurance, [Pt. 2]," *Southern Journal of Medicine and Pharmacy* 2 (March 1847): 137.

8. Samuel A. Cartwright, "The Diseases and Physical Peculiarities of the Negro Race," *Charleston Medical Journal and Review* 6 (September 1851): 649; Samuel A. Cartwright, "Editorial: Cartwright on the Diseases and Physical Peculiarities of the Negro Race," *Oglethorpe Medical and Surgical Journal* 4 (January 1861): 278.

9. A. P. Merrᵢll, "An Essay on Some of the Distinctive Peculiarities of the Negro Race, No. II," *Southern Medical and Surgical Journal* 12 (February 1856): 84–85.

10. Sophie D Belle, in George P. Rawick, gen. ed., *The American Slave: A Composite Autobiography*, 19 vols. (Westport, CT: Greenwood, 1974), vol. 8, *Arkansas Narratives*, 1:139.

11. J. Dawson. "The Substance of Some Remarks Made before the Columbus Scientific Association, on Ethnology," *Oglethorpe Medical and Surgical Journal* 2 (November 1859): 249.

12. H. L. B[yrd], "Editorial: African Race—Re-Opening of the Slave Trade, &c.," *Oglethorpe Medical and Surgical Journal* 1 (August 1858): 194.

13. A. P. Merrill, "An Essay on Some of the Distinctive Peculiarities of the Negro Race, No. III," *Southern Medical and Surgical Journal* 12 (March 1856): 155.

14. Merrill, "An Essay on Some of the Distinctive Peculiarities of the Negro Race, No. II," 85.

15. [D. F. Nardin], "The Cholera—No. II," *Southern Botanic Journal* 1 (29 April 1837): 97.

16. "Reviews: Cartwright on the Diseases and Physical Peculiarities of the Negro Race, Concluded," *Charleston Medical Journal and Review* 7 (January 1852): 92.

17. On interracial sexual relationships, see Joshua D. Rothman, *Notorious in the Neighborhood: Sex and Families across the Color Line in Virginia, 1787–1861* (Chapel Hill: University of North Carolina Press, 2003); Martha Hodes, *White Women, Black Men: Illicit Sex in the Nineteenth Century* (New Haven, Conn.: Yale University Press, 1997); Victoria Bynum, *Unruly Women: The Politics of Sexual Control in the Old South* (Chapel Hill: University of North Carolina Press, 1992).

18. W. L. Sutton, "Miscellany: A Case of Doubtful Paternity," *Southern Medical and Surgical Journal* 8 (December 1852): 760–63.

19. Ibid.

20. A. F. Attaway, "A Case of Twins of Different Color," *Southern Medical and Surgical Journal* 10 (June 1854): 348.

21. Tho[ma]s B. Taylor, "Monthly Periscope: A Case of Superfoetation and Mixed Birth," *Southern Medical and Surgical Journal* 5 (February 1849): 114–15; see also W. C. Sankford, "Superfoetation" *Medical Journal of North Carolina* 2 (April 1859): 435.

22. Winthrop D. Jordan, *White over Black: American Attitudes toward the Negro, 1550–1812* (Chapel Hill: University of North Carolina Press, 1968), 239–52.

23. A. Harvey, "On the Foetus in Utero, as Inoculating the Maternal with the Peculiarities of the Paternal Organism," *Charleston Medical Journal and Review* 5 (March 1850): 255–62.

24. Those boundaries and the issues raised by them have been of interest to medical historians as well; see, for example, Alice Domurat Dreger, *Hermaphrodites and the Medical Invention of Sex* (Cambridge, Mass.: Harvard University Press, 1998); Alice Domurat Dreger, "'Ambiguous Sex'—Or Ambivalent Medicine?" in Arthur L. Caplan, James J. McCartney, and Dominic A. Sisti, eds., *Health, Disease, and Illness: Concepts in Medicine* (Washington, DC: Georgetown University Press, 2004), 137–52; Anne Fausto-Sterling, *Sexing the Body: Gender Politics and the Construction of Sexuality* (New York: Basic Books, 2000).

25. J. P. Maygrer, *Midwifery Illustrated*, 5th ed., tr. from the French by A. Sidney Doane (New York: J. S. Redfield, Clinton Hall, 1845), xiv–xv.

26. F. Le Jau Farker, "Hermaphrodism: Description of a Supposed Case," *Charleston*

*Medical Journal and Review* 14 (January 1859): 57–63. In spite of Parker's pronouncement, I have chosen to refer to Jacob using male pronouns, because he identified himself as male.

27. In this single instance, Parker used the male pronoun for Jacob, perhaps because he could not imagine the phrase "her wife."

28. Parker, "Hermaphrodism," 57–63.

29. [S. H.] Harris, "Monthly Periscope: Case of Doubtful Sex," *Southern Medical and Surgical Journal* 3 (August 1847): 504–5.

30. S. H. Harris, "Case of Doubtful Sex," *Southern Medical and Surgical Journal* 3 (November 1847): 676–78. This is a somewhat different and longer version of the piece in the previous note, both apparently reprinted from the *American Journal of the Medical Sciences*. Ned and Harris are also discussed in Todd L. Savitt, *Medicine and Slavery: The Diseases and Health Care of Blacks in Antebellum Virginia* (Urbana: University of Illinois Press, 1978), 304–5.

31. S. D. Gross, "Case of Hermaphrodism, Involving the Operation of Castration and Illustrating a New Principle in Juridical Medicine," *Southern Medical and Surgical Journal* 8 (December 1852): 753–56.

32. Ibid.

33. Wm. James Barry, "Case of Doubtful Sex," *Southern Medical and Surgical Journal* 3 (February 1847): 118–19.

34. Paul F. Eve, "A Case of Probable Absence of the Uterus," *Southern Medical and Surgical Journal* 2 (December 1846): 724–25; see also "Review of *An Elementary Treatise on Midwifery*," *Southern Medical and Surgical Journal* 3 (October 1838): 50–51. For examples of double vaginas, another form of biological anomaly, see [Charles] Meigs, "Two Cases of Double Vagina," *Southern Medical and Surgical Journal* 3 (February 1847): 170–72.

35. See also "Review of Charles Meigs, *Females and Their Diseases*," *Charleston Medical Journal and Review* 3 (March 1848): 186, 188.

36. John S. Holliday, "A Case of Self-Castration," *Southern Medical and Surgical Journal* 4 (June 1848): 343–44.

37. John Stainback Wilson, *Woman's Home Book of Health* (Philadelphia: J. B. Lippincott, 1860), 238.

38. Hugh A. Blair, "A Case of Attempted Vicarious Menstruation, Attended with Conjunctivitis and Opacity of the Cornea," *Oglethorpe Medical and Surgical Journal* 1 (April 1858): 11–15.

39. Sanious refers to a thin, bloody discharge; purulent refers to pus.

40. E. C. Baker, "A Case of Vicarious Menstruation from an Ulcer on the Right Mamma," *Southern Journal of Medicine and Pharmacy* 2 (March 1847): 152–55.

41. S. B. R. Finley, "Case of Menstruation from the Mammae," *Carolina Journal of Medicine, Science, and Agriculture* 1 (July 1825): 263–64.

42. D. T. Tayloe, "A Case of Strangulated Umbilical Hernia without a Sac," *Medical Journal of North Carolina* 3 (October 1860): 527.

43. [Prof. Boring,] "Vicarious Menstruation," *Southern Medical and Surgical Journal* 12 (June 1856): 358–60; see also R. T. Dismukes Medical Notebook, "Menstrual Ulcers," 73, Duke University.

44. Gunning S. Bedford, *Clinical Lectures on the Diseases of Women and Children,* 2nd ed. (New York: Samuel S. and William Wood, 1855), 80, 207.

45. Tomlinson Fort, *A Dissertation on the Practice of Medicine* (Milledgeville, Ga.: Federal Union Office, 1849), 277, 429, also 600.

46. "Rape—Pregnancy," *Southern Medical and Surgical Journal* 2 (July 1838): 749–59.

47. Ibid.

48. T. L. Ogier, "A Case of Conception, with Occlusion of the Vagina," *Charleston Medical Journal and Review* 8 (November 1853): 811–14.

49. Ariel Hunton, "Cases of 'Spurious Pregnancy,'" *Southern Medical Reformer* 4 (December 1854): 315–16.

50. Joseph F. Wright, *A Practical Treatise on the Management and Diseases of Infants and Children, with Some of the Diseases Peculiar to Females, and Their Treatment* (Macon, Ga.: Joseph Clisby, 1859), 151.

51. Hydatids, a kind of tapeworm, form a mass in the body they invade; dropsical symptoms refers to dropsy, or edema, and means swelling due to retained fluid.

52. George C. Smith, "A Case of Uterine Hydatids," *Southern Medical and Surgical Journal* 1 (May 1845): 250–51.

53. George C. Smith and Joseph A. Eve, "A Case of Probable Extra-Uterine Pregnancy," *Southern Medical and Surgical Journal* 1 (October 1845): 573–76; see also John Challice, "Abdominal Tumor Mistaken for Pregnancy," *Southern Medical and Surgical Journal* 4 (February 1848): 416–20.

54. Smith and Eve, "A Case of Probable Extra-Uterine Pregnancy," 573–76.

55. W. Spillman, "A Remarkable Case of Foetation," *Charleston Medical Journal and Review* 7 (February 1852): 157–59.

56. G. Harrison, "Medical and Medico-Legal Notes of a Case of Extra-Uterine Pregnancy," *Southern Medical and Surgical Journal* 14 (October 1858): 676–80.

57. Melton A. McLaurin, *Celia, a Slave* (New York: Avon, 1991).

58. Bedford, *Clinical Lectures on the Diseases of Women and Children,* 48–49, 53.

59. Robert Gooch, *A Practical Compendium of Midwifery* (Philadelphia: E. L. Carey and A. Hart, 1832), 100–101, 104; see also *American Lady's Medical Pocket-Book, and Nursery Adviser* (Philadelphia: James Kay, Jun. and Brother; Pittsburgh: John I. Kay, 1833), 114–15.

60. The midcentury was marked by growing efforts by physicians to claim childbirth as part of their domain for a variety of reasons, squeezing out midwives in the process; see, for example, Judith Walzer Leavitt, *Brought to Bed: Childbearing in America 1750–1950* (New York: Oxford University Press, 1986).

61. W. P. L. Jennings, "Curious Case of Foetation," *Charleston Medical Journal and Review* 7 (February 1852): 173–75.

62. R. H. McIlvain, "Case of Prolonged Gestation, in Which the Date of Conception Was Accurately Ascertained," *Southern Medical and Surgical Journal* 4 (February 1848): 560–61.

63. S. N. Harris, "Cases in Obstetric Practice," *Charleston Medical Journal and Review* 7 (November 1852): 774.

64. J. Douglass, "Ergot in Placenta Praevia—Abortion at Three Months, Delivery of Another Child Six Months After," *Charleston Medical Journal and Review* 15 (May 1860): 229.

65. Elias Horlbeck, "Expulsion of Two Foetuses of Unequal Size at the Same Time, with Remarks on Superfoetation," *Charleston Medical Journal and Review* 3 (January 1848): 28–33.

66. The debate about maternal influences had a long history; see, for example, Herman W. Roodenburg, "The Maternal Imagination: The Fears of Pregnant Women in Seventeenth-Century Holland," *Journal of Social History* 21 (1988): 701–16; Susan M. Stabile, "A 'Doctrine of Signatures': The Epistolary Physicks of Esther Burr's Journal," in Janet Moore

Lindman and Michele Lise Tarter, eds., *A Centre of Wonders: The Body in Early America* (Ithaca, N.Y.: Cornell University Press, 2001), 109–26.

67. See, for example, Lucy Brown, *The American Slave*, vol. 14, 1:154; unnamed woman, *The American Slave*, 18:194; unnamed woman, *The American Slave*, 19:215. Such comments are ubiquitous in the narratives; see also Dorothy Roberts, *Killing the Black Body: Race, Reproduction, and the Meaning of Liberty* (New York: Vintage, 1997).

68. "Appendix to Our Sermon in the Last Number," *Southern Botanic Journal* 1 (April 29, 1837): 103.

69. "Evils of Tight Lacing," *Southern Botanico-Medical Journal* 1 (October 15, 1841): 473, reprinted from the *Southern Literary Messenger*.

70. "Dr. Thomson's Materia Medica, No. 3," *Southern Botanic Journal* 1 (November 11, 1837): 325.

71. J. R. Lasseter, "A Lesson to Mothers," *Southern Medical Reformer and Review* 5 (June 1855): 65–66.

72. Ibid.

73. Masters regularly advised overseers and one another to attend to the needs of nursing mothers and babies, including allowing women time to cool down from work before nursing; see James O. Breeden, ed., *Advice among Masters: The Ideal in Slave Management in the Old South* (Westport, Conn.: Greenwood Press, 1980), 166, 168, 205.

74. Dr. Turck, "On the Power of the Maternal Imagination in the Production of Monsters," *Southern Medical Reformer* 9 (April 1859): 120–23.

75. T. L. Ogier, "Hereditary Predisposition," *Charleston Medical Journal and Review* 3 (May 1848): 265–67.

76. Antony, "An Essay on the Subject of Maternal Influence on the Foetus in Utero," 65–76.

77. Ibid.

78. William Hauser, "Pre-Natal Influences," *Oglethorpe Medical and Surgical Journal* 2 (November 1859): 217–19.

79. Charles Atkins, "Description of a Case of Neuralgia Congenita," *Carolina Journal of Medicine, Science, and Agriculture* n.s. 1 (May 1826): 123–24.

80. F. P. Porcher, "Case of St. Vitus's Dance, (Chorea Sancti Viti,) with Large Number of Supernumerary Toes and Fingers," *Charleston Medical Journal and Review* 3 (March 1848): 162–63.

81. E. V. Culver, "On a Case of Monstrosity," *Southern Medical and Surgical Journal* 8 (October 1852): 604–5.

82. O. C. Gibbs, "Summary: Mental Influence on the Products of Conception," *Southern Medical and Surgical Journal* 15 (November 1859): 784–85.

83. Alexander Y. Nicoll and Richard D. Arnold, "Account of an Anencephalus, or Human Monstrosity without a Brain and Spinal Marrow," *Southern Medical and Surgical Journal* 2 (August 1837): 10, 18.

84. H. V. M. Miller, "Account of a Case of Double Monstrosity," *Southern Medical and Surgical Journal* 10 (February 1854): 79–81.

85. W[illia]m W. Morland, "Physiology: Extracts from the Records of the Boston Society for Medical Improvement," *Charleston Medical Journal and Review* 8 (May 1853): 404–10.

86. W. H. Coffin, *The Art of Medicine Simplified, or a Treatise on the Nature and Cure of Diseases, for the Use of Families and Travelers* (Wellsburg, Va.: W. Barnes, 1853), 154.

87. Wilson, *Woman's Home Book of Health*, 277, 310; see also *American Lady's Medical*

*Pocket-Book,* 122–24; Thomas Denman, *An Introduction to the Practice of Midwifery,* 6th London ed., 3rd American ed. (New York: Carvill, 1829), 370.

88. James Campbell to David Campbell, August 1, 1834, Campbell Family Papers, Duke University.

89. Carolyn Elizabeth Burgwin Clitherall Reminiscences, *American Women's Diaries: Southern Women,* vol. 6 (New Canaan, Conn.: Readex Film Products, 1988).

90. September 30, 1862, Meta Morris Grimball Diary, *Records of Ante-Bellum Southern Plantations,* ser. J, pt. 3.

91. Peninnah Minnir to Phereby P. Philips, July 10, 1854, James Jones Philips Papers, *Records of Ante-Bellum Southern Plantations,* ser. J, pt. 12.

92. Easter Sudie Campbell, *The American Slave,* vol. 16, *Kentucky,* 91–92.

93. Henrietta King, in Charles L. Perdue Jr., Thomas E. Barden, and Robert K. Phillips, eds., *Weevils in the Wheat: Interviews with Virginia Ex-Slaves* (Charlottesville: University of Virginia Press, 1976), 190.

94. "Application of Physiology and Phrenology, in the Formation of Marriages," *Southern Botanico-Medical Journal* 1 (April 15, 1841): 186–87.

95. W. Byrd Powell, "Physiological Incompatibility between the Sexes in Relation to Progeny," *Southern Medical Reformer* 9 (January 1859): 2–3.

96. Antony, "An Essay on the Subject of Maternal Influence on the Foetus in Utero," 73–74.

97. Larkin G. Jones, "On the Peculiarities of the Female: The Physiological Changes Produced by Conception and the Treatment of Some of the Most Important Diseases Consecutive to Parturition," MD thesis, Medical College of South Carolina, 1829, Waring Medical Library, Medical University of South Carolina, Charleston.

## Chapter 5. The Examined Body

1. Physicians as well as laypeople today continue to debate the connections between mind and body; it has remained an important area of inquiry for historians as well. The literature on the history of mental illness as it relates to issues of race, sex, and place is vast; see, for example, Sander Gilman, *Disease and Representation: Images of Illness from Madness to AIDS* (Ithaca, N.Y.: Cornell University Press, 1988); Michael Sappol, *A Traffic of Dead Bodies: Anatomy and Embodied Social Identity in Nineteenth Century America* (Princeton, N.J.: Princeton University Press, 2001); Sander Gilman, *Difference and Pathology: Stereotypes of Sexuality, Race, and Madness* (Ithaca, N.Y.: Cornell University Press, 1985), Thomas Szasz, "The Sane Slave: A Historical Note on the Use of Medical Diagnosis," *American Journal of Psychotherapy* 25 (1971): 228–39; Robert Whitaker, *Mad in America: Bad Science, Bad Medicine, and the Enduring Mistreatment of the Mentally Ill* (Cambridge, Mass.: Perseus, 2002); Peter McCandless, *Moonlight, Magnolias, and Madness: Insanity in South Carolina from the Colonial Period to the Progressive Era* (Chapel Hill: University of North Carolina Press, 1996); see also Roy Porter, *Flesh in the Age of Reason: The Modern Foundations of Body and Soul* (New York: Norton, 2003).

2. "[Review of] *Elements of Health, and Principles of Female Hygiene,* by E. J. Tilt," *Charleston Medical Journal and Review* 8 (September 1853): 660.

3. Dr. Burdon, "Influence of the Mother's Imagination upon the Production of Monstrous Children," *Southern Medical and Surgical Journal* 5 (August 1849): 482.

4. For example, Thompson McGown prescribed remedies for what he called neuralgic

affections based on the "general condition of the system," such as "leucophlegmatic"; Thompson McGown, *A Practical Treatise on the Most Common Diseases of the South* (Philadelphia: Grigg, Elliot, 1849), 158, also 161, 175.

5. Dyspepsia refers to a range of stomach disorders, including from what would today likely be considered heartburn to more serious ailments.

6. Samuel K. Jennings, *A Compendium of Medical Science* (Tuscaloosa, Ala.: Marmaduke J. Slade, 1847), 451.

7. On the history of menstruation, see Vern Bullough and Martha Voght, "Women, Menstruation, and Nineteenth-Century Medicine," *Bulletin of the History of Medicine* 47 (1973): 66–82.

8. H. R. Easterling, "The Effects of Uterine Diseases on the Constitution," *Charleston Medical Journal and Review* 10 (July 1855): 469.

9. James M. Green, "Cases of Inflammation and Ulceration of the Cervix Uteri," *Charleston Medical Journal and Review* 8 (January 1853): 43; see also Tomlinson Fort, *A Dissertation on the Practice of Medicine* (Milledgeville, Ga.: Federal Union Office, 1849), 627.

10. John Douglass, "Ovarian Dropsy, Cured by a Simple Operation," *Charleston Medical Journal and Review* 6 (September 1851): 369–70.

11. Obstructed menstruation referred to the failure of menses to appear at the appointed time in a woman who was neither pregnant nor menopausal, usually because of some mechanical difficulty such as a prolapsed uterus. Women who claimed to suffer from either retained or suppressed menstruation could easily have been pregnant, a possibility doctors warned one another to take into consideration, especially when the woman who complained of them was not married.

12. M. Antony, "On Menstrual Irregularities," *Southern Medical and Surgical Journal* 1 (May 1837): 720. Antony is credited with founding and acting as the driving force behind the Medical College of Georgia; see Phinizy Spalding, *The History of the Medical College of Georgia* (Athens: University of Georgia Press, 1987), ch. 1–3.

13. Dysmenorrhea refers to painful menstruation.

14. J. A. Hamilton, "Medical Electricity," *Southern Medical and Surgical Journal* 3 (September 1839): 766.

15. Eben Hillyer, "An Essay on the Physiology of Menstruation," *Southern Medical and Surgical Journal* 14 (December 1858): 797.

16. Amenorrhea was yet another term used to refer to the absence of menstruation in women neither pregnant nor menopausal.

17. Sampson Eagon, "Epilepsy Succeeding a Suppression of the Menstrual Discharge, Cured by the Supervention of Dysentery, and the Restoration of the Catamenia," *Southern Medical and Surgical Journal* 15 (November 1859): 778.

18. Epilepsy was poorly understood throughout the nineteenth century and earlier as well. In women, it was frequently linked to reproductive disorders. On the history of epilepsy, including changes in its definition, diagnosis, and treatment, see Owesi Temkin, *The Falling Sickness: A History of Epilepsy from the Greeks to the Beginnings of Modern Neurology*, 2nd ed. (Baltimore: Johns Hopkins University Press, 1971).

19. W. H. Coffin, *The Art of Medicine Simplified, or a Treatise on the Nature and Cause of Diseases, for the Use of Families and Travelers* (Wellsburg, Va.: W. Barnes, 1853), 147; Ralph Schenck, *The Family Physician, Treating of the Diseases Which Assail the Human System* (Fincastle, Va.: Oliver Callaghan and Wm. E. M. Word, 1842), 419.

20. John Stainback Wilson, *Woman's Home Book of Health* (Philadelphia: J. B. Lippincott, 1860), 237.

21. J. Hume Simons, *The Planter's Guide and Family Book of Medicine* (Charleston, S.C.: M'Carter and A.len, 1848), 147.

22. Joseph F. Wright, *A Practical Treatise on the Management and Diseases of Infants and Children, with Some of the Diseases Peculiar to Females, and Their Treatment* (Macon, Ga.: Joseph Clisby, 1859), 134, 136–37, 142–43; see also Wilson, *Woman's Home Book of Health*, 237.

23. W[illia]m B. Atkinson, "Puerperal Insanity," *Medical Journal of North Carolina* 3 (May 1861): 295.

24. Green, "Cases of Inflammation and Ulceration of the Cervix Uteri," 45.

25. W. C. Horlbeck, "A Case of Tubal Pregnancy, with Rupture of the Fallopian Tube," *Charleston Medical Journal and Review* 5 (May 1850): 309.

26. Wright, *A Practical Treatise on the Management and Diseases of Infants and Children*, 173–74.

27. M. Antony, "An Essay on the Subject of Maternal Influence on the Foetus in Utero," *Southern Medical and Surgical Journal* 3 (November 1838): 72.

28. Wilson, *Woman's Home Book of Health*, 276, 289–94, 303–5, 277.

29. J. H. Lasseter, "A Lesson to Mothers," *Southern Medical Reformer and Review* 5 (June 1855): 67; see also *The American Lady's Medical Pocket-Book, and Nursery-Advisor* (Philadelphia: James Kay, Jun. and Brother; Pittsburgh: John I. Kay, 1833), 115, 123–24.

30. E. James Mims, "General Dropsey," *Oglethorpe Medical and Surgical Journal* 1 (October 1858): 246–47.

31. Tyler Smith, "The Uterus," *Medical Journal of North Carolina* 1 (October 1858): 157.

32. T. Gaillard Thomas, "A Lecture on the Prevention of Post-partum Haemorrhage," *Charleston Medical Journal and Review* 14 (May 1859): 340.

33. Samuel D. Gamble, "On the Influence of Pain in the Production of Death," *Southern Medical and Surgical Journal* 2 (July 1838): 707–8.

34. M. Antony, "Contributions from the Obstetric Record of M. Antony," *Southern Medical and Surgical Journal* 2 (January 1838): 333.

35. J. A. Eve, "Medical Intelligence: Letter to the Editor on the Use of Chloroform in Obstetric Practice," *Southern Medical and Surgical Review* 4 (April 1848): 253.

36. Syncope refers to fainting.

37. J. J. Robertson, "Successful Employment of Chloroform during Labor," *Southern Medical and Surgical Journal* 4 (August 1848): 471–72; "Successful Employment of Chloroform during Labor [Part 2]," *Southern Medical and Surgical Journal* 4 (October 1848): 590–91. For another nineteenth-century reference as well as a useful discussion of body-mind connections, see Charles E. Rosenberg, "Body and Mind in Nineteenth-Century Medicine: Some Clinical Origins of the Neurosis Construct," in *Explain Epidemics and Other Studies in the History of Medicine* (New York: Cambridge University Press, 1992), 74–89, esp. 83.

38. Protheroe Smith, "On the Employment of Ether by Inhalation in Obstetric Practice, with Cases and Observations," *Southern Medical and Surgical Journal* 3 (September 1847): 549, 551. On the use of anesthesia in obstetrics, see Mary Poovey, "'Scenes of an Indelicate Character': The Medical 'Treatment' of Victorian Women," in Catherine Gallagher and Thomas Laqueur, eds., *The Making of the Modern Body: Sexuality and Society in the Nineteenth Century* (Berkeley: University of California Press, 1987), 137–68.

39. Wilson, *Woman's Home Book of Health*, 311.

40. Jesse Beck, "Report of Anolalous and Complicated Cases," *Southern Medical Reformer and Review* 6 (December 1856): 181.

41. J. H. Hand, "Statistics of Obstetrical Cases," *Southern Medical Reformer and Review* 8 (August 1858): 241–42, 245.

42. James M. Gordon, "Contributions to Practical Midwifery, with Cases Occurring in Obstetrical Practice," *Southern Medical and Surgical Journal* 3 (December 1847): 704–5.

43. Jennings, *A Compendium of Medical Science,* 273.

44. Atkinson, "Puerperal Insanity," 292–96.

45. Thomas, "A Lecture on the Prevention of Post-partum Haemorrhage," 340, 346.

46. Alfred M. Folger, *The Family Physician, Being a Domestic Medicine Work, Written in Plain Style* (Spartanburg C.H., S.C.: Z. D. Cottrell, 1845), 54–55.

47. Simons, *The Planter's Guide and Family Book of Medicine,* 201.

48. Puerperal (or childbed) fever killed many women shortly after they gave birth.

49. John P. Mettauer, "The Prophylactic Treatment of Puerperal Fever," *Charleston Medical Journal and Review* 6 (January 1851): 41.

50. [Combe], "Treatment of Infants," *Southern Botanico-Medical Journal* 1 (June 1, 1841): 248; [Combe], "Warning to Nurses," *Southern Botanico-Medical Journal* 1 (July 15, 1841): 327; see also Lasseter, "A Lesson to Mothers," 66; Jay Mechling, "Advice to Historians on Advice to Mothers," *Journal of Social History* 9 (1975): 44–63; and the discussion of maternal influences in chapter 4.

51. T. Bullard, "Ought a Physician to Tell a Patient That He Is Going to Die," *Oglethorpe Medical and Surgical Journal* 2 (November 1859): 267.

52. Antony, "An Essay on the Subject of Maternal Influence on the Foetus in Utero," 73.

53. A. G. Goodlett, *The Family Physician, or Every Man's Companion* (Nashville, Tenn.: Smith and Nesbit, 1838), 18.

54. Doctors and slaveholders did notice that slave infants had a far higher mortality rate than white infants and in particular were far more likely to be smothered in bed by their mothers, which they attributed to the slave mothers' carelessness; see Michael P. Johnson, "Smothered Slave Infants: Were Slave Mothers at Fault?" *Journal of Southern History* 47 (November 1981): 493–520; Todd L. Savitt, "Smothering and Overlaying of Virginia Slave Children: A Suggested Explanation," *Bulletin of the History of Medicine* 49 (Fall 1975): 400–404; see also John Campbell, "Work, Pregnancy, and Infant Mortality among Southern Slaves," *Journal of Interdisciplinary History* 14 (Spring 1984): 793–812; Wilma King, *Stolen Childhood: Slave Youth in Nineteenth-Century America* (Bloomington: Indiana University Press, 1995); Marie Jenkins Schwartz, *Born in Bondage: Growing Up Enslaved in the Antebellum South* (Cambridge, Mass.: Harvard University Press, 2000).

55. Gunning S. Bedford, *Clinical Lectures on the Diseases of Women and Children,* 2nd ed. (New York: Samuel S. and William Wood, 1855), 34–35.

56. Robert Gooch, *An Account of Some of the Most Important Diseases Peculiar to Women,* 2nd ed. (Philadelphia: Ed. Barington and Geo. D. Haswell, 1848), 107.

57. W. L., "Aphorisms on the Hygiene and Nursing of Infants," *Southern Medical Reformer and Review* 9 (December 1859): 378.

58. "Reviews: *On Diseases of Menstruation and Ovarian Inflammation, in Connexion with Sterility, Pelvic Tumours and Affections of the Womb,* by Edward John Tilt," *Charleston Medical Journal and Review* 6 (July 1851): 534, 536, 542; see also Charles E. Rosenberg, "Sexuality, Class, and Role in Nineteenth-Century America," *American Quarterly* 25 (May 1975): 131–53.

59. The pessary was a device inserted into the vagina in order to support a sagging uterus.

60. Paul F. Eve, "An Essay on the Question, Ought Not the Use of Pessaries to Be Now Abandoned?" *Southern Medical and Surgical Journal* 1 (April 1837): 649.

61. Joseph A. Eve, "A Report on Diseases of the Cervix Uteri, Concluded," *Southern Medical and Surgical Journal* 13 (November, 1857): 645.

62. Wright, *A Practical Treatise on the Management and Diseases of Infants and Children,* 148; Robert Gooch, *A Practical Compendium of Midwifery; Being the Course of Lectures on Midwifery, and on the Diseases of Women and Infants* (Philadelphia: E. L. Carey and A. Hart, 1832), 50. On the history of onanism, or masturbation, see Thomas W. Laqueur, *Solitary Sex: A Cultural History of Masturbation* (New York: Zone Books, 2003).

63. Wilson, *Woman's Home Book of Health,* 221.

64. "Extirpation of the Clitoris," *Carolina Journal of Medicine, Science, and Agriculture* 1 (October 1825): 384–85.

65. J. A. Long, "A Case of Onanism, Presenting Great Difficulty of Diagnosis," *Southern Medical and Surgical Journal* 8 (April 1852): 208–10.

66. Prof. Trousseau, "Lecture on Impotence," *Southern Medical and Surgical Journal* 12 (October 1856): 605–13.

67. R. T. Dismukes, Medical Notebook, 290–92, Duke University.

68. "Review of Edward Rigsby, MD, *On the Constitutional Treatment of Female Diseases,*" *Charleston Medical Journal and Review* 12 (March 1857): 244.

69. [L. A. Dugas], "Editorial and Miscellany: Remarks upon the Use of Pessaries in the Treatment of Prolapsus Uteri," *Southern Medical and Surgical Journal* 10 (September 1854): 573.

70. J. McF. Gaston, "Ovarian Tumor and Ovarian Irritation," *Charleston Medical Journal and Review* 8 (September 1853): 610–11.

71. McGown, *A Practical Treatise on the Most Common Diseases of the South,* 431.

72. Moral treatment had a quite specific meaning in the nineteenth century, linked to more humane ways of treating the insane than previously practiced; see chapter 7.

73. Alexander H. Stevens, "On the Diagnosis of Nervous Diseases," *Southern Medical and Surgical Journal* 3 (June 1847): 352–53.

74. "Reviews and Editorial," *Medical Journal of North Carolina* 3 (May 1861): 316–17.

75. William R. King, "A Report on the Diseases of Franklin County," *Medical Journal of North Carolina* 1 (October 1858): 113–14.

76. [Simon Saunders,] "Monthly Periscope: Prolapsus Uteri," *Southern Medical and Surgical Journal* 3 (April 1839): 431; see also Wilson, *Woman's Home Book of Health,* 266.

77. John Lake, "Cases of Episioraphy," *Southern Medical and Surgical Journal* 1 (March 1845): 114–15.

78. This meant that she had tears between her rectum and vagina, usually called fistula, which "afforded a free transmission of fecal matter through the lower part of the vagina, and out at the vulva." Prolapse itself could often cause urine to leak uncontrollably throughout the vagina and vulval areas, leading to irritated and infected tissue and what many sufferers and physicians described as an almost unbearable stench, to say nothing of extreme pain.

79. Antony, "On Menstrual Irregularities," 724–27.

80. Ibid.

81. Joseph A. Eve, "A Report on Diseases of Cervix Uteri [Part I]," *Southern Medical and Surgical Journal* 13 (September 1857): 526–27.

82. Wright, *A Practical Treatise on the Management and Diseases of Infants and Children,* 160.

83. In addition to sources on the history of mental illness, see Elaine Showalter, *The*

*Female Malady* (New York: Viking Penguin, 1985); Elaine Showalter, *Hystories: Hysterical Epidemics and Modern Culture* (New York: Columbia University Press, 1997); Ilza Veith, *Hysteria: The History of a Disease* (Chicago: University of Chicago Press, 1965).

84. Wilson, *Woman's Home Book of Health,* 295–96.

85. Coffin, *The Art of Medicine Simplified,* 150–51.

86. W. Camps, "Hysteria Considered as a Connecting Link between Mental and Bodily Diseases," *Southern Medical and Surgical Journal* 15 (October 1859): 701–3. The article, which credits W. Camps as the author, is in fact an anonymously written summary of his views published in the *British Medical Journal.*

87. "Rape—Pregnancy," *Southern Medical and Surgical Journal* 2 (July 1838): 750–51.

88. Joseph Eve, "A Report on Diseases of the Cervix Uteri [Part I]," 525.

89. Albert W. Henley, "Remarkable Case of Hysterical Convulsions," *Southern Medical and Surgical Journal* 13 (November 1857): 656–61.

90. Camps, "Hysteria Considered as a Connecting Link between Mental and Bodily Diseases," 702–3.

91. "Reviews: *On Diseases of Menstruation and Ovarian Inflammation,*" 537–38.

92. Called "the whites" from the color of the discharge, this would today most likely be diagnosed as a yeast or other vaginal infection and not linked to menstruation.

93. John P. Miller, "Fluor Albus," *Southern Medical Reformer and Review* 10 (September 1860): 266–68.

94. McGown, *A Practical Treatise on the Most Common Diseases of the South,* 165–66.

95. Joseph A. Eve, "Cases of Convulsions and Other Nervous Affections, during Pregnancy, Parturition and the Puerperal State," *Southern Medical and Surgical Journal* 4 (February 1848): 76–77; see also Green, "Cases of Inflammation and Ulceration of the Cervix Uteri," 53–54.

96. E. Y. Harris, "Anomalous Cases," *Southern Medical and Surgical Journal* 8 (October 1852): 592–95.

97. See chapter 4.

98. F. P. Porcher, "Case of St. Vitus's Dance, (Chorea Sancti Viti), with Large Number of Supernumerary Toes and Fingers," *Charleston Medical Journal and Review* 3 (March 1848): 162–65.

99. Joseph A. Eve, "Cases of Convulsions and Other Nervous Affections, during Pregnancy, Parturition and the Puerperal State," *Southern Medical and Surgical Journal* 3 (September 1847): 513, 519.

100. Fort, *A Dissertation on the Practice of Medicine,* 613–17.

101. E. Miller, "Observations from Cases of Hysteria," *Oglethorpe Medical and Surgical Journal* 2 (November 1859): 221–23. On insanity in slaves, see Todd L. Savitt, *Medicine and Slavery: The Diseases and Health Care of Blacks in Antebellum Virginia* (Urbana: University of Illinois Press, 1978), ch. 8.

102. Miller, "Observations from Cases of Hysteria," 221–23.

103. Ibid.

104. Miller would not, of course, have used this term; see chapter 4.

105. Green, "Cases of Inflammation and Ulceration of the Cervix Uteri," 54–55.

106. "Review of *Females and Their Diseases; a Series of Letters to His Class,* by Charles D. Meigs," *Charleston Medical Journal and Review* 3 (March 1848), 195; see also Gail Pat Parsons, "Equal Treatment for All: American Medical Remedies for Male Sexual Problems: 1850–1900," *Journal of the History of Medicine and Applied Sciences* 32, no. 1 (1977): 55–71.

107. Gunning S. Bedford, *Clinical Lectures on the Diseases of Women and Children*, 2nd ed. (New York: Samuel S. and William Wood, 1855), 371.

108. Schenck, *The Family Physician*, 358–59; see also Fort, *A Dissertation on the Practice of Medicine*, 521–26.

109. Jennings. *A Compendium of Medical Science*, 212–13.

110. Schenck, *The Family Physician*, 358–59.

111. J. Y. DuPre, "Case of Hysteria in the Male," *Charleston Medical Journal and Review* 7 (February 1852): 159–64.

112. Ibid.

113. Folger, *The Family Physician*, 182; Folger did not agree with this diagnosis.

## Chapter 6. The Unexamined Body

1. Although historians have discussed laypeople's caregiving responsibilities, particularly those of women, few have focused on their efforts to explain sickness or the bodies that suffered from it. For an important exception, see Steven Stowe, "Writing Sickness: A Southern Woman's Diary of Cares," in Anne Goodwyn Jones and Susan V. Donaldson, eds., *Haunted Bodies: Gender and Southern Texts* (Charlottesville: University Press of Virginia, 1997), 257–84.

2. I am indebted to Kristin Langellier for helping me think through these issues.

3. Joseph Milligan to Elizabeth Camfield Milligan, August 20, 1844, Milligan Family Papers, *Southern Women and Their Families in the 19th Century: Papers and Diaries*, ser. A, *Holdings of the Southern Historical Collection, University of North Carolina, Chapel Hill*; pt. 5, *Alabama, South Carolina, Georgia, and Florida Collections*, consulting ed. Anne Firor Scott (Bethesda, Md.: University Publications of America, 1991).

4. August 7, 1853, Carolyn Elizabeth (Eliza) Burgwin Clitherall Diary, Southern Historical Collection, University of North Carolina, Chapel Hill; *American Women's Diaries: Southern Women* (New Canaan, Conn.: Readex Film Products, 1988).

5. Carol Bleser, ed., *Tokens of Affection: The Letters of a Planter's Daughter in the Old South* (Athens: University of Georgia Press, 1996), 75, 104, 175.

6. Virginia Campbell to Margaret Campbell, May 1, 1845, Campbell Family Papers, Special Collections, William Perkins Library, Duke University.

7. September 7, 1859, Mary Jeffreys Bethell Diary, *Records of Ante-Bellum Southern Plantations from the Revolution through the Civil War*, ser. J, *Selections from the Southern Historical Collection, Manuscripts Department, Library of the University of North Carolina at Chapel Hill*, pt. 13, *Piedmont North Carolina*, gen. ed. Kenneth M. Stampp (Frederick, Md.: University Publications of America, 1992).

8. M. Blanks to Eliza Blanks, September 21, 1833, Elizabeth J. Holmes Blanks Papers, Duke University.

9. Virginia Campbell to Margaret Campbell, May 1, 1845, Campbell Family Papers, Duke University.

10. Lizzie to Sallie J. Lenoir, September 8, 1855, Lenoir Family Papers, Southern Historical Collection, Wilson Library, University of North Carolina at Chapel Hill.

11. E[liza DeRosset] to Mary and Ashley Curtis, January 1, 1850, Moses Ashley Curtis Family Papers, University of North Carolina.

12. Carolyn Elizabeth (Eliza) Burgwin Clitherall, family reminiscences, vol. 2.

13. Bleser, *Tokens of Affection*, 24, 141.

14. Martha Dupree Treadwell to E. W. Treadwell, December 14, 1859, E. W. Treadwell Papers, Duke University.

15. Christine Jacobson Carter, ed., *The Diary of Dolly Lunt Burge, 1848–1879* (Athens: University of Georgia Press, 1997), 135.

16. E[lizabeth] J. [Camfield] Milligan to Joseph A. S. Milligan, April 4, 1848, Milligan Family Papers.

17. M. T. to unnamed person, May 4, [1861?], William Eliza (Rhodes) Terrell Papers, Duke University.

18. April 25, 1864, January 1, 1863, Margaret Ann "Meta" Morris Grimball Diary, *Records of Ante-Bellum Southern Plantations,* ser. J, pt. 3.

19. August 1822, Ann A. Turner Diary, Duke University. Turner would live until at least 1837.

20. Bleser, *Tokens of Affection,* 182.

21. Michael O'Brien, ed., *An Evening When Alone: Four Journals of Single Women in the South, 1827–67* (Charlottesville: University Press of Virginia, 1993), 143.

22. Judith Walzer Leavitt, *Brought to Bed: Childbearing in America 1750 to 1950* (New York: Oxford University Press, 1986); Sally McMillen, *Motherhood in the Old South: Pregnancy, Childbirth, and Infant Rearing* (Baton Rouge: Louisiana State University Press, 1990); Steven M. Stowe, "Obstetrics and the Work of Doctoring in the Mid-Nineteenth-Century American South," *Bulletin of the History of Medicine* 64 (Winter 1990): 540–66; Marie Jenkins Schwartz, "Medical Men and Midwives: Managing Pregnancy and Childbirth in the Slave South," paper presented at the American Seminar, John Nicholas Brown Center, Providence, Rhode Island, May 10, 2000. For slaves, see John Campbell, "Work, Pregnancy, and Infant Mortality among Southern Slaves," *Journal of Interdisciplinary History* 14 (Spring 1984): 793–812.

23. April 21, 1828, July 12, 1828, September 15, 1828, early November 1833, March 5, 1834, December 1, 1834, January 4, 1835, August 22, 1829, Sarah Haynesworth Gayle Diary, *American Women's Diaries: Southern Women* (New Canaan, Conn.: Readex Film Products, 1988). We know little about any southern women's deliberate efforts to reduce their fertility, although doctors and others sometimes accused slave women of doing so; see Jan Lewis and Kenneth A. Lockridge, "'Sally Has Been Sick': Pregnancy and Family Limitation among Virginia Gentry Women, 1780–1830," *Journal of Social History* 229 (1988): 5–19.

24. Penelope Skinner Warren to Thomas Warren, August 9, 1840, August 16, 1840, August 22, 1840; Penelope Skinner Warren to Mrs. William D. Warren, September 11, 1840, Skinner Family Papers, *Records of Ante-Bellum Southern Plantations,* ser. J, pt. 12, *Tidewater and Coastal Plains North Carolina.*

25. February 6, 1844, February 22, 1845, Frances Bumpas Journal, University of North Carolina.

26. Bleser, *Tokens of Affection,* 173.

27. Sarah McCulloh Lemmon, ed., *The Pettigrew Papers,* vol. 2, *1819–1843* (Raleigh: North Carolina Department of Cultural Resources, Division of Archives and History, 1988), 228, 98.

28. July 20, 1861, Meta Morris Grimball Diary.

29. Penelope Skinner Warren to Thomas Warren, August 8, 1840, Skinner Family Papers.

30. August 15, 1844, September 9, 1844, Bumpas Family Papers, University of North Carolina.

31. Bleser, *Tokens of Affection,* 318; interpolation Bleser's.

32. Margaret Devereux to Ellen Mordecai, October 6, 1847, Margaret Mordecai Devereux Papers, *Records of Ante-Bellum Southern Plantations,* ser. J, pt. 12.

33. Sophia Peck to Mary Peck, April 25, 1841, Henry Watson Jr. Papers, *Records of Ante-Bellum Southern Plantations,* ser. F, *Selections from the Manuscript Department, Duke University,* pt. 1 *The Deep South.*

34. April 30, 1857, John Berkley Grimball Diary.

35. Lemmon, *The Pettigrew Papers,* 179. For Pettigrew's care of his slaves, see Bennett H. Wall, "Medical Care of Ebenezer Pettigrew's Slaves," *Mississippi Valley Historical Review* 37 (1950): 451–70.

36. Lemmon, *The Pettigrew Papers,* 297, 615.

37. O'Brien, *An Evening When Alone,* 118.

38. Bleser, *Tokens of Affection,* 289.

39. Ulrich B. Phillips, ed., *Plantation and Frontier Documents: 1649–1863: Illustrative of Industrial History in the Colonial and Ante-Bellum South,* 2 vols. (Cleveland: Arthur H. Clark Co., 1909), 1:120.

40. January 31, 1851, Carolyn Clitherall Diary.

41. July 22, 1849, July 29, 1849, Tristrim Skinner to Joseph Skinner, Skinner Family Papers.

42. Sophia Watson to Henry Watson, August 31, 1848, Henry Watson Jr. Papers. Only ten days earlier, Sophia wrote nearly the same thing about a white man: "Dr. Kittrell is now very sick—dangerously so I was told this morning—but such things are generally so much exaggerated—there is no telling how much truth there is in it"; Sophia Watson to Henry Watson, August 21, 1848.

43. Bleser, *Tokens of Affection,* 228.

44. March 9, 1830, John Peyre Thomas Diary, Thomas Family Papers, *Records of Ante-Bellum Southern Plantations,* ser. A, *Selections from the South Caroliniana Library, University of South Carolina,* pt. 2, *Miscellaneous Collections.*

45. Margaret Devereux to Ellen Mordecai, February 16, 1851, Margaret Mordecai Devereux Papers.

46. Among the most useful explications of slaves' views is Sharla Fett, *Working Cures: Healing, Health, and Power on Southern Slave Plantations* (Chapel Hill: University of North Carolina Press, 2002); see also Todd Savitt, *Medicine and Slavery: The Diseases and Health Care of Blacks in Antebellum Virginia* (Urbana: University of Illinois Press, 1978).

47. Unnamed woman, *The American Slave: A Composite Autobiography,* vol. 19, *God Struck Me Dead* (Fisk University), gen. ed. George P. Rawick (Westport, Conn.: Greenwood, 1971), 206–7 214–15.

48. Unnamed woman, *The American Slave,* vol. 18, *Unwritten History of Slavery* (Fisk University), 135, 138–39. The fourth slave was apparently killed by soldiers, although it is not clear from the testimony whether they were Northern or Southern.

49. Sophia Word *The American Slave,* vol. 16, *Kansas, Kentucky, Maryland, Ohio, Virginia, and Tennessee Narratives,* Kentucky, 67.

50. Unnamed woman, *The American Slave,* 18:213–14.

51. Amanda Jackson, *The American Slave,* vol. 18, 2:292.

52. George Womble, *The American Slave,* vol. 8, 4:188; see also Ronald Killion and Charles Waller, eds., *Slavery Time When I was Chillun Down on Marster's Plantation: Interviews with Georgia Slaves,* (Savannah, Ga.: Beehive Press, 1973), 120.

53. Emmaline Heard, *The American Slave,* vol. 12, 2:151.

54. Temple Pitts, *The American Slave,* 15:174.

55. Fleming Clark, *The American Slave,* vol. 16, Ohio, 24.

56. Jennie Kendricks and Amanda McDaniel, *The American Slave,* vol. 13, 3:4, 74; Isiah Green, *The American Slave,* vol. 12, 2:53.

57. Elsie Clews Parsons, *Folk-Lore of the Sea Islands, South Carolina* (Chicago, Afro-Am Press, 1969; reprint of Cambridge, Mass.: American Folk-Lore Society, 1923), 62.

58. Charles Grandy, in Charles L. Perdue Jr., Thomas E. Barden, and Robert K. Phillips, eds., *Weevils in the Wheat: Interviews with Virginia Ex-Slaves* (Charlottesville: University Press of Virginia, 1976), 119.

59. Ambrose E. Gonzales, *The Black Border: Gullah Stories of the Carolina Coast* (Columbia, S.C.: State Company, 1922), 130.

60. Ibid., 132–33; interpolation mine.

61. Parsons, *Folk-Lore of the Sea Islands,* 8, 44, 53–54. These stories appear in similar versions in other collections; various stories of animals' shamming are ubiquitous in all of the collections of African American folklore, suggesting widespread concern about the practice.

62. Charles C. Jones Jr., *Negro Myths from the Georgia Coast, Told in the Vernacular* (Columbia, S.C.: State Company, 1925), 55–58; interpolation mine.

63. Joel Chandler Harris, *The Complete Tales of Uncle Remus,* comp. Richard Chase (Boston: Houghton Mifflin, 1955), 504–7.

64. Cicely Cawthon, in Killion and Waller, *Slavery Time When I Was Chillun Down on Marster's Plantation,* 39; see also Cicely Cathon, *The American Slave,* suppl. 1, vol. 3, 1:189. On the importance of slaves' diet, see Sam Bowers Hilliard, *Hog Meat and Hoecake: Food Supply in the Old South, 1840–1860* (Carbondale: Southern Illinois University Press, 1972); Kenneth Kiple and Virginia H. King, *Another Dimension to the Black Diaspora: Diet, Disease, and Racism* (New York: Cambridge University Press, 1981).

65. David Blount, *The American Slave,* 14:112.

66. Rev. W. B. Allen, *The American Slave,* suppl. ser. 1, vol. 3, Georgia Narratives, 1:6, also 14.

67. Genia Woodberry, *The American Slave,* vol. 3, 4:221.

68. Unnamed woman, *The American Slave,* 18:213.

69. Ike Derricote, *The American Slave,* vol. 12, 1:275.

70. Virginia Hayes Shepherd, in Barden and Phillips, *Weevils in the Wheat,* 262.

71. Orland Kay Armstrong, *Old Massa's People: The Old Slaves Tell Their Story* (Indianapolis: Bobbs-Merrill, 1931), 65.

72. Buckruh (or buckrah) was a term many slaves used for white people.

73. Gonzales, *The Black Border,* 260.

74. Georgia Baker, *The American Slave,* vol. 12, 1:49.

75. Neal Upson, *The American Slave,* vol. 13, 4:62.

76. Robert Shepherd, *The American Slave,* vol. 13, 3:251.

77. Sally Brown, *The American Slave,* vol. 12, 1:145–46. Such comments are common in the narratives.

78. Unnamed man, *The American Slave,* 18:294.

79. Savitt, *Medicine and Slavery;* Fett, *Working Cures.*

80. See esp. Newbell Niles Puckett, *Folk Beliefs of the Southern Negro* (Chapel Hill: University of North Carolina Press, 1926).

81. Sally Brown, *The American Slave,* vol. 12, 1:143.

82. Shang Harris, *The American Slave,* vol. 12, 2:123.

83. Mason Crum, *Gullah: Negro Life in the Carolina Sea Islands* (New York: Negro Universities Press, 1968; reprint of Durham: Duke University Press, 1940), 95; see also Puckett, *Folk Beliefs of the Southern Negro,* 99.

84. Alec Pope, *The American Slave,* vol. 13, 3:176; Green Willbanks, *The American Slave,* vol. 13, 4:145.

85. Mrs. Moore, *The American Slave,* 18:39. This belief was repeated in many of the folklore accounts of behaviors to avoid.

86. Mary Wright, *The American Slave,* vol. 16, Kentucky, 64; see also Cora Torian, *The American Slave,* vol. 16, Kentucky, 106; Annie B. Boyd, *The American Slave,* vol. 16, Kentucky, 58; Emma Coker, *The American Slave,* suppl. 1, vol. 3, 1:209; Julia Henderson, *The American Slave,* suppl. 1, vol. 3, 1:323.

87. Betty Cofer, *The American Slave,* 14:170.

88. Sam Rawls, *The American Slave,* vol. 3, 4:6.

89. Penny Williams, *The American Slave,* 15:405.

90. William McWhorter, *The American Slave,* vol. 13, 3:100.

91. Jones, *Negro Myths from the Georgia Coast,* 92.

92. Puckett, *Folk Beliefs of the Southern Negro,* 154, 168, 259–61.

93. Anna Grant, *The American Slave,* suppl. 1, vol. 3, 1:265–66; see also Lula Pyron, *The American Slave,* suppl. 1, vol. 4, 2:495.

94. Mary Colbert, *The American Slave,* vol. 12, 1:222.

95. George White, in Barden and Phillips, *Weevils in the Wheat,* 310.

96. Unnamed person, *The American Slave,* 19:76.

97. David Goodman Gullins, *The American Slave,* vol. 12, 2:85–86.

98. Marrinda Jane Singleton, in Barden and Phillips, *Weevils in the Wheat,* 267–68. Singleton attributed responsibility for conjure's teachings to "the Negroes who were from the Indies and other Islands," adding "much of it was handed down from the wilds of Africa."

99. Virginia Hayes Shepherd, in Barden and Phillips, *Weevils in the Wheat,* 263.

100. E. Geddings, "Case of Extraordinary Enlargement and Ossific Transformation of the Ovaria," *Southern Medical and Surgical Journal* 2 (May 1838): 580.

101. Armstrong, *Old Massa's People,* 249–50.

102. Unnamed woman, *The American Slave,* 18:139.

103. Unnamed man, *The American Slave,* 18:100; see also Julia Henderson, *The American Slave,* suppl. 1, vol. 3, 1:322.

104. Jones, *Negro Myths from the Georgia Coast,* 75–76. Another version of this story, but without the references to conjure, appears in Harris, *The Complete Tales of Uncle Remus,* 494–96.

105. Ellen Trell, *The American Slave,* 15:361.

106. Patsy Mitchner, *The American Slave,* 15:121.

107. Henry C. Davis, "Negro Folk-Lore in South Carolina," *Journal of American Folk-Lore* 27 (July–September 1914): 247, n. 2.

108. [H. J. Nott], "Superstitions and Traditions of the Backwoods of South Carolina, Number One," *Southern Literary Journal and Monthly Review* 3 (September 1836–March 1837): 258–62.

109. David Goodman Gullins, *The American Slave,* vol. 12, 2:86.

110. Unnamed woman, *The American Slave,* 18:273; see also Lu, *The American Slave,* 19:202.

111. Unnamed woman, *The American Slave,* 18:110.

## Chapter 7. *The Diseased Body*

1. "Code of Medical Ethics, Adopted at the Late Meeting of the National Medical Convention," *Southern Medical and Surgical Journal* 3 (September 1847): 538.

2. Carol Bleser, ed., *Tokens of Affection: The Letters of a Planter's Daughter in the Old South* (Athens: University of Georgia Press, 1996), 315.

3. Simon B. Abbott, *The Southern Botanic Physician* (Charleston: for the author, 1844), ix.

4. "Editorial and Miscellaneous: *The People's Medical Gazette,*" *Charleston Medical Journal and Review* 9 (January 1854): 121, 126.

5. T. Bullard, "Ought a Physician to Tell a Patient That He Is Going to Die," *Oglethorpe Medical and Surgical Journal* 2 (November 1859): 265–68; see also Gail E. Henderson et al., *The Social Medicine Reader* (Durham, N.C.: Duke University Press, 1997), pt. 4.

6. "Review of *Females and their Diseases,*" *Southern Medical and Surgical Journal* 4 (May 1848): 287–88.

7. S. M. Meek, "An Essay on Female Diseases, and the Use of the Pessary in Uterine Displacements," *Southern Medical and Surgical Journal* 2 (August 1837): 33–34. For the case of a woman whose hysterical convulsions were caused by an injury to her knee and who survived, see George D. Cullender, "Singular Case of Hysteria," *Southern Medical and Surgical Journal* 5 (July 1849): 400.

8. Meek, "An Essay on Female Diseases," 33–34.

9. For a fuller discussion of consent, see later sections in this chapter.

10. E. C. Baker, "A Case of Vicarious Menstruation from an Ulcer on the Right Mamma," *Southern Journal of Medicine and Pharmacy* 2 (March 1847): 152–53.

11. [L. A. Dugas], "Editorial and Miscellany: Remarks upon the Use of Pessaries in the Treatment of Prolapsus Uteri," *Southern Medical and Surgical Journal* 10 (September 1854): 572.

12. "Inflammation and Ulceration of the Neck of the Uterus in the Virgin Female," *Southern Medical and Surgical Journal* 3 (November 1847): 667, also 670–71.

13. "[Review of] *Females and Their Diseases,*" *Charleston Medical Journal and Review* 3 (March 1848): 191.

14. [Charles] Meigs, "Two Cases of Double Vagina," *Southern Medical and Surgical Journal* 3 (March 1847): 171.

15. H. R. Easterling, "The Effects of Uterine Diseases on the Constitution—Their Diagnosis and Treatment—With Remarks on the Importance of Instituting a Physical Exploration as a Means of Diagnosis," *Charleston Medical Journal and Review* 10 (July 1855): 473.

16. W. F. Barr, "Cases of Ulceration and Induration of the Cervix Uteri," *Charleston Medical Journal and Review* 6 (January 1851): 59–60.

17. John Stainback Wilson, *Woman's Home Book of Health* (Philadelphia: J. B. Lippincott, 1860), 255.

18. Joseph A. Eve, "A Report on Diseases of the Cervix Uteri [Part I]," *Southern Medical and Surgical Journal* 13 (September 1857): 525.

19. Joseph A. Eve, "Notes to a Report on Diseases of the Cervix Uteri," *Southern Medical and Surgical Journal* 14 (February 1858): 101–3.

20. Joseph A. Eve, "A Case of Pregnancy and Parturition during the Existence of Cancer of the Uterus," *Southern Medical and Surgical Journal* 3 (April 1847): 199–200; see also editor's note to Alf. A. L. M. Velpeau, "An Elementary Treatise on Midwifery, or Principles of Tokology and Embryology," *Southern Medical and Surgical Journal* 3 (October 1838): 50–51.

21. James M. Green, "Cases of Inflammation and Ulceration of the Cervix Uteri, Continued," *Charleston Medical Journal and Review* 9 (May 1854): 290–92.

22. Polypus was a form of tumor, usually described as emerging on a stalklike neck from the organ from which it grew. They were nearly always diagnosed on the uterus or other reproductive organ. The most common method of treatment was tying off the polypus with a thread or wire, in an effort to cut off the blood supply, although various drugs were also regularly employed.

23. Z. P. Landrum, "Case of Uterine Polypus," *Southern Medical and Surgical Journal* 15 (May 1859): 316–22.

24. The pessary was a device worn partly inside and partly outside the body, designed to support a prolapsed uterus by applying mechanical pressure to it. Most consisted of a ring or cup-shaped device designed to hold the cervix in place, plus a series of straps, braces, and bandages designed to hold the contraption in place.

25. Dugas, "Editorial and Miscellany: Remarks upon the Use of Pessaries in the Treatment of Prolapsus Uteri," 572–73.

26. Paul F. Eve, "Essay on the Question, Ought Not the Use of Pessaries to Be Now Abandoned," *Southern Medical and Surgical Journal* 1 (April 1837): 649. Eve was the son of Joseph Eve, one of the founders of the Medical College of Georgia. Paul studied at the University of Pennsylvania and in Paris, then taught at the Medical College of Georgia; in Louisville, Kentucky; and at the Nashville Medical College in Tennessee. He became president of the American Medical Association in 1857; Phinizy Spaulding, *The History of the Medical College of Georgia* (Athens: University of Georgia Press, 1987), 17, 22–25, 67.

27. "Reviews and Editorial," *Medical Journal of North Carolina* 3 (May 1861): 318. Other sorts of technological intervention could be similarly problematic; see Lawrence D. Longo, "Electrotherapy in Gynecology: The American Experience," *Bulletin of the History of Medicine* 60 (1986): 343–66; Dixon Burns and Lisa Calache, "An Evaluation of Some Early Obstetrical Instruments," *Caduceus* 3 (Spring 1987): 32–39.

28. "Review of *Females and Their Diseases*," *Southern Medical and Surgical Journal*, 291.

29. "Monthly Periscope: Medical Society of Augusta," *Southern Medical and Surgical Journal* 1 (April 1837): 694.

30. Joseph F. Wright, *A Practical Treatise on the Management and Diseases of Infants and Children, with Some of the Diseases Peculiar to Females, and Their Treatment* (Macon, Ga.: Joseph Clisby, 1859), 160–61.

31. Rob[er]t S. Bailey, "Observations on the Death of the Foetus in Utero," *Charleston Medical Journal and Review* 7 (September 1852): 599.

32. "Monthly Periscope: Prolapsus Uteri," *Southern Medical and Surgical Journal* 3 (April 1839): 432.

33. D. C. O'Keefe, "Extracts from the Records of the Physicians' Society for Medical Observation, of Greene and Adjoining Counties, Georgia," *Southern Medical and Surgical Journal* 8 (March 1852): 149–50.

34. Steven M. Stowe, ed., *A Southern Practice: The Diary and Autobiography of Charles A. Hentz, M.D.* (Charlottesville: University Press of Virginia, 2000), 322–23.

35. P. C. Carsten, "Case of Laceration of the Perinaeum by the Glans Penis," *Charleston Medical Journal and Review* 7 (November 1852): 778–80.

36. Placenta previa refers to births in which the placenta blocks the opening from the dilating cervix to the vagina, thus preventing the baby from descending and being born.

37. John H. Grant, "My First Case of Placenta Previa," *Charleston Medical Journal and Review* 13 (March 1858): 184; see also "Dr. Lindsly's Case of Retained Placenta," *Southern Medical and Surgical Journal* 1 (April 1837): 698–701.

38. W. A. Beasley, "Retained Placenta," *Southern Medical Reformer* 7 (September 1857): 260–61.

39. T. Gaillard Thomas, "Midwifery: Lecture on Parturient Hemorrhage," *Medical Journal of North Carolina* 3 (October 1860): 590.

40. Joseph Milligan to Joseph A. S. Milligan, July 9, 1846, Milligan Family Papers, *Southern Women and Their Families in the Nineteenth Century: Papers and Diaries,* ser. A, *Holdings of the Southern Historical Collection, University of North Carolina, Chapel Hill,* pt. 5, *Alabama, South Carolina, Georgia, and Florida Collections,* consulting ed. Anne Firor Scott (Bethesda, Md.: University Publications of America, 1991).

41. J. Dickson Smith, "Adherent Placenta; the Use of Chloroform in Its Removal," *Oglethorpe Medical and Surgical Journal* 1 (October 1858): 221–22.

42. In addition to general works on the history of insanity, see Peter McCandless, *Moonlight, Magnolias, and Madness: Insanity in South Carolina from the Colonial Period to the Progressive Era* (Chapel Hill: University of North Carolina Press, 1996), 36–39 and passim.

43. Wilson, *Woman's Home Book of Health,* 324.

44. W. Camps, "Hysteria Considered as a Connecting Link between Mental and Bodily Disease," *Southern Medical and Surgical Journal* 15 (October 1859): 701–3. The article, which credits W. Camps as the author, is in fact an anonymously written summary of his views published in the *British Medical Journal.*

45. Wright, *A Practical Treatise on the Management and Diseases of Infants and Children,* 157.

46. Joseph Milligan to Joseph A. S. Milligan, June 4, 1846, Milligan Family Papers, *Southern Women and Their Families,* ser. A, pt. 5.

47. Alfred M. Folger, *The Family Physician, Being a Domestic Medicine Work, Written in Plain Style* (Spartanburg C.H., S.C.: Z. D. Cottrell, 1845), 62–63.

48. Stowe, *A Southern Practice,* 375, 524. The diary contains multiple references to Dr. Telfair's drinking and the irresponsible way it caused him to behave toward his patients; see also Carol Bleser, ed., *Secret and Sacred: The Diaries of James Henry Hammond, a Southern Slaveholder* (Columbia: University of South Carolina Press, 1988), 71.

49. Salivation was the result of dosing the patient with calomel, which was mercurous chloride, a preparation of mercury. It was widely used to treat many types of illnesses, including most fevers.

50. Autobiography of Charles A. Hentz, *Southern Women and Their Families,* ser. A, pt. 5.

51. "Monthly Periscope: Medical Society of Augusta," 695.

52. E. M. Pendleton, "Case of Parturition, with Deformed Pelvis and Abscess of the Womb," *Charleston Medical Journal and Review* 5 (November 1850): 735–36.

53. February 7, 1849, Charles A. Hentz Diary 1848–1851, *Southern Women and Their Families,* ser. A, pt. 5; see also Autobiography of Charles A. Hentz, 165.

54. Joseph Milligan to Jane Milligan, April 13, 1835, Milligan Family Papers, *Southern Women and Their Families,* ser. A, pt. 5.

55. "Monthly Periscope: Carbonic Acid Gas in Dysmenorrhoea," *Southern Medical and Surgical Journal* 3 (December 1838): 185.

56. [Milton M. Antony and Joseph A. Eve], "Reviews and Extracts: *The Young Mother's Guide, and Nurses Manual . . .,* by Richard S. Kissam," *Southern Medical and Surgical Journal* 2 (August 1837): 35–36.

57. John Challice, "Abdominal Tumor Mistaken for Pregnancy," *Southern Medical and Surgical Journal* 4 (July 1848): 420.

58. Eve, "Notes to a Report on Diseases of the Cervix Uteri," 99.

59. "Code of Medical Ethics," 575–76.

60. Folger, *The Family Physician,* 218–19; see also W. H. Coffin, *The Art of Medicine Simplified; or a Treatise on the Nature and Cause of Diseases, for the Use of Families and Travelers* (Wellsburg, Va.: W. Barnes, 1853), 5.

61. Wilson, *Woman's Home Book of Health,* 216–17.

62. "Code of Medical Ethics," 540.

63. John G. Roberts, "Obstetrics," *Southern Botanic Journal Devoted to the Dissemination and Support of the Thomsonian System of Medical Practice* 2 (26 May 1838): 110.

64. John Stainback Wilson, "Female Medical Education," *Southern Medical and Surgical Journal* 10 (January 1854): 5–17. Wilson was a prolific medical writer who was the editor of the "Health Department" of *Godey's Lady's Book* for several years in the 1850s. He also wrote a series of articles on "The Peculiarities and Diseases of Negroes" and announced a book to be titled "The Plantation and Family Physician: A Work for Families Generally and Southern Slaveholders Especially . . ." whose publication was halted by the Civil War; Weymouth T. Jordan, "Plantation Medicine in the Old South," *Alabama Review* 3 (April 1950): 92–95 and passim.

65. Wilson, "Female Medical Education."

66. William Hauser, "Pre-Natal Influences," *Oglethorpe Medical and Surgical Journal* 2 (November 1859): 217.

67. A. P. Merrill, "An Essay on Some of the Distinctive Peculiarities of the Negro Race, No. II," *Southern Medical and Surgical Journal* 12 (February 1856): 90.

68. A. P. Merrill, "An Essay on Some of the Distinctive Peculiarities of the Negro Race [No. I]," *Southern Medical and Surgical Journal* 12 (January 1856): 35.

69. Merrill, "An Essay on Some of the Distinctive Peculiarities of the Negro Race, No. II," 88, 90.

70. H. W. Moore, "A Thesis on Plantation Hygiene," Medical College of the State of South Carolina, February 1856, 31, Waring Medical Library, Medical University of South Carolina, Charleston.

71. M. Antony, "On Menstrual Irregularities," *Southern Medical and Surgical Journal* 1 (May 1837): 721.

72. W[illia]m M. Boling, "An Essay on the Mechanism and Management of Parturition, in the Shoulder Presentation," *Charleston Medical Journal and Review* 8 (November 1853): 797.

73. Wilson, *Woman's Home Book of Health,* 331.

74. "Monthly Periscope: Spontaneous Rupture of the Uterus during Delivery," *Southern Medical and Surgical Journal* 3 (November 1838): 118.

75. William M. Post, "Report of a Case of Placenta Praevia," *Charleston Medical Journal and Review* 12 (March 1857): 198–200.

76. E. R. Feild, "Rupture of the Uterus Occurring during Natural Labor—Escape of the Child into the Peritoneal Cavity—Sectio Abdominis—Recovery of the Mother," *Charleston Medical and Surgical Journal* 6 (May 1851): 360–63.

77. Bellinger describes four such cases but says nothing about consent in his discussion of the fourth woman; John Bellinger, "Operations for the Removal of Abdominal Tumors," *Southern Journal of Medicine and Pharmacy* 2 (May 1847): 241–45.

78. H. Steele, "The Pessary and Other Mechanical Means in Prolapsus Uteri," *Oglethorpe Medical and Surgical Journal* 1 (October 1858): 209.

79. [Dugas], "Editorial and Miscellany: Remarks upon the Use of Pessaries in the Treatment of Prolapsus Uteri," 575.

80. Stowe, *A Southern Practice*, 286. On another occasion, while he was still studying medicine, Hentz wanted to pull a tooth for a black woman, but she refused; September 30, 1846, Charles A. Hentz Diary, *Southern Women and Their Families*.

81. W. Michael Boyd and Linda A. Clayton, *An American Health Dilemma*, vol. 1, *A Medical History of African Americans and the Problem of Race: Beginnings to 1900* (New York: Routledge, 2000); Susan M. Reverby, ed., *Tuskegee's Truths: Rethinking the Tuskegee Syphilis Study* (Chapel Hill: University of North Carolina Press, 2000); Todd L. Savitt, "The Use of Blacks for Medical Experimentation and Demonstration in the Old South," *Journal of Southern History* 48 (August 1982): 331–48.

82. Susan E. Lederer, *Subjected to Science: Human Experimentation in America Before the Second World War* (Baltimore: Johns Hopkins University Press, 1995); Allen M. Hornblum, *Acres of Skin: Human Experiments at Holmesburg Prison: A True Story of Abuse and Exploitation in the Name of Medical Science* (New York: Routledge, 1999).

83. See, for example, Edwin Black, *War against the Weak: Eugenics and America's Campaign to Create a Master Race* (New York: Four Walls Eight Windows, 2003).

84. On Sims, see Deborah Kuhn McGregor, *From Midwives to Medicine: The Birth of American Gynecology* (New Brunswick, N.J.: Rutgers University Press, 1998). After perfecting his techniques, Sims moved to the North and became a celebrated and wealthy physician, much in demand by the elite; see also L. Lewis Wall, "Did J. Marion Sims Deliberately Addict His First Fistula Patients to Opium?" *Journal of the History of Medicine and Allied Sciences* 62 (July 2007): 336–56.

85. See, for example, Kirsten Emmott, "1852: J. Marion Sims Perfects a Repair for Vesicovaginal Fistula," in Robert Coles et al., eds., *A Life in Medicine: A Literary Anthology* (New York: New Press, 2002), 28–30.

86. Joseph A. Eve, "Cases of Convulsions and Other Nervous Affections, during Pregnancy, Parturition and the Puerperal State," *Southern Medical and Surgical Journal* 4 (February 1848): 524, 526. On sources for cadavers used in medical schools, which in the South were almost exclusively those of slaves, see David C. Humphrey, "Dissection and Discrimination: The Social Origins of Cadavers in America, 1760–1915," *Bulletin of the New York Academy of Medicine* 49 (September 1973): 819–27; Robert L. Blakely and Judith M. Harrington, *Bones in the Basement: Post-Mortem Racism in Nineteenth Century Medical Training* (Washington, DC: Smithsonian Institution Press, 1997).

87. P. W. Harper, "Cases Occurring in the Practice of P. W. Harper," *Southern Medical and Surgical Journal* 5 (December 1849): 716–17.

88. Cha[rle]s Witsell, "Case of Enormous Polypus of the Uterus Treated with the Muriated Tincture of Iron," *Charleston Journal of Medicine and Pharmacy* 15 (May 1860): 227.

89. Myddleton Michel, "On the Dependence of Menstruation upon the Development and Expulsion of Ova," *Charleston Medical Journal and Review* 3 (January 1848): 26–27.

90. Samuel A. Cartwright, "Remarks on Dysentery among Negroes," *New Orleans Medical and Surgical Journal* 11 (September 1854): 145–63.

91. Ibid.

92. Ibid.

93. W[illia]m A. Brown, "A Curious Case of Malingering—A Woman Passes 'Black Balls' from Her Vagina, and Simulates Convulsions, in Order to Get Opium," *Medical Journal of North Carolina* 3 (May 1860): 375–78.

94. Tomlinson Fort, *A Dissertation on the Practice of Medicine* (Milledgeville, Ga.: Federal Union Office, 1849), 430.

95. Joseph Quattlebum, "Case of Ovarian Pregnancy," *Charleston Medical Journal and Review* 5 (May 1850): 315–18.

96. Stowe, *A Southern Practice,* 323–24.

97. January 10, 11, 12, 1861, Charles A. Hentz Medical Journal, Hentz Family Papers, *Southern Women and Their Families.*

98. M. D. McLoud, "Hints on the Medical Treatment of Negroes," medical thesis submitted to the Medical College of South Carolina, March 1850, 1.

99. Ibid., 2–3.

100. Ibid., 3–5.

101. Ibid., 5–6.

102. Ibid., 6–7.

103. Ibid., 7–12.

## Conclusion

1. T. S. Hopkins, "A Remarkable Case of Feigned Disease," *Charleston Medical Journal and Review* 8 (March 1853): 173.

2. Ibid., 174.

3. Ibid.

4. Cephalalgia refers to pains in the head.

5. The meatus auditorius refers to the opening of the ear.

6. Hopkins, "A Remarkable Case of Feigned Disease," 174–75.

7. Ibid., 173–76.

8. Ibid., 175.

# INDEX

Abbott, Simon, 184
acclimation to southern climate. *See* geography and medicine
Agassiz, Louis, 16
*American Lady's Medical Pocket-Book, The,* 53
American Medical Association, 183
animal folklore, 173–74
Antony, Milton: on black female slave sensibilities, 202; on emotions and childbirth, 131; on fear and women's physical problems, 128; on mind-body relationship and pregnancy, 129; on nervous disease and gynecological disorders, 141–42; on prenatal influences, 116, 121; on prolapsed uterus dangers, 141
Armstrong, Orland, 179
Arnold, Richard, 118
Atkins, Charles, 117
Atkinson, William B., 132
Attaway, A. F., 100
Auntie Rachel, 175
autopsies, 205–6

Bailey, Robert, 191–92
Baker, E. C., 107, 187
Baker, Georgia, 175
Bampas, Frances, 164
Barr, W. F., 188
Battey, Robert, 52
Beasley, W. A., 192
Beck, Jessie, 132
Bedford, Gunning: on civilization as debilitating influence on women, 48–50; on diagnostic caution, 6; female vulnerability diagnoses, 44–45; on lactation implications, 134; on male hysteria diagnosis, 150; on pregnancy complications, 111–12; on vicarious menstruation, 108
Beecher, Catharine, 49
Bellamy, William C., 1
Belle, Sophie D., 97
Bellinger, John, 203–4

Ben's case, 1–3
Bethell, Mary Jeffries, 87, 89, 160
black diseases, 28–29, 169. *See also* diseases
black folklore, 36–41, 172–73, 177–82
blackness, 36–41
black women. *See* women, black
Blair, Hugh, 106–7
Blanks, Eliza, 160
Blount, David, 174
Boling, William, 202
Bolton, Arabella, 89
botanic medicine, 156
Boyd, Annie, 39
brain size theories, 16–17
Breeden, James O., 64
Brer Rabbit, 37
Brown, Frank C., 39
Brown, Sally, 175, 176
Bryan, James, 88
Bryan, Maria: on childbirth and home environment, 90; on disappointment and illness, 161; on distress and health, 159; on doctor's assistance with female medical problems, 183–84; on emotions and convalescence, 165; on emotions and illness, 161, 167; on pregnancy and childbirth fears, 164; on slave illness, 169
Bullard, T., 185
Bumpas, Frances, 164, 165
Burge, Dolly Lunt, 56, 161
Byrd, H. R., 33

cachexia Africana (dirt eating), 25–27, 226n48, 226n53. *See also* diseases
Campbell, Easter Sudie, 120
Campbell, James, 119
Campbell, Virginia, 159–60
Camps, W., 142, 194
*Carolina Journal of Medicine, Science and Agriculture,* 79, 136
Carpenter, W. M., 25–27
Cartwright, John, 97

MARLI F. WEINER (1953–2009) was Adelaide and Alan Bird Professor of History at the University of Maine and the author of several books, including *Place and Gender: Women in Maine History* and *Plantation Women: South Carolina Mistresses and Slaves, 1830–1880*. **Mazie Hough** is an assistant professor of history and women's studies and the associate director of the Women in the Curriculum and Women's Studies program at the University of Maine. She is the author of *Rural Unwed Mothers: An American Experience, 1870–1950*.

The University of Illinois Press
is a founding member of the
Association of American University Presses.

---

Composed in 10.5/13 Minion Pro
by Celia Shapland
at the University of Illinois Press
Manufactured by Sheridan Books, Inc.

University of Illinois Press
1325 South Oak Street
Champaign, IL 61820-6903
www.press.uillinois.edu